Asthma Epidemiology

Asthma Epidemiology
Principles and Methods

NEIL PEARCE

RICHARD BEASLEY

CARL BURGESS

JULIAN CRANE

Wellington Asthma Research Group
Department of Medicine
Wellington School of Medicine
Wellington, New Zealand

New York   Oxford

OXFORD UNIVERSITY PRESS

1998

Oxford University Press

Oxford   New York
Athens   Auckland   Bangkok   Bogota   Bombay
Buenos Aires   Calcutta   Cape Town   Dar es Salaam
Delhi   Florence   Hong Kong   Istanbul   Karachi
Kuala Lumpur   Madras   Madrid   Melbourne
Mexico City   Nairobi   Paris   Singapore
Taipei   Tokyo   Toronto   Warsaw

and associated companies in
Berlin   Ibadan

Copyright © 1998 by Oxford University Press

Published by Oxford University Press, Inc.
198 Madison Avenue, New York, New York 10016

Oxford is a registered trademark of Oxford University Press

Library of Congress Cataloging-in-Publication Data
Asthma epidemiology : principles and methods /
Neil Pearce . . . [et al.]
p.   cm.   Includes bibliographical references and index.
ISBN 0-19-508016-5
1. Asthma—Epidemiology.   I. Pearce, Neil.
[DNLM: 1. Asthma—epidemiology.   2. Epidemiologic Methods.
WA   950   A853   1998]
RA645.A83A84   1998   614.5'9238—dc21
DNLM/DLC for Library of Congress   97-17577

9   8   7   6   5   4   3   2   1

Printed in the United States of America
on acid-free paper

To Eru Pomare

Preface

Asthma epidemiology is currently undergoing the same type of rapid expansion that occurred in cardiovascular and cancer epidemiology several decades ago. This growth of interest in asthma epidemiology is occurring in the context of major concerns about asthma mortality and the increasing burden of asthma morbidity, and major developments in the understanding and management of asthma.

Although many factors are known to trigger asthma attacks, relatively little is known about the underlying causes of asthma. A necessary first step in studying this issue is the development of international comparisons of asthma prevalence, similar to those that were conducted several decades ago for mortality from cancer and cardiovascular disease. However, preliminary evidence suggests that asthma is becoming more common, in a number of Western countries. In addition, there were major epidemics of asthma deaths in six countries in the 1960s and a second epidemic in New Zealand in the 1970s, and asthma mortality has increased gradually in a number of other countries in the last few decades, although mortality has now begun to decline again in some countries. Accordingly, attention has focused on the possible causes of these changes, including changes in environmental factors, an increase in asthma prevalence, and the possible hazards of some modern asthma drugs.

There have also been major developments in the way in which the management of asthma has been approached. Increasingly, it has been realized that the informed patient is the most appropriate person to be in control of his or her management, and self-management plans have been developed, based on the interpretation of symptoms and peak-flow measurements.

Epidemiology is integral to all of these developments, but the various epidemiological principles and methods have not previously been assembled in a single text. Although asthma epidemiology has many features in common with other types of epidemiological research, there are also many features that are relatively unique or that receive special emphasis. Most fields of epidemiological research involve the study of healthy populations, in order to ascertain which factors increase the risk of developing disease.

Asthma epidemiology has another layer of complexity in that it involves the study not only of healthy populations (to determine risk factors for developing asthma), but also of populations with asthma (to determine factors that increase the risk of worsening asthma or asthma death). The latter group may be exposed not only to environmental risk factors, but also to pharmacological and nonpharmacological interventions that are intended to be beneficial but that may also be hazardous. Accordingly, there are some issues and complexities in asthma epidemiology that rarely occur in other areas of epidemiology. It is these aspects of asthma epidemiology that receive particular attention in this text.

The book begins with a historical overview of the field. Part I involves a brief review of the general principles of asthma epidemiology studies; although many of these principles are "generic" to all epidemiology studies, particular emphasis is given to those methods and issues that are relatively unique to asthma epidemiology. Part II discusses studies of asthma morbidity; it thus concentrates on the study of factors that increase the risk of developing asthma or that increase the severity of asthma. It reviews current knowledge of the diagnosis and etiology of asthma as well as methods for measuring asthma prevalence. The latter include symptom questionnaires, physiologic measurements, and other field survey techniques, and particular emphasis is given to the standardization of techniques for international comparisons. This is followed by reviews of methods for measuring asthma severity and control. Methods for measuring asthma risk factors are also reviewed, including measures of the indoor and outdoor environment, early life events, and atopy.

In Part III the focus is on asthma mortality and in particular the study of factors that can increase the risk of asthma death in people who already have asthma. A review of principles and methods for studies of international time trends in asthma mortality is followed by a discussion of epidemiological methods for studying the causes of asthma mortality, including case-control studies of pharmacological and nonpharmacological risk factors.

We should also stress what this book is not. Although we have attempted to use a wide and representative range of studies as examples, the book is not intended to be a comprehensive review of current knowledge from substantive epidemiological studies. The focus of the book is on epidemiological principles and methods, and readers should consult other sources for state-of-the-art reviews of specific substantive issues (e.g., genetics and asthma, air pollution and asthma). Furthermore, the book is intended as a general introduction to the field not an advanced treatise for a single specialized audience. Thus, most readers will find some material with which they are very familiar and other material that is relatively new to them. The general approach we have followed throughout the book is a reflection of our own research program in which epidemiology is part of a multidisciplinary program involving biomedical, clinical, and epidemiological studies. The book will therefore interest not only epidemiologists, but also respiratory physicians, allergists, and pediatricians who are involved in asthma epidemiology. We hope that the book will stimulate further interdisciplinary research efforts into the causes and management of this major public health problem.

Wellington, New Zealand   N.P.
August 1997   R.B.
                                                             C.B.
                                                             J.C.

Acknowledgments

The Wellington Asthma Research Group is funded by a Type I Programme Grant and Julian Crane and Neil Pearce are funded by Professorial Research Fellowships of the Health Research Council of New Zealand. The Wellington Asthma Research Group is also supported by a major grant from the Guardian Trust (Trustee of the David and Cassie Anderson Medical Charitable Trust). We are grateful to Audrey Hayman and Tania Slater for technical assistance, to Sander Greenland for his comments on the drafts of several chapters, and to David Fishwick for his comments on the draft of Chapter 6.

Contents

Asthma Epidemiology

1

Introduction

Asthma

We begin this introductory chapter with a brief historical overview of the concepts of asthma definition and diagnosis, and the causative factors that contribute to this condition. Then we briefly mention some recent and current controversies in which epidemiological observations have played an important role. The discussion is not intended to be comprehensive, but rather to highlight some aspects of asthma epidemiology that will be considered in more depth in the rest of the book. In this context, we discuss some of the methodological features of asthma epidemiology that distinguish it from other disease-based areas of epidemiology, such as cancer or cardiovascular disease. These distinctive features will receive emphasis in the following chapters.

Formal epidemiological studies of asthma started barely fifty years ago and in many respects they have failed to deliver the insight or testable hypotheses that have derived from studies of other common diseases. The roots of this failure lie in the problem of definition and the consequent difficulty of reproducible and conclusive case ascertainment, in the transient nature of the principal symptom, and in the absence of simple, sensitive, and specific markers for the condition. For these reasons it is important to focus on the problems of definition and the underlying pathology and physiology before considering the distinctive features of asthma epidemiology.

Historical aspects

Asthma has puzzled and confused physicians from the time of Hippocrates to the present day. The word "asthma" comes from a Greek word meaning "panting" (Keeney, 1964), but reference to asthma can also be found in ancient Egyptian, Hebrew, and Indian medical writings (Ellul-Micallef, 1976; Unger and Harris, 1974). There were clear observations of patients experiencing attacks of asthma in the second century and evidence of disordered anatomy in the lung as far back as the seventeenth century (Willis, 1678).

Aretaeus of Cappadocia, a Greek physician in Rome in the second century A.D. and a contemporary of Galen, provided the first accurate written description of an attack of asthma (Unger and Harris, 1974):

> If from running and exercise, and labour of any kind, a difficulty of breathing follows, it is termed asthma, and the disease of orthopnoea, itself is likewise called asthma. . . . The precursory symptoms of this disease are weight at the chest, an unwillingness to attend to one's ordinary vocation, or to business altogether, an uneasiness of respiration in running, or going uphill. . . . Under increasing disorder the cheeks flush, the eyes are prominent as in cases of strangulation, a snoring is heard while they are awake and the evil is much augmented during the sleep. The voice indicates the presence of mucus, is feeble and indistinct . . . when the disease takes a favourable turn the cough is longer, though less frequent, with an excretion of humid matter in great quantity . . . the breathing becomes rare, gentle, but there is asperity of the voice . . .

Thus, many important signs and symptoms of a severe attack of asthma were recognized some 1800 years ago. The knowledge of asthma progressed during the ancient and medieval period, as illustrated by the observations of Maimonides, a Spanish physician who practiced in Cairo in the twelfth century (Unger and Harris, 1974), and who recognized that viral respiratory tract infections are an important cause of exacerbations of severe asthma:

> This disorder starts with a common cold, especially in the rainy season, and the patient is forced to gasp for breath day and night, depending on the duration of the onset, until the phlegm is expelled, the flow completed and the lung well cleared. This is all I know about the prodromal phases of this illness.

In the Renaissance, the role of atopy was increasingly recognized, not only as a cause for the development of asthma, but also as a potential factor for prevention. For example, in the sixteenth century, when Gerolamo Cardano was called from Italy to Edinburgh to treat John Hamilton, the Archbishop of St Andrews, his treatment included the substitution of unspun silk for feathers in the mattress, a regimen that succeeded in keeping Hamilton alive long enough to be hanged by the Scottish Reformers (Keeney, 1964).

During the Renaissance, the increased interest in anatomy and physiology led to a better understanding of asthma and its causation. Van Helmont in the seventeenth century observed that asthma involved "a drawing together of the smallest terminal bronchi" (Ellul-Micallef, 1976) and described asthma attacks induced by exposure to dust and by eating fish (Stolkind, 1933).

Willis (1678) described two forms of asthma: "pneumonick" asthma involved obstruction of the bronchi by thick humors, swelling of the walls, and obstruction from without; "convulsive" asthma was due to "cramps of the moving fibres of the bronchi" and also of the vessels of the lung, diaphragm, and muscles of the breast. These descriptions encompass the concepts of airways inflammation and bronchospasm, which more recently have come to be recognized as two of the characteristic pathophysiological features of asthma.

The concept of bronchial hyperreactivity, the exaggerated bronchoconstrictor response to a wide variety of nonspecific and allergic stimuli, was later developed. Floyer appreciated the importance of this response to nonspecific stimuli by ascribing asthma to "the straitness, compression or constriction of the bronchia" in response to London air or strong odors (Unger and Harris, 1974). This enhanced response to atopic stimuli was described by Salter (1860):

> The cause of this asthma is the proximity of a common domestic cat. The asthmatic spasm is immediate and violent, accompanied with sneezing and a burning and watery condition of the eyes and nose. . . . After removal of the cause the symptoms I have described begin immediately to subside and, if the paroxysm is not very severe, the cure is effective in five or ten minutes, leaving, as in all other cases of asthmatic spasm, a tendency to mucus at the top of the windpipe, which being repeatedly removed, in the ordinary way, the last symptom disappears, and the lungs and throat resume their normal condition.

The role of airways inflammation in asthma was increasingly recognized in the late 1800s, with the study of asthmatic sputum. Curschmann (1883) described spiral mucoid casts in asthmatic sputum and proposed that mucus within airways can cause airflow obstruction. At about the same time, Vierrordt noticed that large clusters of epithelial cells were present in the sputum of asthmatics, reflecting extensive damage to, and denudation of, the respiratory epithelium (Naylor, 1962). The presence of Charcot-Leyden crystals (composed of eosinophils and products) in the sputum of asthmatics provided evidence for eosinophil activation in asthmatic airways (Leyden, 1872; Dor et al, 1984).

Further progress in the understanding of asthma was made when Meltzer (1910) noted the similarity between bronchospasm in guinea pigs dying of anaphylactic shock and bronchospasm in humans during asthma attacks; on this basis he suggested that asthma was an allergic phenomenon (Unger and Harris, 1974).

In the early 1920s a series of postmortem studies demonstrated the presence of widespread airways inflammation as a prominent feature of death from asthma. These studies established the importance of airways inflammation in severe asthma, although clinicians had difficulties relating these pathological features to the clinical and physiological indices of less severe forms of the disease. However, the recent application of fiber-optic bronchoscopy to obtain mucosal lavage and biopsy samples has provided evidence for the central role of airways inflammation in the pathogenesis of childhood and adult asthma of varying degrees of severity (Beasley et al, 1993). Mast cells and eosinophils have been identified as key effector cells of the inflammatory response, through their capacity to secrete a wide range of preformed and newly generated mediators that act on airways directly and indirectly through neural mechanisms. The T lymphocyte is recognized as a pivotal cell in orchestrating the inflammatory responses through the release of cytokines (Lord and Lamb, 1996); other cells, such as fibroblasts and endothelial and epithelial cells, may also be important in maintaining the inflammatory response.

What is asthma?

It is clear from the early historical accounts of asthma that the essential clinical features were observed and described. With the advent of anatomic pathology, the differing factors leading to airway obstruction were observed. It was noted that exogenous factors could induce attacks, and the similarities with anaphylaxis prompted consideration of asthma as an allergic disease. This evolution in understanding has been reflected in many attempts to define asthma, and such definitions have steadily evolved from clinical descriptions to encompass physiological and pathological features. Nevertheless, the definition and classification of asthma has continued to be a subject of controversy (Howell, 1995); Salter (1860, *On Asthma: Its Pathology and Treatment,* quoted by Unger and Harris, 1974) observed that:

> The circumstances under which asthma may occur are so various and the features of different causes so peculiar, and impart to those cases such an individuality, that all writers are tempted with more or less success to make some classification of its different varieties. . . . It seems to me a subject in which authors have done more in the way of reading each other's books than in scrutinising their own patients.

In modern times, the cardinal clinical feature of asthma, reversible airflow obstruction, has formed the basis of the definition of asthma. For example, Barnes et al (1995) define asthma as "a syndrome comprising a spectrum of disorders characterized by widespread airway obstruction, varying spontaneously and with treatment."

Similarly, the definition initially proposed at the Ciba Foundation conference in 1959 (Ciba Foundation Guest Symposium, 1959) and endorsed by the American Thoracic Society in 1962 (American Thoracic Society Committee on Diagnostic Standards, 1962) is that "Asthma is a disease characterized by wide variation over short periods of time in resistance to flow in the airways of the lung."

In elaborating this definition, the American Thoracic Society introduced the characteristic of hyperreactivity of the airways as a feature that would usually (but not always) be present in asthma. Subsequently it has been proposed that this phenomenon of bronchial hyperreactivity might be the unifying mechanism underlying all subjects with the range of disorders encompassed by the term asthma. However, it has been demonstrated that subjects with clinical asthma may have normal bronchial reactivity, that subjects without clinical asthma may have enhanced bronchial reactivity, and that there is a poor correlation between current asthma severity and the degree of bronchial hyperreactivity (Josephs et al, 1989). As a result, although bronchial hyperreactivity may be present in many asthmatics, it is no longer considered to be synonymous with asthma.

Recently the major clinical and physiological characteristics of asthma have been incorporated in an operational definition, which also recognizes the underlying disease mechanisms. In this way the International Consensus Report on the Diagnosis and Treatment of Asthma (DHHS, 1992) defines asthma as

> . . . . a chronic inflammatory disorder of the airways in which many cells play a role, including mast cells and eosinophils. In susceptible individuals this inflammation causes symptoms which are usually associated with widespread, but variable airflow obstruction that is often reversible either spontaneously or with treatment, and causes an associated increase in airway responsiveness to a variety of stimuli.

These three components—chronic airways inflammation, reversible airflow obstruction, and enhanced bronchial reactivity—form the basis of this current definition of asthma. They also represent the major pathophysiological events leading to the symptoms of wheezing, breathlessness, chest tightness, cough, and sputum production by which physicians clinically diagnose this disorder.

Is asthma becoming more common?

Given the difficulties with diagnosing and classifying asthma, it is not surprising that there are also difficulties with determining the prevalence of the disease and whether this has changed over time (Burr, 1987). However, recent studies in the United Kingdom (Burr et al, 1989), Finland (Haahtela et al, 1990), Australia (Robertson et al, 1991), New Zealand (Mitchell, 1983; Shaw et al, 1990), Japan (Nishima, 1993), Taiwan (Hsieh and Shen,

1988), the United States (Weitzman et al, 1992), and many other countries (Balfe et al, 1996) have indicated that asthma prevalence has increased in recent decades (Global Initiative for Asthma, 1995). Methods of measuring asthma prevalence are discussed in Chapter 4.

Is asthma becoming more severe?

There is some evidence that the prevalence of severe asthma, especially, is on the increase (methods for measuring asthma severity are discussed in Chapter 5). In particular, hospital admission rates are increasing in many different countries (Mitchell, 1985). Anderson (1989) reviewed data on hospital admissions for childhood asthma in the United Kingdom and concluded that the increase in admissions could not be explained by changes in medical practice alone, and that it appeared that severe asthma attacks were occurring more frequently in asthmatic children. Similarly, a New Zealand study (Dawson et al, 1987) found that the recent increase in hospital admissions for asthma in children was not due to less severe asthmatics being admitted, but that the severity of acute attacks seemed to have actually increased.

The reasons for this apparent increase in severe asthma are unclear. It is possible that exposures to some risk factors for asthma may have increased, and there has been a great deal of concern about various risk factors such as outdoor and indoor air pollution, other aspects of the indoor environment (particularly house dust mites), and familial factors (methods for measuring such risk factors are discussed in Chapter 6).

A more worrying possibility is that asthma drugs themselves may have had a more direct role in the increase in asthma severity and deaths; beta agonists have come into greater use since the end of the 1970s (Keating et al, 1984), and there is evidence that regular use of some beta agonists may make asthma more severe (Mitchell, 1989; Sears et al, 1990; Taylor and Sears, 1994). In considering the possible causes of this apparent increase in severe asthma, it is important to emphasize that disease prevalence depends on both disease incidence and disease duration. Thus, an increase in the prevalence of severe asthma may be due to factors that prolong or exacerbate asthma (in people who already have the disease) as well as factors that cause people to develop asthma in the first place.

Asthma deaths

Osler observed that asthma deaths were very rare and that "the asthmatic pants into old age." Although this observation was consistent with mortality statistics at the time, there has been much concern about the increases in asthma mortality that have occurred since the advent of modern asthma treatments in the 1940s (Beasley et al, 1990; Speizer and Doll, 1968). Virtually all reviewers have concluded that the increases are real and are not solely due to changes in the diagnosis or classification of asthma. Although the problems of diagnosing and classifying asthma should not be underestimated, death from asthma in a young person is unlikely to be confused with alternative diagnoses. The evidence of increasing mortality observed in many countries at a time of increasing awareness and treatment of the condition has underlined the need for more extensive and systematic epidemiological studies.

In addition to the gradual increase in asthma deaths that has occurred over the past few decades, six countries experienced sudden epidemics of asthma deaths in the 1960s (Jackson et al, 1988). These epidemics coincided with the marketing of a high-dose preparation of a beta agonist known as isoprenaline forte (Stolley, 1972). A second mortality epidemic occurred in New Zealand in the 1970s (Jackson et al, 1982). This has been attributed to fenoterol, another potent full beta agonist that was marketed as a high-dose preparation. This was heavily used in New Zealand but not in most other countries (Beasley et al, 1991; Pearce et al, 1991, 1995a), and the epidemic ended abruptly when the availability of fenoterol was restricted in 1989 (Pearce et al, 1995b). The epidemiological studies investigating the role of beta agonist therapy in asthma mortality are reviewed in Part III (Chapters 7 and 8).

Asthma management

In the past, treatments for asthma have included fox lungs, syrup of garlick, tincture of lavender, saffron lozenges and smoked amber with tobacco (seventeenth century), bloodletting and gentle vomits (eighteenth century), and whiffs of chloroform, lobelia, and morphine (nineteenth century). A variety of other asthma drugs were also available in the nineteenth and early twentieth century, including marijuana, petroleum, oil, and various "asthma powders" including extracts of plants such as datura. In some countries these were sold without restriction in shops and on street corners.

More recently, concerns about the possible role of beta agonists in asthma morbidity and mortality, and the increasing realization of the central role of the airways inflammation underlying the disorder, have prompted a general reexamination of asthma management. Thus, emphasis is currently shifting from the use of beta-agonist drugs and oral theophylline therapy, and more emphasis is being placed on the use of inhaled corticosteroid drugs. More generally, it has been increasingly recognized in recent years that the key person in the long-term management of asthma is the informed patient. More emphasis has therefore been given to self-management of asthma and asthma education; this trend follows the approach established several decades earlier for other major chronic diseases such as diabetes. This in turn requires the use of epidemiological methods, or related methods from clinical trials, to assess whether particular interventions such as novel pharmacologic agents or education programs, have led to a decrease in asthma severity for elimination of the disease itself is rarely, if ever, a realistic option (methods for measuring asthma severity are discussed in Chapter 5).

Asthma Epidemiology

Thus, there have been continuing difficulties not only with the diagnosis and classification of asthma, but also with determining the causes of the recent trends of increasing prevalence, morbidity, and mortality from this common disorder. Although epidemiological studies have contributed to our understanding of these issues, they have not always been coherent or systematic. In many ways, the epidemiology of asthma is in a situation similar to that of cancer epidemiology or cardiovascular disease epidemiology before the major advances in understanding of the causes of these diseases in the 1960s (e.g., Doll et al, 1996). Asthma epidemiology is poised to make similar major advances, provided that the discipline can be placed on a more coherent and rigorous basis, and provided that international comparisons and national and regional studies can be conducted in a more standardized and systematic manner. In the case of cancer and heart disease, this has involved a "top down" approach (Pearce, 1996) in which international comparisons (e.g., Doll et al, 1966) have revealed striking international differences in disease incidence and have suggested hypotheses concerning the possible reasons for these international differences. These hypotheses have then been specifically assessed in more in-depth studies in particular populations. Such an approach is now being followed for asthma, with the first phases involving international comparisons of asthma prevalence in children (Asher et al, 1995; Pearce et al, 1993) and adults (Burney, 1994; ECRHS, 1996).

In the rest of this section, we briefly consider the distinctive characteristics of asthma epidemiology, which have prompted the development of the methods presented in this book. In fact, all epidemiology studies are conceptually the same, insofar as the objective is to examine the relationship between one or more exposures and one or more health outcomes (Checkoway et al, 1989). However, different branches of epidemiology differ as to the exposures or health outcomes under study, which may require specific techniques or particular emphasis on techniques that are not widely used in other areas of epidemiology. Epidemiology can thus be divided on two axes; subdisciplines such as occupational epidemiology are oriented toward particular exposures, whereas subdisciplines such as cancer epidemiology are oriented toward particular outcomes. Asthma epidemiology falls into the latter category of disease-oriented subdisciplines, but it has some distinctive characteristics.

First, asthma epidemiology involves two major fields of research: (1) the investigation of factors that may cause a "healthy" person to develop asthma and (2) the investigation of factors that affect prognosis in persons who have developed asthma. In the former case, the source population comprises initially healthy persons, some of whom develop asthma as they are followed over time. In the latter case, the source population comprises persons who have already developed asthma, which may regress or deteriorate (sometimes resulting in death) as they are followed over time; this latter aspect of epidemiology is essentially a form of clinical epidemiology in that it is a clinical population that is under study. These two branches of asthma epidemiology can be referred to as *population-based* studies and *patient-based* studies.

Second, there are the well-known problems of measuring the prevalence of asthma or related symptoms or conditions of interest such as wheezing or bronchial hyperreactivity (BHR). These problems are not only practical but also theoretical, in that there is considerable dispute as to what asthma is and how it can be diagnosed and classified, both clinically and in epidemiological studies (Samet, 1987). Most definitions involve the occurrence of symptoms (e.g., reversible airflow obstruction, wheezing) over an extended period of time, rather than just on a particular day. Thus, the prevalence of asthma in a population may vary greatly depending on what operational definition is used, and what measurement techniques are employed. Unfortunately, until recently there has been little standardization of prevalence studies, making it impossible to create a coherent synthesis (Gregg, 1983).

A third, and related, problem is that it is usually very difficult to measure asthma *incidence* in population-based studies because it is very difficult to determine the precise date on which a particular person becomes "asthmatic" without very intensive follow-up.

Fourth, there are analogous problems with measuring asthma *morbidity* in patient-based studies. Although particular events (e.g., hospital admissions for asthma) can be ascertained accurately, these may reflect access to health services and asthma management policies as much as they reflect real asthma morbidity. Thus, for studies of small patient groups, one is forced to rely on other methods of measuring asthma morbidity, such as the occurrence of symptoms or variations in objective measures of lung function such as peak flow rates. Once again, there is considerable debate concerning the appropriate measures to use, and these often require very intensive follow-up.

Fifth, although there are fewer problems with studying asthma *mortality*, asthma deaths are very rare and are only suitable for studies of large populations rather than small patient groups. Furthermore, in studies of this type, attention needs to be confined to persons aged 5 to 34 years because the diagnosis of asthma, as distinct from other chronic obstructive respiratory disorders, is more firmly established in this age group (Sears et al, 1986). Deaths from bronchitis and emphysema may also need to be examined in order to assess the possible contribution of shifts in diagnostic fashion because they are most likely to involve a shift within the chronic obstructive respiratory disease categories (Jackson, 1993).

Finally, although there is much debate as to whether a child with asthma ever completely "loses" the disease, many children who develop the disease certainly go through periods in later life when they no longer have the disease according to many of the operational definitions (Gergen and Weiss, 1995). Furthermore, some people develop asthma late in life (e.g., following sensitization in occupational asthma), without significant previous childhood respiratory illness. Thus, asthma is a disease that can occur, regress, and reoccur, and this poses particular problems for epidemiological studies.

It is these distinctive features of asthma epidemiology that make it both challenging and stimulating and that have prompted the development of the methods presented in this book.

References

American Thoracic Society Committee on Diagnostic Standards (1962). Definitions and classification of chronic bronchitis, asthma and pulmonary emphysema. Am Rev Respir Dis 85: 762–8.

Anderson HR (1989). Increase in hospital admissions for childhood asthma: trends in referral, severity, and readmissions from 1970 to 1985 in a health region of the United Kingdom. Thorax 44: 614–9.

Asher I, Keil U, Anderson HR, et al (1995). International study of asthma and allergies in childhood (ISAAC): rationale and methods. Eur Respir J 8: 483–91.

Balfe D, Crane J, Beasley R, Pearce N (1996). The worldwide increase in the prevalence of asthma in children and young adults. Continuing Med Education J 14: 433–42.

Barnes PJ, Djukanovic R, Holgate ST (1995). Pathogenesis. In: Brewis RAL, Corrin B, Geddes DM, Gibson GJ (eds). Respiratory Medicine. 2nd ed. London: WB Saunders, pp 1108–53.

Beasley R, Smith K, Pearce NE, et al (1990). Trends in asthma mortality in New Zealand, 1908–1986. Med J Aust 152: 570–3.

Beasley R, Pearce NE, Crane J, et al (1991). Asthma mortality and inhaled beta agonist therapy. Aust N Z J Med 21: 753–63.

Beasley R, Burgess C, Crane J, et al (1993). The pathology of asthma and its clinical implications. J Allergy Clin Immunol 92: 148–54.

Burney PGJ, Luczynska C, Chinn S, Jarvis D (1994). The European Community Respiratory Health Survey. Eur Respir J 7: 954–60.

Burr ML (1987). Is asthma increasing? J Epidemiol Community Health 41: 185–9.

Burr ML, Butland BK, King S, et al (1989). Changes in asthma prevalence: two surveys 15 years apart. Arch Dis Child 64: 1452–6.

Checkoway H, Pearce NE, Crawford-Brown DJ (1989). Research Methods in Occupational Epidemiology. New York: Oxford University Press.

Ciba Foundation Guest Symposium (1959). Terminology definitions, classification of chronic pulmonary emphysema and related conditions. Thorax 14: 286–99.

Curschmann H (1883). Uber Bronchiolitis exsudativa und ihr Verhaltnis zum Asthma nervosum. Deutsche Arch Klin Med (Leipzig) 32: 1–34.

Dawson KP (1987). The severity of acute asthma attacks in children admitted to hospital. Aust Paed J 23: 167–8.

Department of Health and Human Services (DHHS) (1992). International Consensus Report on Diagnosis and Treatment of Asthma. Washington, DC: DHHS.

Doll R, Payne P, Waterhouse J (eds) (1966). Cancer Incidence in Five Continents: A Technical Report. Berlin: Springer-Verlag (for UICC).

Dor PJ, Ackerman SJ, Gleich GJ (1984). Charcot-Leyden crystal protein and eosinophil granule major basic protein in sputum of patients with respiratory disease. Am Rev Respir Dis 130: 1072–7.

European Community Respiratory Health Survey (ECRHS) (1996). Variations in the prevalence of respiratory symptoms, self-reported asthma attacks, and use of asthma medication in the European Community Respiratory Health Survey (ECRHS). Eur Respir J 9: 687–95.

Ellul-Micallef R (1976). Asthma: a look at the past. Br J Dis Chest 70: 112–6.

Gergen PJ, Weiss KB (1995). Epidemiology of asthma. In: Holgate S, Busse W. Asthma and Rhinitis. Oxford: Blackwell Scientific, pp 15–31.

Global Initiative for Asthma (GINA) (1995). Global strategy for asthma management and prevention. NHLBI/WHO Workshop Report. Washington, DC: NIH.

Gregg I (1983). Epidemiological aspects. In: Clark TJH, Godfrey S (eds). Asthma. 2nd ed. London: Chapman and Hall.

Haahtela T, Lindholm H, Bjorksten F, et al (1990). Prevalence of asthma in Finnish young men. BMJ 301: 266–8.

Howell JBL (1995). Asthma: clinical descriptions and definitions. In: Busse W, Holgate S. Asthma and Rhinitis. Oxford: Blackwell Scientific, pp 3–5.

Hsieh KH, Shen JJ (1988). Prevalence of childhood asthma in Taipei, Taiwan, and other Asian Pacific countries. J Asthma 25: 73–82.

Jackson RT, Beaglehole R, Rea HH, et al (1982). Mortality from asthma: a new epidemic in New Zealand. BMJ 285: 771–4.

Jackson R, Sears MR, Beaglehole R, Rea HH (1988). International trends in asthma mortality: 1970 to 1985. Chest 94: 914–8.

Jackson R (1993). A century of asthma mortality. In: Beasley R, Pearce NE (eds).

The Role of Beta Agonist Therapy in Asthma Mortality. New York: CRC Press, pp 29–47.

Josephs LK, Gregg I, Mullee MA, Holgate ST (1989). Nonspecific bronchial reactivity and its relationship to the clinical expression of asthma. Am Rev Respir Dis 140: 350–7.

Keating G, Mitchell EA, Jackson R, et al (1984). Trends in sales of drugs for asthma in New Zealand, Australia, and the United Kingdom, 1975–81. BMJ 289: 348–51.

Keeney EL (1964). The history of asthma from Hippocrates to Meltzer. J Allergy 35: 215–26.

Leyden E (1872). Zur kentniss des bronchial asthma. Arch Pathol Anat 54: 324.

Lord CJM, Lamb JR (1996). TH$_2$ cells in allergic inflammation: a target of immunotherapy. Clin Exp Allergy 26: 756–65.

Meltzer SJ (1910). Bronchial asthma as a phenomenon of anaphylaxis. JAMA 55: 1021.

Mitchell EA (1983). Increasing prevalence of asthma in children. N Z Med J 96: 463–4.

Mitchell EA (1985). International trends in hospital admission rates for asthma. Arch Dis Child 60: 376–8.

Mitchell EA (1989). Is current treatment increasing asthma mortality and morbidity? Thorax 44: 81–4.

Naylor B (1962). The shedding of the mucosa of the bronchial tree in asthma. Thorax 17: 69–72.

Nishima S (1993). A study of the prevalence of bronchial asthma in school children in western districts of Japan: comparison between the studies in 1982 and 1992 with the same methods and the same districts. Arerugi 42: 192–204.

Pearce NE, Crane J, Burgess C, et al (1991). Beta agonists and asthma mortality: déjà vu. Clin Exp Allergy 21: 401–10.

Pearce NE, Weiland S, Keil U, et al (1993). Self-reported prevalence of asthma symptoms in children in Australia, England, Germany and New Zealand: an international comparison using the ISAAC written and video questionnaires. Eur Respir J 6: 1455–61.

Pearce NE, Beasley R, Crane J, Burgess C (1995a). Epidemiology of asthma mortality. In: Busse W, Holgate S. Asthma and Rhinitis. Oxford: Blackwell Scientific, pp 58–69.

Pearce N, Beasley R, Crane J, et al (1995b). End of the New Zealand asthma mortality epidemic. Lancet 345: 41–4.

Pearce N (1996). Traditional epidemiology, modern epidemiology, and public health. Am J Public Health 86: 678–83.

Robertson CF, Heycock E, Bishop J, et al (1991). Prevalence of asthma in Melbourne schoolchildren: changes over 26 years. BMJ 302: 1116–8.

Salter HH (1860). On asthma; Its pathology and treatment. London.

Samet JM (1987). Epidemiologic approaches for the identification of asthma. Chest 91: 74S–78S.

Sears MR, Rea HH, de Boer G, et al (1986). Accuracy of certification of deaths due to asthma: a national study. Am J Epidemiol 124: 1004–11.

Sears MR, Taylor DR, Print CG, et al (1990). Regular inhaled beta-agonist treatment in bronchial asthma. Lancet 336: 1391–6.

Shaw RA, Crane J, O'Donnell TV, et al (1990). Increasing asthma prevalence in a rural New Zealand adolescent population: 1975–89. Arch Dis Child 63: 1319–23.

Speizer FE, Doll R (1968). A century of asthma deaths in young people. Br Med J 3: 245–6.

Stolkind E (1933). The history of bronchial asthma and allergy. Proc R Soc Med 26: 1120.

Stolley PD (1972). Why the United States was spared an epidemic of deaths due to asthma. Am Rev Respir Dis 105: 883–90.

Taylor DR, Sears MR (1994). Regular beta-adrenergic agonists: evidence, not reassurance, is what is needed. Chest 106: 552–9.

Unger L, Harris MC (1974). Stepping stones in allergy. Ann Allergy 32: 214–30.

Weitzman M, Gortmaker SL, Sobol AM, et al (1992). Recent trends in the prevalence and severity of childhood asthma. JAMA 268: 2673–7.

Willis T (1678). Practice of Physick, Pharmaceutice Rationalis or the Operations of Medicine in Humane Bodies. London.

Part I

BASIC PRINCIPLES
OF ASTHMA EPIDEMIOLOGY

2

Study Design Options

This chapter is a brief overview of the general study design options (and related methods of data analysis) in asthma epidemiology. Although these various study designs are to some extent generic to all epidemiology studies, the emphasis here is on methods that are particularly relevant to asthma epidemiology. The chapter is not intended to be a substitute for more general epidemiology texts (e.g., Breslow and Day, 1980, 1987; Kleinbaum et al, 1982; Schlesselman, 1982; Miettinen, 1985a; Rothman and Greenland, 1997; Hennekens and Buring, 1987; Ahlbom and Norell, 1990; Clayton and Hills, 1993; MacMahon and Trichopolous, 1996). In particular, we present only the most basic methods for the statistical analysis of epidemiological data and readers are encouraged to consult these standard texts for a more comprehensive review.

All epidemiologic studies are (or should be) based on a particular population (the study population, source population, or base population) followed over a particular period of time (the study period or risk period). The different epidemiological study designs differ only in the manner in which the source population is defined, and the manner in which information is drawn from this population (Checkoway et al, 1989). When a dichotomous outcome is under study (e.g., having or not having asthma or bronchial hyperresponsiveness [BHR]) four main types of studies can be identified (Table 2.1): incidence studies, incidence case-control studies, prevalence studies, and prevalence case-control studies (Morgenstern and Thomas, 1993; Pearce and Crane, 1995). These various study types differ according to whether they involve incidence or prevalence data and whether or not they involve sampling on the basis of the outcome under study. Cross-sectional studies (of which prevalence studies are a subgroup) can also include continuous measurements of the health outcome at a particular time (e.g., lung function measurements). Longitudinal studies (of which incidence studies are a subgroup) involve repeated observation of study participants over time and may also include a series of cross-sectional measurements. Time series studies are a particular type of longitudinal study in which each subject serves as his or her own control.

Table 2.1. The four basic study types in studies involving a dichotomous health outcome

| | | Sampling on outcome | |
		No	Yes
Study outcome	Incidence	Incidence studies	Incidence case-control studies
	Prevalence	Prevalence studies	Prevalence case-control studies

Background

Randomized trials

Randomized trials have particular applicability in patient-based studies, in which the aim is to evaluate changes in asthma severity or control over time (Chapter 5). Randomized trials have been conducted to evaluate new treatments (e.g., use of inhaled steroids), treatment regimens (e.g., regular versus on-demand use of beta agonists), management strategies (e.g., asthma action plans), education programs (e.g., community-based asthma education), or other interventions (e.g., dust mite avoidance programs).

Randomized trials are usually considered to fall outside the discipline of epidemiology, which is inherently nonexperimental; in fact, epidemiological techniques were developed because it is unethical or impractical to conduct randomized trials for many major causes of disease. For example, it would be unethical to randomize healthy nonsmoking volunteers into smoking and nonsmoking groups. Similar considerations apply to most important hypotheses in population-based asthma epidemiology.

Nevertheless, in many instances the appropriate paradigm for asthma epidemiology is the randomized double-blind controlled trial, in that an aim of any epidemiological study investigating a specific hypothesis should be to simulate as closely as possible the kind of experimental controls that can be used in such a trial. For example, in an epidemiological study of the effects of tobacco smoking on asthma severity, an aim is to obtain comparisons among groups (smokers and nonsmokers) that are as valid as would have been obtained from a well-conducted randomized controlled trial. On the other hand, it should be stressed that there are limitations to this paradigm in that the ultimate goal of asthma epidemiology is (or should be) to ascertain the major influences on asthma prevalence and severity, and the overall picture (and the relative importance of various factors) may be obscured in studies that focus on a single risk factor (Pearce, 1996).

A related issue is that entire populations may be exposed to a particular risk factor and there is usually a continuum of disease risk (rather than a clear distinction between the "sick" and the "healthy") across the population; thus, small improvements in the health of a "sick population" may be more effective than attempts to treat or prevent illness in "sick individuals" (Rose, 1992). It may therefore be necessary to do studies of geographic patterns and time trends if these (despite their methodological limitations—Greenland and Robins, 1994) are most appropriate to the question at issue. The randomized controlled trial may be an appropriate paradigm in many epidemiological studies of specific risk factors but will often be inadequate in studies that require a consideration of the historical and social context (Dean, 1994; Wing, 1994).

Thus, although we will refer to the principles of design and conduct of randomized controlled trials (e.g., Meinert, 1990) in describing the general principles of epidemiological study design, it should be emphasized that there are many major determinants of asthma incidence, morbidity, and mortality, such as socioeconomic differences, ethnic differences, and international patterns, which are difficult to conceptualize within a randomized controlled trial paradigm.

Case series

The simplest asthma epidemiology study is the case series report. Such reports are of very limited value because it is usually unclear how the cases were identified, which source population they represent, whether case ascertainment has been complete, and whether the cases reported actually represent an excess disease occurrence. Furthermore, asthma is a common disease, whereas case series reports have generally been most useful in studies of rare diseases. For example, the occurrence of several cases of asthma in a particular population (e.g., a factory workforce) may not be unusual, and it is very difficult to know whether such cases represent an excess unless a formal epidemiological study is conducted with an appropriate comparison group. Even if a statistically significant excess of asthma is then found to exist, this may merely represent a chance "cluster" rather than a true increase in risk (Schulte, 1987). More generally, a case series is usually of little value if a control series is not also collected.

Example 2.1

Hjortsberg et al (1986) report a series of asthma cases in workers exposed to potassium aluminum-tetrafluoride at an assembly plant. Seven of 14 workers were in daily contact with the aluminum-fluoride compound; five of these seven workers had developed clinical bronchial asthma and/or bronchial hyperreactivity (BHR); two of these workers had their BHR tested before and after provocation with the aluminum-fluoride flux, and they showed increased hyperreactivity several weeks after the provocation.

The limitations of case series reports are typified by the case series of asthma deaths that have been reported in various countries including Australia (e.g., Robertson et al, 1990), New Zealand (e.g., Sears et al, 1985), the United Kingdom (e.g., Ormerod and Stableforth, 1980), and the United States (e.g., Barger et al, 1988). Although such studies provide some useful information, it has not been possible in each instance to draw firm conclusions as to the causes of the asthma deaths because of the absence of a control series (see Chapters 7 and 8). Nevertheless, case series reports have played a valuable role in indicating the possible role of many environmental causes of asthma, which have then been investigated further in more formal studies.

Example 2.2

The advantages of using a control series are illustrated by a very small Austrian study (Zach and Karner, 1989) that involved a case series of two girls who died suddenly of asthma, and a control series of 37 children who had asthma of the same clinical severity and who were taking the same medication. In comparison with the control series, the two girls who died showed a high degree of bronchial reactivity, incomplete recovery of function after bronchodilation, and appreciably reduced perception of severe lung function impairment. The authors concluded that regular assessment of lung function, bronchial reactivity, and perception of breathlessness might help to identify the patient who is prone to a fatal attack of asthma.

For example, Abramson et al (1989) reviewed the epidemiological evidence concerning aluminum smelting and lung disease and noted that case series reports have established the clinical features of pot room asthma but that few studies have involved random samples of exposed workers, and even fewer have included an unexposed comparison group. They concluded that case series reports had played an important role in identifying the existence of pot room asthma, but that future research should concentrate on cohort studies employing standardized respiratory questionnaires and lung-function measurements.

Epidemiological study designs

A case series report may therefore be an important first step in the research process, but it is usually just a precursor, or a stimulant, for formal epidemiological studies. In the rest of this chapter, we review the various formal epidemiological study designs. We start by considering the possible study designs when a dichotomous outcome is under study (e.g., having or not having asthma or BHR). We next consider continuous measurements of the health outcome (e.g., lung function measurements) and then discuss longitudinal studies, which may comprise a series of observations, involving different types of health outcome measure, of the study participants over time.

Incidence Studies

The most comprehensive approach to studying the causes of asthma involves collecting data on the experience of an entire population over time in order to estimate asthma incidence (the development of asthma for the first time). Figure 2.1 shows the experience of a source population in which all persons are followed from birth. For simplicity, we will initially assume that the source population is confined to persons born in a particular year—that is, a *birth cohort.* In the hypothetical study shown in Figure 2.1, the outcome under study is the "event" of developing asthma. However, the concept of incidence applies equally to studies of other health events, such as hospitalization for asthma or death from asthma; the key feature of incidence studies is that they involve an event (e.g., developing asthma for the first time)

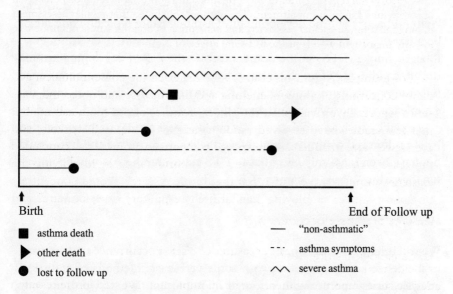

Figure 2.1. Occurrence of asthma in a hypothetical population followed from birth.

that occurs at a particular point in time, rather than a prevalent state (e.g., having asthma), which can exist over an extended period of time.

In this hypothetical study, people enter the study when they are born, and some of them subsequently develop asthma. Of these, some subsequently "lose" their asthma (although they may regain it at a later date), and some have the condition all their lives; some persons die of asthma, but most eventually die of another cause. However, the information is "censored" because the study cannot last indefinitely; that is, follow-up stops by a particular age, at which time some members of the study population have died, and some have been lost to follow-up for other reasons (e.g., emigration).

Example 2.3

Taussig et al (1989) established a cohort study of 1246 infants whose mothers used the services of a Health Maintenance Organisation in Tucson and who were born from May 1980 to October 1984. A questionnaire on demographic factors and parental history of asthma and allergies was completed at the time of enrollment. Blood samples were taken at birth (from cord blood), nine months, and six years of age. Parents were instructed to take their child to their pediatrician if he or she developed symptoms of lower respiratory tract illness (LRI). Follow up for LRI continued for the first three years of life, and reports by the paediatricians were used to classify LRIs as wheezing or non-wheezing. Atopy was determined by skin prick testing at six years of age (Martinez et al, 1995).

In some circumstances, such a study might be conducted to study the "natural history" of the development of asthma. More typically, one might be interested in a particular hyopthesis, such as "exposure to environmental tobacco smoke (ETS) in the home increases the risk of developing asthma during childhood." The children under study would therefore be grouped into those who were exposed to ETS and those who were not, and the experience of the two groups over time would be compared. The data generated by such an incidence study could appear similar to that generated by a randomized controlled trial. Nevertheless, because the children would not have been randomly allocated to ETS exposure, there would be potential for various biases (Chapter 3).

Measures of disease occurrence

We will briefly review the basic measures of disease occurrence that are used in incidence studies, together with some very basic methods of statistical analysis, using the notation depicted in Table 2.2. We will present only "large sample" methods of analysis, which have sample size requirements

Table 2.2. Notation for data for stratum i in studies of asthma incidence and prevalence

	Exposed	Nonexposed	Total
Asthma cases	a_i	b_i	M_{1i}
Non-cases	c_i	d_i	M_{0i}
Initial population size	N_{1i}	N_{0i}	T_i
Person-years	Y_{1i}	Y_{0i}	T_i
Incidence rate	I_{1i}	I_{0i}	
Incidence proportion	R_{1i}	R_{0i}	
Incidence odds	O_{1i}	O_{0i}	

for valid use. More complex techniques are required for analyses of studies involving very small numbers. Once again, readers are referred to standard texts (particularly Rothman and Greenland, 1997) for a more comprehensive review of these methods. There has been considerable discussion regarding the benefits of interval estimation rather than significance testing (Rothman, 1978; Gardner and Altman, 1986; Poole, 1987; Pearce and Jackson, 1988) and we will therefore emphasize confidence intervals. However, we will also present methods for significance testing because the results of significance tests can be used to calculate confidence intervals.

Table 2.3 shows the findings of a hypothetical incidence study of 10,000 children who are exposed from birth to a particular risk factor (e.g., passive smoking), and 10,000 children who are not exposed; both groups are followed until age 10 years.

Three measures of disease incidence are commonly used in incidence studies.

Perhaps the most common measure of disease occurrence is the person-time *incidence rate* (or incidence density; Miettinen, 1985a) which is a measure of the disease occurrence per unit time and has the reciprocal of time as its dimension. In this example, there were 952 cases of asthma diagnosed in the nonexposed group during the 10 years of follow-up, which involved a total of 95,163 person-years; this is less than the total possible person-time of

Table 2.3. Findings from a hypothetical study of 20,000 persons followed for 10 years

	Exposed	Nonexposed	Ratio
Asthma cases	1813 (a)	952 (b)	
Non-cases	8187 (c)	9048 (d)	
Initial population size	10,000 (N_1)	10,000 (N_0)	
Person-years	90,635 (Y_1)	95,163 (Y_0)	
Incidence rate	0.0200 (I_1)	0.0100 (I_0)	2.00
Incidence proportion	0.1813 (CI_1)	0.0952 (CI_0)	1.90
Incidence odds	0.2214 (O_1)	0.1052 (O_0)	2.11

100,000 person-years because children who developed asthma before the end of the 10-year period stopped contributing person-years at that time (for simplicity we will ignore the problem of children whose asthma disappears and then reoccurs over time, and we will assume that we are studying the incidence of the first occurrence of asthma). Thus, the incidence rate in the nonexposed group (b/Y_0) was $952/95,163 = 0.0100$ (or 1000 per 100,000 person-years).

The observed *incidence rate* in the nonexposed group has the form:

$$I_0 = \frac{\text{cases}}{\text{person-time}} = \frac{b}{Y_0}$$

the natural logarithm of I_0 has an approximate standard error (under the Poisson model for random variation in b) of:

$$SE[\ln(I_0)] = (1/b)^{0.5}$$

and an approximate 95% confidence interval for the incidence rate is thus:

$$I_0 e^{\pm 1.96\,SE}$$

A second measure of disease occurrence is the *incidence proportion* or average *risk*, which is the proportion of study subjects who experience the outcome of interest at any time during the follow-up period (the incidence proportion is commonly called the "cumulative incidence" but the latter term is also used to refer to cumulative hazards; Breslow and Day, 1987). Because it is a proportion, it is dimensionless, but it is necessary to specify the time period over which it is being measured. In this instance, there were 952 incident asthma cases among the 10,000 children in the nonexposed group, and the incidence proportion (b/N_0) was therefore $952/10,000 = 0.0952$ over the 10-year follow-up period.

When the outcome of interest is rare over the follow-up period (e.g., an incidence proportion of less than 10%), then the incidence proportion is approximately equal to the incidence rate multiplied by the length of time that the population has been followed (in the example this product is 0.1000 whereas the incidence proportion is 0.0952). In this example we have assumed, for simplicity, that no children died or were lost to follow-up during the study period (and therefore stopped contributing person-years to the study); when this assumption is not valid (i.e., when a significant proportion of children have died or have been lost to follow-up), then the incidence proportion cannot be estimated directly but must be estimated indirectly from the incidence rate (which takes into account that follow-up was not complete) or from life tables (which stratify on follow-up time).

The observed *incidence proportion* in the nonexposed group has the form:

$$R_0 = \frac{cases}{persons} = \frac{b}{N_0}$$

Its logarithm has an approximate standard error (under the binomial model for random variation in b) of:

$$SE[\ln(R_0)] = (1/b - 1/N_0)^{0.5}$$

and an approximate 95% confidence interval for the incidence proportion is thus:

$$R_0 e^{\pm 1.96\,SE}$$

A third possible measure of disease occurrence is the *incidence odds* (Greenland, 1987), which is the ratio of the number of subjects who experience the outcome (b) to the number of subjects who do not experience the outcome (d); as for the incidence proportion, the incidence odds is dimensionless, but it is necessary to specify the time period over which it is being measured. In this example, the incidence odds (b/d) is $952/9,048 = 0.1052$. When the outcome is rare over the follow-up period, then the incidence odds is approximately equal to the incidence proportion; once again, if loss to follow-up is significant, then the incidence odds cannot be estimated directly but must be estimated indirectly from the incidence rate (via the incidence proportion, or via life-table methods). The incidence odds is not of intrinsic interest in incidence studies, but it is presented here both for completeness and because the incidence odds is used to calculate the incidence odds ratio that is estimated in certain case-control studies (see below).

The observed *incidence odds* in the nonexposed group has the form:

$$O_0 = \frac{cases}{non\text{-}cases} = \frac{b}{d}$$

The natural log of the incidence odds ($\ln(O_0)$) has (under a binomial model) an approximate standard error of:

$$SE(\ln(O_0)) = (1/b + 1/d)^{0.5}$$

and a 95% confidence interval for O_0 is:

$$O_0 e^{\pm 1.96\, \text{SE}}$$

These three measures of disease occurrence all involve the same numerator: the number of incident cases of asthma (b). They differ in whether their denominators represent person-years at risk (Y_0), persons at risk (N_0), or survivors (d).

Example 2.4

Anderson et al (1992) analyzed data from the British National Child Development Study, which has followed a British national cohort of over 17,414 children born during one week in March 1958. Reports of asthma or wheezy bronchitis were obtained by interview of parents of children at ages 7, 11, and 16 years, and of cohort members at age 23 years. Linked data from all four interviews were available on 7225 subjects (43% of the original birth cohort). The incidence proportion for asthma was 18.2% (1311/7225) by the age of 7 years, 21.8% (1572/7225) by age 11, 24.5% (1773/7225) by age 16 years, and 28.6% (2064/7225) by age 23 years. Over the four periods examined (0–7 years, 8–11 years, 12–16 years, 17–23 years) the average annual incidence of new cases was 2.6%, 1.1%, 0.7%, and 0.8%; these incidence rates were calculated for each period by excluding those who had developed asthma during the previous period.

Measures of effect in incidence studies

Corresponding to these three measures of disease occurrence, there are three principal ratio measures of effect that can be used in incidence studies. The measure of interest is often the *rate ratio* (incidence density ratio), the ratio of the incidence rate in the exposed group (a/Y_1) to that in the nonexposed group (b/Y_0). In the example in Table 2.3, the incidence rates are 0.02 per person-year in the exposed group and 0.01 per person-year in the nonexposed group, and the rate ratio is therefore 2.00.

The observed incidence *rate ratio* has the form:

$$RR = \frac{I_1}{I_0} = \frac{a/Y_1}{b/Y_0}$$

An approximate p-value for the null hypothesis that the rate ratio equals the null value of 1.0 can be obtained using the person-time version of the

Mantel-Haenszel chi-square (Breslow and Day, 1987). This test statistic compares the observed number of exposed cases with the number expected under the null hypothesis that $I_1 = I_0$:

$$\chi^2 = \frac{[\text{Obs}(a) - \text{Exp}(a)]^2}{\text{Var}(\text{Exp}(a))} = \frac{[a - Y_1 M_1/T]^2}{[M_1 Y_1 Y_0/T^2]}$$

where M_1, Y_1, Y_0, and T are as depicted in Table 2.2.

The natural logarithm of the rate ratio has (under a Poisson model for a and b) an approximate standard error of:

$$\text{SE}[\ln(\text{RR})] = (1/a + 1/b)^{0.5}$$

An approximate 95% confidence interval for the rate ratio is then given by (Rothman and Greenland, 1997):

$$\text{RR } e^{\pm 1.96 \text{ SE}}$$

A second commonly used effect measure is the *risk ratio* (incidence proportion ratio or cumulative incidence ratio), which is the ratio of the incidence proportion in the exposed group (a/N_1) to that in the nonexposed group (b/N_0). In this example, the risk ratio is $0.1813/0.0952 = 1.90$. When the outcome is rare over the follow-up period, the risk ratio is approximately equal to the rate ratio.

The *risk ratio* has the form:

$$\text{RR} = \frac{R_1}{R_0} = \frac{a/N_1}{b/N_0}$$

An approximate p-value for the null hypothesis that the risk ratio equals the null value of 1.0 can be obtained using the Mantel-Haenszel chi-square (Mantel and Haenszel, 1959):

$$\chi^2 = \frac{[\text{Obs}(a) - \text{Exp}(a)]^2}{\text{Var}(\text{Exp}(a))} = \frac{[a - N_1 M_1/T]^2}{[M_1 M_0 N_1 N_0/T^2(T - 1)]}$$

where M_1, M_0, N_1, N_0, and T are as depicted in Table 2.2.

The natural logarithm of the risk ratio has (under a binomial model for a and b) an approximate standard error of:

$$\text{SE}[\ln(\text{RR})] = (1/a - 1/N_1 + 1/b - 1/N_0)^{0.5}$$

An approximate 95% confidence interval for the risk ratio is then given by:

$$RR\ e^{\pm 1.96\ SE}$$

A third possible effect measure is the incidence *odds ratio*, which is the ratio of the incidence odds in the exposed group (a/c) to that in the nonexposed group (b/d). In this example, the odds ratio is $0.2214/0.1052 = 2.11$. Once again, when the outcome is rare over the study period, the incidence odds ratio is approximately equal to the incidence rate ratio.

The *odds ratio* has the form:

$$OR = \frac{O_1}{O_0} = \frac{a/c}{b/d} = \frac{ad}{bc}$$

An approximate p-value for the hypothesis that the odds ratio equals the null value of 1.0 can be obtained from the Mantel-Haenszel chi-square (Mantel and Haenszel, 1959):

$$\chi^2 = \frac{[Obs(a) - Exp(a)]^2}{Var(Exp(a))} = \frac{[a - Y_1 M_1/T]^2}{[M_1 M_0 N_1 N_0/T^2(T - 1)]}$$

where M_1, M_0, N_1, N_0, and T are as depicted in Table 2.2.

The natural logarithm of the odds ratio has (under a binomial model) an approximate standard error of:

$$SE[\ln(OR)] = (1/a + 1/b + 1/c + 1/d)^{0.5}$$

An approximate 95% confidence interval for the odds ratio is then given by:

$$OR\ e^{\pm 1.96\ SE}$$

These three multiplicative effect measures are sometimes referred to under the generic term of *relative risk*. Each involves the ratio of a measure of disease occurrence in the exposed group to that in the nonexposed group. The various measures of disease occurrence all involve the same numerators (incident asthma cases), but differ in whether their denominators are based on person-years, persons, or survivors (children who do not develop asthma at any time during the follow-up period). They are all approximately equal when the disease is rare during the follow-up period (e.g., an incidence proportion of less than 10%). However, the odds ratio has been severely criticized as an effect measure (Greenland, 1987; Miettinen and Cook, 1981) and has little intrinsic meaning in incidence studies, but it is presented here because it is the standard effect measure in incidence case-control studies (see below).

Finally, it should be noted that an analogous approach can be used to calculate measures of effect based on the differences rather than ratios, in particular the *rate difference* and the *risk difference*. Ratio measures are usually of greater interest in etiologic research, because they have more convenient statistical properties, and it is easier to assess the strength of effect and the possible role of various sources of bias when using ratio measures (Cornfield et al, 1959). Thus, we will concentrate on the use of ratio measures in the remainder of this text. However, difference measures may be of value in certain circumstances, such as evaluating the public health impact of a particular exposure, and we encourage readers to consult standard texts for a comprehensive review of these measures.

Example 2.5

In the study of Anderson et al (1992) described in Example 2.4, there were some differences in incidence between males and females. For example, during the 0–7 years period, 716 (20.0%) of the 3583 males developed asthma, compared with 595 (16.3%) of the 3642 females. The risk ratio for males compared with females can be calculated as follows:

	Males	Females	Risk ratio	95% CI
Cases	716	595		
Person-years	22,575	23,412		
Incidence rate per 10,000 person-years	317	254	1.18	1.07–1.31

Thus, asthma incidence was slightly higher in males than in females during the first 7 years of life.

Incidence Case-Control Studies

Incidence studies are the most comprehensive approach to studying the causes of asthma because they use all of the information about the source population over the risk period. However, they are usually very expensive in terms of time and resources. For example, the hypothetical study presented in Table 2.3 would involve enrolling 20,000 children and collecting exposure information (e.g., on past and present exposure to passive smoking) for all of them. The same findings can be obtained more efficiently by using a case-control design.

An asthma incidence case-control study involves studying all the incident cases of asthma that occurred in the source population over the risk period, and a control group sampled from the same population over the same period (the possible methods of sampling controls are described in the next section).

Table 2.4 shows the data from a hypothetical case-control study, which involved studying all 2765 incident asthma cases that would have been identified in the full incidence study, and a sample of 2765 controls (one for each case). Such a case-control study would achieve the same findings as the full incidence study but would be considerably more efficient because it would involve ascertaining the exposure history of 5530 children (2765 cases and 2765 controls) rather than 20,000. When the outcome under study is very rare, an even more remarkable gain in efficiency can be achieved with only a minimal reduction in the precision of the effect estimate.

Measures of Effect in Incidence Case-Control Studies

In case-control studies, the relative risk is estimated using the *odds ratio*. The statistical aspects of the estimation, testing, and calculation of confidence intervals for odds ratios, are exactly the same as presented above for incidence studies.

Suppose that a case-control study is conducted in the study population shown in Table 2.3; such a study might involve all 2765 incident asthma cases and a group of 2765 controls (Table 2.4). The effect measure that the odds ratio obtained from this case-control study will estimate depends on the manner in which controls are selected. Once again, there are three main options (Miettinen, 1985a; Pearce, 1993).

One option, called *cumulative* (or cumulative incidence) sampling, is to select controls from those who do not experience the outcome during the follow-up period, that is, the *survivors* (those who did not develop asthma at

Table 2.4. Findings from a hypothetical case-control study based on the population represented in Table 2.2

	Exposed	Nonexposed	Odds ratio
Asthma cases	1813 (a)	952 (b)	
Controls			
from survivors (cumulative sampling)	1313(c)	1452 (d)	2.11
from base population (case-base sampling)	1383(c)	1383 (d)	1.90
from person-years (density sampling)	1349(c)	1416 (d)	2.00

any time during the follow-up period). In this instance, the ratio of exposed to nonexposed controls will estimate the exposure odds (b/d) of the survivors, and the odds ratio obtained in the case-control study will therefore estimate the incidence odds ratio in the source population over the study period (2.11). Early presentations of the case-control approach were usually presented in this context (Cornfield, 1951), and it was emphasized that the odds ratio was approximately equal to the risk ratio when the disease was rare.

It was later recognized that controls can be sampled from the entire *source population* (those at risk at the beginning of follow-up), rather than just from the survivors (those at risk at the end of follow-up). This approach, which was previously used by Thomas (1972) and Kupper et al (1975), has more recently been termed *case-base sampling* (Miettinen, 1982), or the case-cohort approach (Prentice, 1986). In this instance, the ratio of exposed to nonexposed controls will estimate the exposure odds in the source population of persons at risk at the start of follow-up (N_1/N_0), and the odds ratio obtained in the case-control study will therefore estimate the risk ratio in the source population over the study period (1.90). In this instance the method of calculation of the odds ratio is the same as for any other case-control study, except that cases who are also selected as controls are excluded from the control group when calculating significance tests and confidence intervals (Greenland, 1986).

The third approach is to select controls longitudinally throughout the course of the study (Sheehe, 1962; Miettinen, 1976); this is sometimes described as risk-set sampling (Robins et al, 1986), sampling from the study base (the person-time experience) (Miettinen, 1985b), or *density sampling* (Kleinbaum et al, 1982). In this instance, the ratio of exposed to nonexposed controls will estimate the exposure odds in the person-time ($Y_1/Y_0 = 1349/1416$), and the odds ratio obtained in the case-control study will therefore estimate the rate ratio in the study population over the study period (2.00).

Although case-control studies have traditionally been presented in terms of cumulative sampling (e.g., Cornfield, 1951), it has been pointed out (Miettinen, 1976) that most case-control studies actually involve density sampling (often with matching on a time variable such as calendar time or age), and therefore estimate the rate ratio without the need for any rare disease assumption (Sheehe, 1962; Miettinen, 1976; Greenland and Thomas, 1982).

Example 2.6

Infante-Rivard (1993) conducted an incidence case-control study of asthma among 3- to 4-year-old children in Québec, Canada. The cases comprised 457 children (whose parents were recruited at a hospital emergency room) with a first-time diagnosis of asthma. Controls were chosen from family allowance files and comprised children of the same age ($\pm$ one month) and the same census tract or postal code as the case at the time of diagnosis and who had not had a previous diagnosis of asthma made by a physician. Thus, controls were selected from population members "at risk" at the time that the case was diagnosed (i.e., they were selected by density sampling).

Prevalence Studies

Studies of asthma incidence involve lengthy periods of follow-up and large resources, in terms of both time and funding. Consequently, although such studies are the ideal (because they involve collecting and analyzing all of the relevant information on the source population), they are conducted infrequently, and it is more common to study a subset of the source population experience, rather than the entire experience of the source population over the risk period. In particular, it is common to study the prevalence of asthma in a particular population at a particular point in time.

The term *prevalence* denotes the number of cases of asthma existing in the population at the time the study was conducted. This can be defined as *point prevalence* estimated at one point in time, or *period prevalence,* which denotes the number of cases that existed during some time interval (e.g., one year). Asthma prevalence studies usually involve specification of a particular time interval (e.g., current BHR and occurrence of symptoms during the previous 12 months; Toelle et al, 1992).

The prevalence is a proportion, and the statistical methods for calculating a confidence interval for the prevalence are identical to those presented above for calculating a confidence interval for the incidence proportion (see above).

In some instances, the aim of a prevalence study may simply be to compare the asthma prevalence among this population with that among children in other communities or countries in order to discover differences in asthma prevalence and to thus suggest possible causes of asthma that warrant further study. These further studies may involve testing specific hypotheses by comparing asthma prevalence in subgroups of children who have or have not been exposed to a particular risk factor (such as passive smoking) in the past.

Example 2.7

Charpin et al (1988) studied asthma prevalence in two towns with contrasted environments: Marseille, located on the seashore, and Briancon, 1350 m in altitude.

The towns were chosen to test the hypothesis that people living in high altitude where house dust mites are known to be uncommon would have a lower prevalence of asthma and allergy to house dust mites. The source population consisted of adults aged 18 to 65 years who were permanent residents in the towns, and the study included 4008 people in Marseille and 1055 in Briancon. The reported prevalence was lower in Briancon for asthma attacks (2.4% and 3.8%), asthma diagnosed by a doctor (2.1% and 3.4%), and house dust mite sensitivity (10.2% and 27.5%). The authors concluded that the findings supported the hypothesis that exposure to environmental factors may have a major influence on developing allergic diseases.

Prevalence studies represent a considerable saving in resources compared with incidence studies because it is only necessary to evaluate asthma prevalence at one point in time, rather than continually searching for incident asthma cases over an extended period of time. On the other hand, this gain in efficiency is achieved at the cost of greater risk of biased inferences because it may be much more difficult to understand the temporal relationship between various exposures and the occurrence of asthma.

For example, it is well known that asthma attacks can be provoked by allergies to household cats; however, a prevalence study might find a relatively low current ownership of cats among children with asthma because the families concerned have identified cats as a factor in the child's asthma and removed the offending cat from the household. This is illustrated by a study of childhood asthma prevalence in Wales, South Africa, New Zealand, and Sweden (Burr et al, 1994) in which cat ownership was positively associated with asthma prevalence across the four countries but was significantly less common in current asthmatics than in nonasthmatics within Sweden, and was only weakly positively associated with current asthma within the other three countries. This phenomenon can be identified only by collecting detailed information on both past and current pet ownership (Brunekreef, 1992), and such information may be more difficult to collect historically in a prevalence study than concurrently in an incidence study. A related problem is that it is usually difficult to ascertain, in a prevalence study, at what age asthma first occurred, and it is therefore difficult to determine which exposures preceded the development of asthma, even when accurate historical exposure information is available.

Measures of Effect in Prevalence Studies

If we denote the prevalence of asthma in the study population by P, and if we assume that the population is in a *steady state* (stationary) over time, in that its distribution with respect to exposure and covariates does not change with time and incidence does not change with time, and suppose also that exposure and disease status are unrelated to the immigration and emigration rates, and that average disease duration (D) does not change over time, then the prevalence odds is equal to the incidence rate (I) times the average disease duration (Alho, 1992):

$$\frac{P}{(1 - P)} = ID$$

Now suppose that we compare two populations (indexed by 1 = exposed and 0 = nonexposed) and that both satisfy the above conditions. Then, the *prevalence odds* is directly proportional to the disease incidence, and the *prevalence odds ratio* (POR) satisfies the equation:

$$POR = \frac{P_1/(1 - P_1)}{P_0/(1 - P_0)} = \frac{I_1 D_1}{I_0 D_0}$$

An increased prevalence odds ratio may thus reflect the influence of factors that increase the duration of disease, as well as those that increase disease incidence. However, in the special case where the average duration of disease is the same in the exposed and nonexposed groups, then the prevalence odds ratio satisfies the equation:

$$POR = I_1/I_0$$

That is, under the above assumptions, the prevalence odds ratio directly estimates the incidence rate ratio. However, it should be emphasized that asthma prevalence depends on both asthma incidence and average disease duration, and a prevalence difference between two groups could entirely depend on differences in disease duration (e.g., because of factors that prolong or exacerbate asthma symptoms) rather than differences in incidence. Changes in incidence rates, disease duration, and population sizes over time can also bias the POR away from the rate ratio, as can migration into and out of the prevalence pool.

The statistical methods for estimation and testing of the prevalence odds ratio are identical to those for odds ratios in the context of an incidence study (see above). Table 2.5 shows data from a prevalence study of 20,000 children at age 10 years. This is based on the incidence study represented in Table 2.3, with the assumptions that, for both populations, the incidence rate and population size is constant over time, that the average duration of disease is 5 years, and that there is no migration of asthmatic children into or out of the population (such assumptions may not be realistic but are

Table 2.5. Findings from a hypothetical asthma prevalence study of 20,000 persons

	Exposed	Nonexposed	Ratio
Asthma cases	909 (a)	476 (b)	
Non-cases	9091 (c)	9524 (d)	
Source population	10,000 (N_1)	10,000 (N_2)	
Prevalence	0.0909 (P_1)	0.0476 (P_0)	1.91
Prevalence odds	0.1000 (O_1)	0.0500 (O_0)	2.00

made here for purposes of illustration). In this situation, the number of asthmatics who "lose" the disease each year is balanced by the number of new cases generated from the source population. For example, in the nonexposed group, there are 476 children who currently have asthma, and 95 (20%) of these lose their asthma each year; this is balanced by the 95 children who develop asthma each year (0.0100 of the susceptible population of 9524 children). With the additional assumption that the average duration of disease is the same in the exposed and nonexposed groups, then the prevalence odds ratio (2.00) validly estimates the incidence rate ratio (see Table 2.4).

Example 2.8

Senthilselvan et al (1992) investigated self-reported asthma and pesticide use in 1939 male farmers in 17 municipalities in Saskatchewan, Canada. Of these, 83 (4.3%) were found to have asthma and 32 (38.6%) reported having used carbamate insecticides, compared with 465 (25.1%) of the 1856 non-asthmatics. Thus, the odds ratio for asthma in those exposed to carbamate insecticides was (32/51)/(465/1391), yielding an odds ratio estimate of 1.88 (95% CI 1.17–2.96). The authors concluded that these findings raise the possibility that exposure to agricultural chemicals could be related to lung dysfunction in farmers.

Prevalence Case-Control Studies

Just as an incidence case-control study can be used to obtain the same findings as a full incidence study, a prevalence case-control study can be used to obtain the same findings as a full prevalence study in a more efficient manner. In particular, if obtaining exposure information is difficult or costly (e.g., if it involves lengthy interviews or serum samples), then it may be more efficient to conduct a prevalence case-control study by obtaining exposure information on all the prevalent cases of asthma and a sample of controls selected at random from the non-cases.

Table 2.6. Findings from a hypothetical prevalence case-control study based on the population represented in Table 2.4

	Exposed	Nonexposed	Ratio
Asthma cases	909 (a)	476 (b)	
Controls	676 (c)	709 (d)	
Prevalence odds	1.345 (O_1)	0.671 (O_0)	2.00

Measures of Effect in Prevalence Case-Control Studies

Suppose that a nested case-control study is conducted in the study population (Table 2.5), involving all 1385 prevalent asthma cases and a group of 1385 controls (Table 2.6). In this instance, the usual option for selecting controls is to select them from the non-cases. In this instance, the ratio of exposed to nonexposed controls will estimate the exposure odds (b/d) of the non-cases, and the odds ratio obtained in the prevalence case-control study will therefore estimate the prevalence odds ratio in the source population (2.00), which in turn estimates the incidence rate ratio, provided that the above assumptions are satisfied in the exposed and nonexposed populations. As in a full prevalence study, the statistical methods for estimation, testing, and calculating confidence intervals for the prevalence odds ratio in a prevalence case-control study are identical to those for the odds ratio in an incidence case-control study (see above).

Example 2.9

Oliveti et al (1996) conducted a prevalence case-control study of risk factors for asthma in inner city African-American children in Cleveland, Ohio. The 131 cases and 131 controls were aged 4–9 years and all resided in a poor urban area and received health care at a local hospital-based clinic. Cases were children who had physician-diagnosed asthma and who had had wheezing or coughing symptoms in the previous 12 months that had resulted in the use of asthma medication. Controls were sampled from patients who had no history of recurrent respiratory problems. Risk factors were ascertained through review of obstetric, perinatal, and pediatric records. It was found that asthmatic cases had significantly lower birthweights and gestational ages that non-asthmatic controls. The authors concluded that pre- and perinatal exposures may increase susceptibility to asthma in inner city children.

Cross-Sectional Studies

In the foregoing sections, the health outcome under study is a "state" (e.g., having or not having asthma), and studies can observe the prevalence of the disease state in the population, or the incidence of the "event" of acquiring the disease state (e.g., the incidence of being diagnosed with asthma). More generally, the health state under study may have multiple categories (e.g., non-asthmatic, mild asthma, moderate asthma, severe asthma) or may be represented by a continuous measurement (e.g., FEV_1). Because these measurements are taken at a particular point in time, such studies are often referred to as *cross-sectional studies;* prevalence studies (see above) are a subgroup of cross-sectional studies in which the disease outcome is dichotomous.

Although cross-sectional studies are sometimes described as studies in which exposure and disease information is collected at the same point in time (e.g., Kramer and Boivin, 1988; Last, 1988), this is not in fact an inherent feature of such studies. In most cross-sectional studies (including prevalence studies), some information on exposure will be physically collected by the investigator at the same time that information on disease is collected. Nonetheless, exposure information may include factors that do not change over time (e.g., gender) or change in a predictable manner (e.g., age) as well as factors that do change over time; the latter may have been measured at the time of data collection (e.g., current levels of airborne dust exposure), or at a previous time (e.g., from historical records on past exposure levels) or integrated over time (e.g., using a job-exposure matrix and work history records). The key feature of cross-sectional studies is that they involve studying disease at a particular point in time; a wide variety of exposure assessment methods can be used within this general category of study.

Just as a prevalence case-control study can be based on a prevalence survey, a cross-sectional study can also involve sampling on the basis of the disease outcome. For example, a cross-sectional study of bronchial hyperresponsiveness (BHR) could involve testing all study participants for BHR and then categorizing the test results into severe BHR, mild BHR, and no BHR, and then obtaining exposure information on all severe BHR cases and from random samples of the other two groups.

Measures of Effect in Cross-Sectional Studies

In a simple cross-sectional study involving continuous outcome data, the basic methods of statistical analysis involve comparing the mean level of the outcome in exposed and nonexposed groups—for example, the mean levels of FEV_1 in exposed and nonexposed workers. Standard statistical methods of analysis for comparing means (perhaps after a suitable transformation to normalize the data), and calculating confidence intervals (and associated p-values) for differences between means, can be used to analyze such studies (Armitage and Berry, 1987; Beaglehole et al, 1993). More generally, regression methods can be used to model the relationship between the level of exposure (measured as a continuous variable) and the level of the outcome measure (also measured as a continuous variable). Such methods are covered by standard statistical texts (e.g., Kleinbaum et al, 1988) and will not be reviewed in detail here. However, measurement of continuous outcome measures (e.g., FEV_1) at a single time is not sufficient to diagnose asthma (see Chapter 4), and such cross-sectional measures are rarely used in asthma epidemiology studies, which require the assessment of changes in these measures over time.

Longitudinal Studies

Longitudinal studies (cohort studies) involve repeated observation of study participants over time (Ware and Weiss, 1996). Incidence studies (described above) are a subgroup of longitudinal study in which the disease measure is dichotomous and disease incidence is measured over time. More generally, longitudinal studies may involve repeated assessment of categorical or continuous disease measures over time (e.g., a series of linked cross-sectional studies in the same population). They thus can involve incidence data, a series of prevalence surveys, or a series of cross-sectional continuous outcome measures.

General longitudinal studies

A simple longitudinal study may involve comparing the disease outcome measure or, more usually, changes in the measure over time (Weiss and Ware, 1996), between exposed and nonexposed groups. For example, rather than comparing the incidence of diagnosed asthma (as in an incidence study), or the prevalence of asthma at a particular time (as in a prevalence study), or the mean FEV_1 at a particular point in time (as in a cross-sectional study), a longitudinal study might involve measuring baseline FEV_1 in exposed and nonexposed persons and then comparing changes in mean FEV_1 (i.e., the change from the baseline measure) over time in the two groups. Such a comparison of means can be made using standard statistical methods for comparing means and calculating confidence intervals and associated p-values for the difference between the means (Armitage and Berry, 1987; Beaglehole et al, 1993). Once again, more generally, regression methods (Clayton and Hills, 1993; Kleinbaum et al, 1988) might be used to model the relationship between the level of

Table 2.7. Regression model relating change in FEV$_1$ over a 1-year period to mother's and child's smoking status

Risk factor	Regression coefficient	Standard error	p-value
Initial level of FEV$_1$ (liters)	0.839	0.015	<0.001
Age (years)	−0.010	0.004	0.006
Sex (male)	0.035	0.011	0.002
Height (cm)	0.085	0.005	<0.001
Change in height at 1 year (cm)	0.084	0.011	<0.001
Child's smoking status	−0.094	0.028	<0.001
Mother's smoking status	−0.028	0.011	0.015

Source: Adapted from Tager et al (1983).

exposure (measured as a continuous variable) and the level of the outcome measure (also measured as a continuous variable, in this instance the change in FEV$_1$).

Example 2.10

Tager et al (1983) studied the effects of maternal cigarette smoking on pulmonary function in a cohort of children and adolescents followed prospectively for 7 years. A 34% random sample was selected from all children aged 5 to 9 years who were enrolled in the public and parochial schools of East Boston, Massachusetts, in September 1974. The children were visited in their homes during the school year for six annual follow-up examinations. These involved standardized questionnaires on respiratory symptoms and illnesses, smoking history, and demographic data, as well as pulmonary function testing. Table 2.7 shows that after adjustment for the previous level of FEV$_1$, age, height, change in height, and cigarette smoking by the child, maternal smoking significantly lowered the average annual increase in FEV$_1$ by 28 mL. The authors concluded that passive smoking due to maternal cigarette smoke may have important effects on the development of pulmonary function in children.

Time series

One special type of longitudinal study is that of "time series" comparisons in which variations in exposure levels and symptom levels are assessed over time with each individual serving as his or her own control (Sherrill and Viegi, 1996). Thus, the comparison of exposed and nonexposed involves the same persons evaluated at different times, rather than different groups of persons being compared (often at the same time) as in other longitudinal studies. The advantage of the time series approach is that it reduces or eliminates confounding (see Chapter 3) by factors that vary among subjects but not over time, or whose day-to-day variation is unlikely to be related to the main exposure (Pope and Schwartz, 1996). On the other hand, time series data often require special statistical technique because any two factors that show a time trend will be correlated; for example, even a 3-month study of peak flow in children will generally show an upward trend due to growth, as well as learning effects (Pope and Schwartz, 1996). A further problem is that the change in a measure over time may depend on the baseline value; for example, changes in FEV_1 over time may depend on the baseline level (Schouten and Tager, 1996).

Time series can involve dichotomous (binary) data, continuous data, or "counts" of events (e.g., hospital admissions) (Pope and Schwartz, 1996), and the changes in these values may be measured over minutes, hours, days, weeks, months, or years (Dockery and Brunekreef, 1996). In many instances, such data can be analyzed using the standard statistical techniques outlined above. For example, a study of daily levels of air pollution and asthma hospital admission rates (e.g., Ponka, 1991) can be conceptualized as a study of the incidence of hospital admission in a population exposed to air pollution compared with that in a population not exposed to air pollution. The key difference is that only a single population is involved, and it is regarded as exposed on high pollution days and as nonexposed on low pollution days. Provided that the person-time of exposure is appropriately defined and assessed, then the basic methods of analysis are not markedly different from other studies involving comparisons of exposed and nonexposed groups.

However, the analysis of time series may be complicated because the data for an individual are not independent and serial data are often correlated (Sherrill and Viegi, 1996); for example, the value of FEV_1 on a particular day may be correlated with the value for the previous day. Furthermore, previous exposure may be as relevant as, or more relevant than, current exposure; for example, the effects of air pollution may depend on exposure on preceding days as well as on the current day (Pope and Schwartz, 1996). Time series analyses will not be considered in depth in this book, but we will use examples from such studies to illustrate the issues involved.

Example 2.11

Roemer et al (1993) conducted a time series study of the effects of ambient winter air pollution on respiratory health of children with chronic respiratory symptoms. The study involved children with chronic respiratory symptoms in the winter of 1990 to 1991 who were selected from all children aged 6 to 12 years in Wageningen and Bennekom in the Netherlands. The children completed daily asthma diaries for a period of 3 months. There was a consistent positive association between levels of air pollution (sulfur dioxide, nitrogen dioxide, black smoke, and particulate matter) and measures of asthma morbidity including wheeze, bronchodilator use, and peak flow

Table 2.8. Prevalence of acute respiratory symptoms in classes defined by daily average concentration (on the same day) of particulate matter less than 10 μm (PM_{10}), Wageningen, 12/25/90 to 3/17/91

Symptom	$\leqq 40$ μm/m^3 (27 days)	40–70 μg/m^3 (32 days)	70–100 μg/m^3 (11 days)	>100 μg/m^3 (9 days)
Attacks of shortness of breath and wheeze	3.1%	3.8%	3.0%	5.1%
Wheeze	8.1%	9.6%	10.1%	13.3%
Woke up with breathing problems	10.6%	11.6%	11.4%	15.2%
Short of breath	12.5%	12.3%	11.3%	15.4%
Cough	44.6%	36.0%	34.9%	39.7%
Runny or stuffed nose	37.2%	40.9%	41.5%	45.6%
Cough with phlegm	21.6%	19.0%	19.0%	20.6%
Bronchodilator use	9.0%	10.3%	11.5%	12.1%
Preventive medication	21.5%	18.8%	18.8%	18.9%
"Cough" medication	4.5%	4.6%	4.8%	5.3%

Source: Roemer et al (1993).

rates. Table 2.8 shows the findings for the prevalence of symptoms and medication use according to daily concentrations of particulate matter. The study found that wheeze and waking with breathing problems, and bronchodilator use were more common on days when the concentration of particulate matter less than 10 μm (PM_{10}) was high. This association was explored further in regression analyses in which levels of atmospheric pollution (as the independent variable) were regressed against medication use (as the dependent variable). Table 2.9 shows that there was a significant association of bronchodilator use with PM_{10} levels on the same day, the previous day, and with the average for the week (the day plus the previous 6 days). The association was weaker for sulfur dioxide (SO_2) and black smoke (BS), and there was little association between atmospheric pollutants and use of preventive "cough" medication.

Table 2.9. Association of prevalence of medication usage with air pollution indices, Wageningen, 12/25/90–3/17/91 (adjusted for ambient temperature)

Pollutant index	Regression coefficient (standard error) Bronchodilator use	Preventive medication	"Cough" medication
PM_{10}	0.023*(0.008)	0.007 (0.007)	−0.005 (0.006)
PM_{10} (previous day)	0.020*(0.008)	−0.008 (0.006)	0.002 (0.006)
PM_{10} (week)	0.034*(0.012)	−0.002 (0.013)	0.005 (0.012)
SO_2	0.013 (0.013)	0.001 (0.009)	0.011 (0.008)
SO_2 (previous day)	0.025*(0.012)	−0.013 (0.008)	0.012 (0.007)
SO_2 (week)	0.053 (0.027)	0.008 (0.018)	0.042 (0.021)*
BS	0.021 (0.012)	0.001 (0.010)	−0.001 (0.009)
BS (previous day)	0.023*(0.011)	−0.007 (0.009)	−0.000 (0.008)
BS (week)	0.058*(0.017)	−0.006 (0.018)	0.020 (0.017)

*$p<0.05$.
BS=Black smoke.
Source: Roemer et al (1993).

Summary

When a dichotomous outcome is under study (e.g., having or not having asthma) four main types of studies can be identified: incidence studies, incidence case-control studies, prevalence studies, and prevalence case-control studies (Morgenstern and Thomas, 1993; Pearce and Crane, 1995). These various study types differ according to whether they involve incidence or prevalence data and whether or not they involve sampling on the basis of the outcome under study. Incidence studies involve collecting and analyzing data on the exposure and disease experience of the entire source population. They may closely resemble clinical trials, but they may involve additional problems of confounding because exposure has not been randomly allocated. The other potential study designs all involve sampling from the source population and may therefore include additional biases arising from the sampling process (Chapter 3). In particular, incidence case-control studies involve sampling on the basis of outcome, that is, they usually involve all incident cases generated by the source population and a control group (of non-cases) sampled at random from the source population. Prevalence studies involve measuring the prevalence of asthma at a particular time, rather than the incidence of asthma over time. Prevalence case-control studies involve sampling on the basis of outcome: they usually involve all prevalent cases in the source population and a control group (of non-cases) sampled from the source population. Cross-sectional studies (of which prevalence studies are a subgroup) can also include continuous measurements of the health outcome (e.g., lung function measurements). Longitudinal studies (of which incidence studies are a subgroup) generally involve incidence data but may also involve a series of cross-sectional measurements. Time series studies are a particular type of longitudinal study in which each subject serves as his or her own control.

References

Abramson MJ, Wlodarczyk JH, Saunders NA, Hensley MJ (1989). Does aluminium smelting cause lung disease? Am Rev Respir Dis 139: 1042–57.

Ahlbom A, Norell S (1990). Introduction to Modern Epidemiology. 2nd ed. Boston: Epidemiology Resources.

Alho JM (1992). On prevalence, incidence, and duration in general stable populations. Biometrics 48: 587–92.

Anderson HR, Pottier AC, Strachan DP (1992). Asthma from birth to age 23: incidence and relation to prior and concurrent disease. Thorax 47: 537–42.

Armitage P, Berry G (1987). Statistical Methods in Medical Research. Oxford: Blackwell.

Barger LW, Vollmer WM, Felt RW, Buist AS (1988). Further investigation into the recent increase in asthma death rates: a review of 41 asthma deaths in Oregon in 1982. Ann Allergy 60: 31–9.

Beaglehole R, Bonita R, Kjellstrom T (1993). Basic Epidemiology. Geneva: WHO.

Breslow NE, Day NE (1980). Statistical Methods in Cancer Research. Vol I: The Analysis of Case-Control Studies. Lyon, France: IARC.

Breslow NE, Day NE (1987). Statistical Methods in Cancer Research. Vol II: The Analysis of Cohort Studies. Lyon, France: IARC.

Brunekreef B, Groot B, Hoek G (1992). Pets, allergy and respiratory symptoms in children. Int J Epidemiol 21: 338–42.

Burr ML, Limb ES, Andrae S, et al (1994). Childhood asthma in four countries: a comparative survey. Int J Epidemiol 23: 341–7.

Charpin D, Kleisbauer J-P, Lanteaume A (1988). Asthma and allergy to house-dust mites in populations living in high altitudes. Chest 93: 758–61.

Checkoway HA, Pearce NE, Crawford-Brown DJ (1989). Research Methods in Occupational Epidemiology. New York: Oxford University Press.

Clayton D, Hills M (1993). Statistical Models in Epidemiology. Oxford: Oxford Scientific Publications.

Cornfield J (1951). A method of estimating comparative rates from clinical data: applications to cancer of the lung, breast and cervix. J Natl Cancer Inst 11: 1269–75.

Cornfield J, Haenszel W, Hammond EC, et al (1959). Smoking and lung cancer: recent evidence and a discussion of some questions. J Natl Cancer Inst 22: 173–203.

Dean J, Dean A, Burton A, Dicker R (1990). Epi Info. Version 5.01. Atlanta, GA: Centers for Disease Control.

Dean K (1994). Creating a new knowledge base for the new public health. J Epidemiol Community Health 48: 217–9.

Dockery DW, Brunekreef B (1996). Longitudinal studies of air pollution effects on lung function. Am J Respir Crit Care Med 154: S250–S256.

Gardner MJ, Altman DG (1986). Confidence intervals rather than p values: estimation rather than hypothesis testing. BMJ 292: 746–50.

Greenland S (1986). Adjustment of risk ratios in case-base studies (hybrid epidemiologic designs). Stat Med 5: 579–84.

Greenland S (1987). Interpretation and choice of effect measures in epidemiologic analyses. Am J Epidemiol 125: 761–8.

Greenland S, Robins J (1994). Ecologic studies—biases, misconceptions, and counterexamples. Am J Epidemiol 139: 747–60.

Greenland S, Thomas DC (1982). On the need for the rare disease assumption in case-control studies. Am J Epidemiol 116: 547–53.

Hennekens CH, Buring JE (1987). Epidemiology in Medicine. Boston: Little, Brown.

Hjortsberg U, Nise G, Orbaek P, et al (1986). Bronchial asthma due to exposure to potassium aluminium-tetrafluoride. Scand J Work Environ Health 12: 223 (letter).

Infante-Rivard C (1993). Childhood asthma and indoor environmental risk factors. Am J Epidemiol 137: 834–4.

Jones DT, Sears MR, Holdaway MD, et al (1987). Childhood asthma in New Zealand. Br J Dis Chest 1987; 81: 332–40.

Kleinbaum DG, Kupper LL, Morgenstern H (1982). Epidemiologic Research: Principles and Quantitative Methods. Belmont, CA: Lifetime Learning Publications.

Kleinbaum DG, Kupper LL, Muller K (1988). Applied Regression Analysis and Other Multivariable Methods. 2nd ed. Belmont, CA: Wadsworth.

Kramer MS, Boivin J-F. The importance of directionality in epidemiologic research design. J Clin Epidemiol 1988; 41: 717–8.

Kupper LL, McMichael AJ, Spirtas R (1975). A hybrid epidemiologic design useful in estimating relative risk. J Am Stat Assoc 70: 524–8.

Last JM (ed). A dictionary of epidemiology. New York: Oxford, 1988.

MacMahon B, Trichopolous D (1996). Epidemiology: Principles and Methods. 2nd ed. Boston: Little, Brown.

Mantel N, Haenszel W (1959). Statistical aspects of the analysis of data from retrospective studies of disease. J Natl Cancer Inst 22: 719–48.

Martinez FD, Stern DA, Wright AL, et al (1995). Association of non-wheezing lower respiratory tract illnesses in early life with persistently diminished serum IgE levels. Thorax 50: 1067–72.

Meinert C (1990). Clinical trials: design, conduct, analysis. New York: Oxford University Press.

Miettinen OS (1976). Estimability and estimation in case-referent studies. Am J Epidemiol 103: 226–35.

Miettinen OS, Cook EF (1981). Confounding: essence and detection. Am J Epidemiol 114: 593–603.

Miettinen O (1982). Design options in epidemiologic research: an update. Scand J Work Environ Health 8(suppl 1): 7–14.

Miettinen OS (1985a). Theoretical epidemiology. New York: Wiley.

Miettinen OS (1985b). The "case-control" study: valid selection of subjects. J Chronic Dis 7: 543–8.

Morgenstern H, Thomas D (1993). Principles of study design in environmental epidemiology. Environ Health Perspect 101: S23–S38.

Olivetti JF, Kercsmar CM, Redline S. Pre- and perinatal risk factors for asthma in inner city African-American children. Am J Epidemiol 143: 570–7.

Ormerod LP, Stableforth DE (1980). Asthma mortality in Birmingham 1975–7: 53 deaths. Br Med J 1: 687–90.

Pearce N (1993). What does the odds ratio estimate in a case-control study? Int J Epidemiol 22: 1189–92.

Pearce N (1996). Traditional epidemiology, modern epidemiology, and public health. Am J Public Health 86: 678–83.

Pearce N, Crane J (1995). Epidemiologic methods. In: Harber P, Schenker M, Balmes J (eds). Occupational and Environmental Respiratory Disease. St Louis, MI: Mosby, pp 13–27.

Pearce NE, Jackson RT (1988). Statistical testing and estimation in medical research. N Z Med J 101: 569–70.

Ponka A (1991). Asthma and low level air pollution in Helsinki. Arch Environ Health 46: 262–70.

Poole C (1987). Beyond the confidence interval. Am J Public Health 77: 195–9.

Pope CA, Schwartz J (1996). Time series for the analysis of pulmonary health data. Am J Respir Crit Care Med 154: S229–S233.

Prentice RL (1986). A case-cohort design for epidemiologic cohort studies and disease prevention trials. Biometrika 73: 1–11.

Robertson CF, Rubinfeld AR, Bowes G (1990). Deaths from asthma in Victoria: a 12 month survey. Med J Aust 152: 511–7.

Robins JM, Breslow NE, Greenland S (1986). Estimation of the Mantel-Haenszel variance consistent with both sparse-data and large-strata limiting models. Biometrics 42: 311–23.

Roemer W, Hoek G, Brunekreef B (1993). Effect of ambient winter air pollution on respiratory health of children with chronic respiratory symptoms. Am Rev Respir Dis 147: 118–24.

Rose G (1992). The Strategy of Preventive Medicine. Oxford: Oxford University Press.

Rothman KJ (1978). A show of confidence. N Engl J Med 299: 1362–3.

Rothman KJ, Greenland S (1997). Modern Epidemiology. 2nd ed. Philadelphia: Lippincott.

Schlesselman JJ (1982). Case-control studies: design, conduct, analysis. New York: Oxford University Press.

Schouten JP, Tager IB (1996). Interpretation of longitudinal studies: an overview. Am J Respir Crit Care Med 154: S278–S284.

Schulte PA (1987). Investigation of occupational cancer clusters: theory and practice. Am J Public Health 77: 52–6.

Sears MR, Rea HH, Beaglehole R (1985). Asthma mortality in New Zealand: a two year national study. N Z Med J 98: 271–5.

Senthilselvan A, McDuffie HH, Dosman JA (1992). Association of asthma with use of pesticides. Am Rev Respir Dis 146: 884–7.

Sheehe PR (1962). Dynamic risk analysis of matched pair studies of disease. Biometrics 18: 323–41.

Sherill D, Viegi G (1996). On modeling longitudinal pulmonary function data. Am J Respir Crit Care Med 154: S217–S222.

Tager IB, Weiss ST, Munoz A, et al (1983). Longitudinal study of the effects of maternal smoking on pulmonary function in children. N Engl J Med 309: 699–703.

Taussig LM, Wright AL, Morgan WJ, et al (1989). The Tucson Children's Respiratory Study: I Design and implementation of a prospective study of acute and chronic respiratory illness in children. Am J Epidemiol 129: 1219–31.

Thomas DB (1972). The relationship of oral contraceptives to cervical carcinogenesis. Obstet Gynecol 40: 508–18.

Toelle BG, Peat JK, Salome CM, et al (1992). Toward a definition of asthma for epidemiology. Am Rev Respir Dis 146: 633–7.

Ware JH, Weiss S (1996). Statistical issues in longitudinal research on respiratory health. Am J Respir Crit Care Med 154: S208–S211.

Weiss KB (1990). Seasonal trends in US asthma hospitalizations and mortality. JAMA 263: 2323–28.

Weiss KB, Wagener DK (1990). Geographic variations in US asthma mortality: small area analyses of excess mortality, 1981–1985. Am J Epidemiol 132: S107–S115.

Weiss ST, Ware JH (1996). Overview of issues in the longitudinal analysis of respiratory data. Am J Respir Crit Care Med 154: S208–S211.

Wing S (1994). Limits of epidemiology. Medicine and Global Survival 1: 74–86.

Zach MS, Karner U (1989). Sudden death in asthma. Arch Dis Child 64: 1446–51.

3

Study Design Issues

As noted in Chapter 2, the general study design options that can be used in asthma epidemiology differ only in the manner and timing of data collection. Incidence studies collect exposure and outcome data on all members of the source population over the time period under study. The other study designs (incidence case-control studies, prevalence studies, prevalence case-control studies, and other cross-sectional studies) all involve sampling from the experience of the source population over time and may therefore include additional biases arising from the sampling process. This chapter gives a brief overview of general study design issues. We start by drawing the distinction between random error (lack of precision) and systematic error (lack of validity); we then discuss the various types of systematic error and the study design issues involved in minimizing, or controlling, the various types of bias. Once again, the emphasis is on issues that are particularly relevant to asthma epidemiology, and the chapter is not intended to be a substitute for more general epidemiology texts.

Precision

Random error will occur in any epidemiologic study, just as it occurs in experimental studies. It is often referred to as "chance," although it can perhaps more reasonably be regarded as ignorance (Checkoway et al, 1989). For example, if we toss a coin 300 times, then ideally we might be able to predict the outcome of each toss based on the speed, spin, and trajectory of the coin. In practice, we do not have all of the necessary information (because of ignorance), or the computing power to use it (because of chaotic behavior), and we therefore regard the outcome of each toss as a chance phenomenon; however, we may note that, on the average, 50% of the tosses are heads, and therefore we may say that a particular toss has a 50% chance of producing a head.

Similarly, suppose that a study of 20,000 children found 300 incident cases of asthma in one year. Then, if half of the children are exposed to a particular factor and half are not exposed, and if we knew that exposure has no influence on the risk of developing asthma, and if we did not know of any association of exposure with other asthma risk factors, then we might expect the two subgroups of 10,000 children to each experience 150 new cases of asthma during the one-year follow-up period. However, just as 300 tosses of a coin will not usually produce exactly 150 heads and 150 tails, rarely in reality would there be exactly 150 incident cases in each group. This occurs because of differences in exposure to other risk factors for asthma, including differences in susceptibility factors between the two groups. Ideally, we should attempt to gather information on all known risk factors, but there will always be other risk factors operating that are unknown, or unmeasurable, and hence the incidence of asthma will not be identical in exposed and nonexposed in particular populations, even if the exposure has no effect on the development of asthma.

Even in an experimental study, in which participants are randomized into exposed and nonexposed groups, there will be "random" differences in background risk between the compared groups, but these will diminish in importance (i.e., the random differences will tend to even out) as the study size grows. In epidemiological studies, because of the lack of randomization, there is no guarantee that differences in baseline (background) risk will even out between the exposure groups as the study size grows, but it is necessary to make this assumption in order to proceed with the study (Greenland and Robins, 1986). Hence, any epidemiological study in which known risk factors have been controlled for involves the assumption that any background fluctuation in incidence or prevalence rates is random in that it arises merely because a subgroup has effectively been sampled "at random" from the overall source population, rather than because of systematic subgroup differences in exposure to unknown risk factors. If random error can be reduced (by increasing the study size), then the precision of the effect estimate will be increased—that is, the confidence intervals will be narrower.

A second factor that can affect precision, given a fixed total study size, is the relative size of the reference group (the unexposed group in a cohort study, or the controls in a case-control study). When exposure has no effect (i.e., the true relative risk is 1.0), and the costs of index and reference subjects are the same, then a 1:1 ratio is most efficient for a given total study size. When exposure increases the risk of the outcome, or referents are cheaper to include in the study than index subjects, then a larger ratio may be more efficient. The optimal reference to index ratio is rarely greater than 2 to 1 for a simple unstratified analysis (Walter, 1977) with equal index and referent costs, but a larger average ratio may be desirable in order to assure an adequate ratio in each stratum for stratified analyses.

The ideal study would be infinitely large, but practical considerations set limits on the number of participants that can be included. Given these limits, it is desirable to find out, before commencing the study, whether it is large enough to be informative. One method is to calculate the "power" of the study. This depends on five factors:

- the cutoff value (i.e., alpha level) below which the p value from the study would be considered statistically significant; this value is almost always 0.05 or 5%
- the disease rate in the nonexposed group in a cohort study or the exposure prevalence of the controls in a case-control study
- the expected relative risk
- the relative size of the two groups
- the total number of study participants.

Once these quantities have been determined, standard formulas are then available to calculate the statistical power of a proposed study (Walter, 1977; Schlesselman, 1982). Nowadays, standard calculator and microcomputer programs—e.g., EPI-INFO (Dean et al, 1990)—incorporating subroutines for power calculations are widely available, and we will therefore not present the detailed procedures here.

The power is not the likelihood that the study will estimate the size of the effect correctly. Rather, it is the likelihood that the study will yield a statistically significant finding when an effect of the postulated size exists. The observed effect could be greater or less than expected, but still be statistically significant. The overemphasis on statistical significance is the source of many of the limitations of power calculations. Many features such as the significance level are completely arbitrary; issues of confounding, misclassification, and effect modification are generally ignored (although appropriate methods are available—see, e.g., Schlesselman, 1982; Greenland, 1983); and the size of the expected effect is often just a guess. Nevertheless, power calculations are an essential aspect of planning a study because, despite all their assumptions and uncertainties, they nevertheless provide a useful general indication as to whether a proposed study will be large enough to satisfy the objectives of the study. On the other hand, once a study has been completed, there is no value in retrospectively performing power calculations because the confidence limits of the observed measure of effect provide the best indication of the range of likely values for the true effect (Smith and Bates, 1992; Goodman and Berlin, 1994).

Estimating the expected precision can also be conceptually useful (Rothman and Greenland, 1997). This can be done by "inventing" the results, based on the same assumptions used in power calculations, and carrying out a standard analysis with effect estimates and confidence limits. It has particular advantages when an exposure is expected to have no effect (i.e., the relative risk is expected to be 1.0), because the concept of power is not applicable but precision is still of concern. However, this approach should be used with caution (Greenland, 1988a) because the results may be misinterpreted as indicating the power of the study. In particular, a study with an expected lower limit equal to a particular value (e.g., 1.0) will have only a 50% chance of yielding an observed lower limit above that value.

Example 3.1

Consider a study involving 3500 exposed children, and 3500 nonexposed children followed for a period of one year. Suppose that the expected incidence of asthma is 20 per 1000 person-years in the exposed group and 10 per 1000 person-years in the nonexposed group (i.e., the exposed group is expected to have twice the incidence rate of the nonexposed group). Then, with a 0.05 alpha level, the study has a power of approximately 92%. This means that if 100 studies of this size were performed that were identical except for the random error (and if the assumptions involved in the power calculations are correct), then we would expect 92 of them to yield a p value of less than 0.05 and 8 of them to yield a p value greater than 0.05. An alternative approach is to carry out a standard analysis of the hypothesized results. If we make the assumptions given above, then the expected rate ratio would be 2.0, with expected 90% confidence limits of 1.3 to 3.0. This approach has only an indirect relationship to the power calculations. For example, if the expected lower 90% confidence limit was 1.0, then the power for a one-tailed test (the probability that $p < 0.05$) would be only 50%. The confidence limit approach nevertheless gives the same general conclusion as the power calculation: that the study will have reasonable power if the true rate ratio is 2.0. It also provides the additional information that if the "true" odds ratio is 2.0, then in a study of this size, it is quite likely that the estimate of the rate ratio could be as large as 3.0 or as low as 1.3.

In practice, the study size depends on the number of available participants and the available resources. Within these limitations it is desirable to make the study as large as possible, taking into account the trade-off between including more participants and gathering more detailed information about a smaller number of participants (Greenland, 1988b). Hence, power calculations can only serve as a rough guide as to whether a feasible study is large enough to be worthwhile. Even if such calculations suggest that a particular study would have very low power, the study may still be worthwhile if exposure information is collected in a form that will permit the study to contribute to the broader pool of information concerning a particular issue.

Validity

Systematic error is distinguished from random error in that it would be present even with an infinitely large study, whereas random error can be reduced by increasing the study size. Thus, systematic error, or *bias,* occurs if there is a systematic difference between what the study is actually estimating and what it is intended to estimate.

There are many different types of bias, but three general forms can be identified (Rothman and Greenland, 1997): confounding, selection bias, and information bias. In general terms, these refer to biases arising from differences in baseline disease risk between the exposed and nonexposed subpopulations (confounding), biases resulting from the manner in which study participants are selected from the source population (selection bias), and biases resulting from the misclassification of these study participants with respect to exposure or disease (information bias).

Confounding

Confounding occurs when the exposed and nonexposed subpopulations of the source population are not comparable, because of inherent differences in background disease risk (Greenland and Robins, 1986) caused by exposure to other risk factors. Similar problems can occur in randomized trials because randomization may fail, leaving the treatment groups with different characteristics (and different baseline disease risk) at the time that they enter the study, and because of differential loss and noncompliance across treatment groups. However, there is more concern about noncomparability in epidemiological studies because of the absence of randomization. The concept of confounding thus generally refers to the source population, although confounding can also be introduced (or removed) by the manner in which study participants are selected from the source population.

If no other biases are present, three conditions are necessary for a factor to be a confounder (Rothman and Greenland, 1997) in asthma epidemiology studies:

First, a confounder is a factor that is predictive of asthma in the absence of the exposure under study. Note that a confounder need not be a genuine cause of asthma, but merely "predictive." Hence, surrogates for causal factors (e.g., age) may be regarded as potential confounders, even though they are rarely directly causal factors.

Second, a confounder is associated with exposure in the source population at the start of follow-up (i.e., at baseline). In case-control studies this implies that a confounder will tend to be associated with exposure among the controls. An association can occur among the cases simply because the study factor and a potential confounder are both risk factors for the disease, but this does not cause confounding in itself unless the association also exists in the source population.

Third, a variable that is affected by the exposure (e.g., an intermediate in the causal pathway between exposure and disease) should not be treated as a confounder because to do so could introduce serious bias into the results (Greenland and Neutra, 1981; Robins, 1987; Weinberg, 1993). Such variables can sometimes be used in the analysis, but special techniques are then required to avoid adding bias (Robins, 1989; Robins et al, 1992; Pearce, 1992).

Example 3.2

In a study of humidity (e.g., from damp housing) and the development of asthma, exposure to environmental tobacco smoke would be a potential confounder if people who lived in humid houses were more likely to have been exposed to environmental tobacco smoke (i.e., if exposure to humidity and exposure to tobacco smoke were coincidentally associated). However, exposure to house dust mites might not be regarded as a confounder if it were considered that one mechanism by which humidity increased the risk of developing asthma was by increasing the population of house dust mites, which in turn increased the risk of developing asthma. In this instance, exposure to house dust mites would be an intermediate factor in the causal pathway between humidity and the development of asthma.

Control of confounding. Confounding can be controlled in the study design, or in the analysis, or both. Control at the design stage involves three main methods (Rothman and Greenland, 1997). The first is randomization, but this is not usually an option (by definition) in epidemiological studies.

A second method of control at the design stage is restriction of the study to narrow ranges of values of the potential confounders—for example, by restricting the study to white females in a particular age group. This approach has some conceptual and computational advantages but may severely restrict the number of potential study participants.

A third method of control involves matching study participants on potential confounders (e.g., matching on age, gender, and ethnicity). This will prevent confounding in a cohort study but is not often done as it may be very expensive. Matching can also be expensive in case-control studies, and does not remove confounding but merely facilitates its control in the analysis. Furthermore, matching may reduce precision in a case-control study if it is done on a factor that is associated with exposure but is not a risk factor for asthma (and hence not a true confounder). However, matching on a strong risk factor will usually increase precision, and matching may also have practical advantages in some situations.

Example 3.3

In the prevalence case-control study of Oliveti et al (1996) discussed in example 2.9, controls were matched to cases on census tract of residence, age ($\pm$ one month), race, and gender. The control chosen for each case was the patient born closest to the subject who met the above criteria for matching.

The most common approach for controlling confounding is control in the analysis. This involves stratifying the data into subgroups according to the levels of the confounder(s) and calculating a summary estimate of the association across strata. For example, controlling for age (grouped into seven categories) and gender (with two categories) might involve grouping the data into the 14 ($=7\times2$) age-gender confounder strata and calculating a summary rate ratio.

In general, control of confounding requires careful use of a priori knowledge, together with assessment of the extent to which the effect estimate changes when the factor is controlled in the analysis. Most epidemiologists prefer to make a decision based on the latter criterion, although it can be misleading, particularly if misclassification is present (Greenland and Robins, 1985b). The decision to control for a presumed confounder can certainly be made with more confidence if there is supporting prior knowledge that the factor is predictive of disease. Misclassification of a confounder leads to a loss of ability to control confounding, although control may still be useful provided that misclassification of the confounder was non-differential (unbiased) (Greenland, 1980). Misclassification of exposure is more problematic, because factors that influence misclassification may appear to be confounders, but control of these factors may increase the net bias (Greenland and Robins, 1985b).

There are two methods of calculating a summary effect measure to control confounding: pooling and standardization (Rothman and Greenland, 1997).

Pooling involves calculating a summary effect estimate assuming stratum-specific effects are equal. There are a number of different methods of obtaining pooled effect estimates, but a commonly used method that is both simple and close to being statistically optimal (even when there are small numbers in all strata) is the method of Mantel and Haenszel (1959).

The Mantel-Haenszel summary *rate ratio* has the form:

$$RR = \frac{\Sigma a_i Y_{0i}/T_i}{\Sigma b_i Y_{1i}/T_i}$$

where

$$T_i = Y_{1i} + Y_{0i}$$

An approximate p-value for the hypothesis that the summary rate ratio is 1.0 can be obtained from the person-time version of the one degree-of-freedom Mantel-Haenszel summary chi-square (Mantel and Haenszel, 1959):

$$\chi^2 = \frac{[\Sigma \, \mathrm{Obs(a)} - \Sigma \, \mathrm{Exp(a)}]^2}{\Sigma \, \mathrm{Var(Exp(a))}} = \frac{[\Sigma \, a_i - \Sigma Y_{1i} M_{1i}/Ti]^2}{[\Sigma M_{1i} Y_{1i} Y_{0i}/T_i^2]}$$

where M_{1i}, Y_{1i}, Y_{0i}, and T_i are as depicted in Table 2.1.

An approximate standard error for the natural log of the rate ratio is (Greenland and Robins, 1985a):

$$SE = \frac{[\Sigma \, M_{1i} Y_{1i} Y_{0i}/T_i^2]^{0.5}}{[(\Sigma a_i Y_{0i}/T_i)(\Sigma b_i Y_{1i}/T_i)]^{0.5}}$$

Thus, an approximate 95% confidence interval for the summary rate ratio is then given by:

$$RR \, e^{\pm 1.96 \, SE}$$

The Mantel-Haenszel summary *risk ratio* has the form:

$$RR = \frac{\Sigma \, a_i N_{0i}/T_i}{\Sigma b_i N_{1i}/T_i}$$

An approximate *P*-value for the hypothesis that the summary risk ratio is 1.0 can be obtained from the one degree-of-freedom Mantel-Haenszel summary chi-square (Mantel and Haenszel, 1959):

$$\chi_2 = \frac{[\Sigma \, \mathrm{Obs(a)} - \Sigma \, \mathrm{Exp(a)}]^2}{\Sigma \, \mathrm{Var(Exp(a))}} = \frac{[\Sigma \, a_i - \Sigma N_{1i} M_{1i}/T_i]^2}{[\Sigma \, M_{1i} M_{0i} N_{1i} N_{0i}/T_i^2]}$$

where M_{1i}, M_{0i}, N_{1i}, N_{0i} and T_i are as depicted in Table 2.1.

An approximate standard error for the natural log of the risk ratio is (Greenland and Robins, 1985a):

$$SE = \frac{[\Sigma \, M_{1i} N_{1i} N_{0i}/T_i^2 - \Sigma a_i b_i/T_i]^{0.5}}{[(\Sigma a_i N_{0i}/T_i)(\Sigma b_i N_{1i}/T_i)]^{9.5}}$$

Thus, an approximate 95% confidence interval for the summary risk ratio is then given by:

$$RR\ e^{\pm 1.96\ SE}$$

The Mantel-Haenszel summary *odds ratio* has the form:

$$OR = \frac{\Sigma\ a_i d_i / T_i}{\Sigma\ b_i c_i / T_i}$$

An approximate p-value for the hypothesis that the summary odds ratio is 1.0 can be obtained from the one degree-of-freedom Mantel-Haenszel summary chi-square (Mantel and Haenszel, 1959):

$$\chi^2 = \frac{[\Sigma\ Obs(a) - \Sigma\ Exp(a)]^2}{\Sigma\ Var(Exp(a))} = \frac{[\Sigma\ a_i - \Sigma\ N_{1i} M_{1i} / T_i]^2}{[\Sigma\ M_{1i} M_{0i} N_{1i} N_{0i} / T_i^2]}$$

where M_{1i}, M_{0i}, N_{1i}, N_{0i} and T_i are as depicted in Table 2.1.

An approximate standard error for the natural log of the odds ratio (under a binomial model) is (Robins et al, 1986):

$$SE = \frac{\Sigma PR}{2R_+^2} + \frac{\Sigma(PS + QR)}{2R_+ S_+} + \frac{\Sigma QS}{2S_+^2}$$

where $P = (a_i + d_i)/T_i$; $Q = (b_i + c_i)/T_i$; $R = a_i d_i / T_i$; $S = b_i c_i / T_i$; $R_+ = \Sigma R$; and $S_+ = \Sigma S$.

Thus, an approximate 95% confidence interval for the summary odds ratio is then given by:

$$OR\ e^{\pm 1.96\ SE}$$

It is usually not possible to control for more than 2 or 3 confounders in a pooled analysis, because finer stratification will often lead to many strata containing either no exposed or no nonexposed persons (or no asthmatics or non-asthmatics). Such strata are uninformative, and such stratification is wasteful of information. This problem can be mitigated, to some extent, by the use of multiple regression methods (see below).

Example 3.4

In the study of Anderson et al (1992) reported in Example 2.3 (Chapter 2), the rate ratio for asthma incidence in males compared with females was slightly different in

Table 3.1. Asthma incidence per 10,000 person-years in a British national cohort of children

Age group	Males	Females	Rate ratio	95% CI
0–7				
Cases	716	595		
Person-years	22,575	23,412		
Rate	317	254	1.25	1.12–1.39
8–11				
Cases	144	117		
Person-years	11,180	11,954		
Rate	129	98	1.32	1.03–1.68
12–16				
Cases	116	85		
Person-years	13,325	14,438		
Rate	87	59	1.47	1.12–1.95
Total (0–16)				
Cases	976	797		
Person-years	47,080	49,804		
Rate	207	160	1.30	1.18–1.43

Source: Adapted from Anderson et al (1992).

different age groups. Table 3.1 shows the rate ratios in each stratum and the overall crude rate ratio (not adjusted for age). It is possible to also calculate an age-adjusted rate ratio by the method of Mantel and Haenszel (described above). This yields an age-adjusted summary rate ratio of 1.28; this is very close to the crude rate ratio of 1.30, indicating that there is very little confounding by age in this data.

Standardization is an alternative approach to obtaining a summary effect measure (Miettinen, 1974a; Rothman and Greenland, 1997). Pooling involves calculating the effect measure under the assumption that the measure (e.g., the rate ratio) would be the same (uniform) across strata if random error were absent. In contrast, standardization involves taking a weighted average of the disease occurrence across strata (e.g., the standardized rate) and then comparing the standardized occurrence measure between exposed and nonexposed (e.g., the standardized rate ratio) with no assumptions of uniformity of effect. Standardization is more prone than pooling to suffer from statistical instability due to small numbers in specific strata; by comparison, pooling with Mantel-Haenszel estimators is robust and in general the statistical stability only depends on the overall numbers rather than the numbers in specific strata. However, direct standardization has practical advantages when more than two groups are being compared—for example, when comparing multiple exposure groups or making comparisons between multiple countries or regions—and does not require the assumption of constant effects across strata.

The *standardized rate* has the form:

$$R = \frac{\Sigma \, w_i R_i}{\Sigma \, w_i}$$

The natural log of the standardized rate has an approximate standard error (under the Poisson model for random error) of:

$$SE = \frac{[\Sigma \, w_i^2 \, R_i/Y_i]^{0.5}}{R\Sigma \, w_i}$$

where Y_i is the person-time in stratum i. An approximate 95% confidence interval for the standardized rate is thus:

$$R \, e^{\pm 1.96 \, SE}$$

The *standardized risk* has the form:

$$R = \frac{\Sigma \, w_i R_i}{\Sigma \, w_i}$$

The natural log of the standardized risk has an approximate standard error (under the binomial model for random error) of:

$$SE = \frac{[\Sigma \, w_i^2 R_i(1-R_i)/N_i]^{0.5}}{R\Sigma \, w_i}$$

where N_i is the number of persons in stratum i. An approximate 95% confidence interval for the standardized rate is thus:

$$R \, e^{\pm 1.96 \, SE}$$

Standardization is not usually used for odds, because the odds is only used in the context of a case-control study, where the odds ratio is the effect measure of interest, but standardized odds ratios can be computed from case-control data (Miettinen, 1985; Rothman and Greenland, 1997).

The most common choice of weights in international comparisons is Segi's World Population (Segi, 1960) shown in Table 3.2. In etiologic studies a better approach is to use the structure of the overall source population as the weights when calculating standardized rates or risks in subgroups of the source population. When one is specifically interested in the effects

Table 3.2. Segi's World Population

Age group	Population
0–4 years	12,000
5–9 years	10,000
10–14 years	9,000
15–19 years	9,000
20–24 years	8,000
25–29 years	8,000
30–34 years	6,000
35–39 years	6,000
40–44 years	6,000
45–49 years	6,000
50–54 years	5,000
55–59 years	4,000
60–64 years	4,000
65–69 years	3,000
70–74 years	2,000
75–79 years	1,000
80–84 years	500
85+ years	500
Total	100,000

Source: Segi (1960).

that exposure had, or would have, on a particular subpopulation, then weights should be taken from that subpopulation.

Example 3.5

In the study of Anderson et al (1992) reported in Example 3.3, and shown in Table 3.3, the incidence rate in males standardized to the age distribution of the overall population (i.e., males and females combined) is 263 per 10,000 person-years, and the corresponding standardized incidence rate in females is 209 per 10,000 person-years. The standardized rate ratio is therefore 263/209 = 1.26, which is very similar to the pooled summary rate ratio of 1.28 (see Example 3.4).

Multiple regression allows for the simultaneous control of more confounders by "smoothing" the data across confounder strata. In particular, rate ratios (based on person-time data) can be modeled using Poisson long-linear rate regression, risk ratios can be modeled using binomial log-linear risk regression, and odds ratios can be modeled using binomial logistic regression (Pearce et al, 1988; Rothman and Greenland, 1997). Similarly, continuous outcome variables (e.g., in a cross-sectional study) can be modeled with standard multiple linear regression methods. These models all have similar forms, with minor variations to take into account the different data types. They provide powerful tools when used appropriately, but are often used

Table 3.3. Asthma incidence per 10,000 person-years in a British national cohort of children

Age group	Males	Females	Total
0–7			
Cases	716	595	1,311
Person-years	22,575	23,412	
Rate	317	254	
8–11			
Cases	144	117	261
Person-years	11,180	11,954	
Rate	129	98	
12–16			
Cases	116	85	201
Person-years	13,325	14,438	
Rate	87	59	
Total (0–16)			
Cases	976	797	1,773
Person-years	47,080	49,804	
Rate	207	160	

Source: Adapted from Anderson et al (1992).

inappropriately, and should always be used in combination with the more straightforward methods presented here (Rothman and Greenland, 1997). Mathematical modeling methods and issues are reviewed in depth in a number of standard texts (e.g., Breslow and Day, 1980, 1987; Checkoway et al, 1989; Kleinbaum et al, 1982; Kleinbaum et al, 1988; Hosmer and Lemeshow, 1989; Clayton and Hills, 1993; Rothman and Greenland, 1997) and will not be discussed in detail here.

Assessment of confounding. When one lacks data on a suspected confounder (and thus cannot control confounding directly) it is still desirable to assess the likely direction and magnitude of the confounding it produces. For example, it may be possible to obtain information on a surrogate for the confounder of interest (for example, social class is associated with many lifestyle factors such as smoking and may therefore be a useful surrogate for some lifestyle-related confounders). Even though confounder control will be imperfect in this situation, it is still possible to examine whether the exposure effect estimate changes when the surrogate is controlled in the analysis, and to assess the strength and direction of the change. For example, if the relative risk actually increases (e.g., from 2.0 to 2.5), or remains stable (e.g., at 2.0) when social class is controlled for, then it is unlikely that the observed excess risk is due to smoking, because social class is correlated with smoking, and control for social class involves partial control for smoking.

Alternatively, it may be possible to obtain accurate confounder information for a subgroup of participants in the study and to assess the effects of confounder control in this subgroup. A related approach, known as two-stage sampling, involves obtaining confounder information for a sample of the source population (or a sample of the controls in a case-control study). For example, in a study of asthma in children, it may not be possible to obtain information on humidity levels in the homes of all the children. However, it may still be possible to obtain humidity measurements for a sample of the exposed and nonexposed groups in order to check that the average level of humidity in the home is similar in the two groups. Such limited information, if taken in all exposure-disease subgroups, can also be used to directly control confounding (White, 1982; Walker, 1982; Rothman and Greenland, 1997).

Finally, even if it is not possible to obtain confounder information for any study participants, it may still be possible to estimate how strong the confounding is likely to be from particular risk factors. For example, this is often done in occupational studies, where tobacco smoking is a potential confounder, but smoking information is rarely available; in fact, although smoking is one of the strongest risk factors for lung cancer, with relative risks of 10 or 20 times, it appears that smoking rarely exerts a confounding effect of greater than 1.5 times in studies of occupational disease (Axelson, 1978). It is very unusual to find extreme differences in smoking between various general population groups, and differences between groups exposed or not exposed to various risk factors, or between occupational groups, are usually very much smaller (e.g., Siemiatycki et al, 1988). Thus, if a study finds strong relative risks (e.g., greater than 2.0), then it is usually very unlikely that they are due to confounding by smoking.

Example 3.6

Table 3.4 shows a hypothetical example of an incidence study in which smokers have twice the risk of developing asthma compared with nonsmokers (40% and 20% respectively) and in which the "exposed" group (e.g., exposed to high levels of house

Table 3.4. Hypothetical data from an incidence study in which there is confounding by tobacco smoking

	Smokers		Nonsmokers		Total	
	Exposed	Non-exposed	Exposed	Non-exposed	Exposed	Non-exposed
Asthma cases	800	400	200	400	1000	800
Non-cases	1200	600	800	1600	2000	2200
Persons	2000	1000	1000	2000	3000	3000
Risk/100	40	40	20	20	33.3	26.7
Risk ratio	1.0		1.0		1.25	

dust mite or high levels of an occupational exposure) are twice as likely to smoke as the "nonexposed" group (two thirds of the exposed group are smokers compared with one third of the nonexposed group). It is also assumed that the exposure under study has no effect on the risk of asthma (within the smokers, and within the nonsmokers, the risk of asthma is the same in exposed and nonexposed persons). Even in this scenario, using extreme assumptions, the confounding effect of smoking only increases the relative risk for the exposure under study from 1.00 to 1.25.

Selection bias

Whereas confounding generally involves biases that would occur even if everyone in the source population were included in the study, selection bias involves biases arising from the procedures by which the study participants are chosen from the source population. Thus, selection bias is not an issue in a cohort study involving complete follow-up, since in this case the study cohort comprises the entire source population. However, selection bias can occur if participation in the study or follow-up is incomplete.

Example 3.7

Crane et al (1994) conducted a postal survey of the prevalence of asthma symptoms in adult New Zealanders during 1991–1992. Participants were chosen from the New Zealand Electoral Roll; there is both a general roll (which includes some Maori but mainly comprises non-Maori New Zealanders) and a Maori roll—the response rate from the Maori roll was only 69%, compared with 85% for the general roll, and there was concern that the findings for the Maori roll may have been biased due to the lower response rate. This would represent a type of selection bias in that it involved a bias arising from the manner in which the study participants were "selected" (or selected themselves) into the study from the source population. Crane et al employed two techniques to attempt to assess the symptom prevalence in the nonresponders. The first method involved contacting a sample of nonresponders by telephone; the prevalence rates for those nonresponders who were contacted were then applied to the whole group of nonresponders in estimating the "adjusted" prevalence in the overall source population. The second approach used the method of Drane (1991): positive responses were compared for each of the three mailouts and an estimate of the fourth (nonresponders) prevalence was calculated by linear regression. Table 3.5 shows that these adjustments made little difference to the

Table 3.5. Prevalence of wheezing in past 12 months in New Zealand, by electoral roll, with adjustment for nonresponse

	General roll ($n = 11,392$)	Maori roll ($n = 586$)	Ratio
Unadjusted	25.0%	38.4%	1.54
Telephone method	24.8%	34.5%	1.39
Drane method	24.7%	35.4%	1.43

Source: Adapted from Crane et al (1994).

findings for study participants from the general roll, but did make some difference to the findings for study participants chosen from the Maori roll. The Maori/general comparison was therefore affected to some extent by selection bias involving selective nonresponse.

Additional forms of selection bias can occur in case-control studies because these involve sampling from the source population. In particular, selection bias can occur in a case-control study (involving either incident or prevalent cases) if controls are chosen in a nonrepresentative manner—for example, if exposed children were more likely to be selected as controls than nonexposed children.

Selection bias can sometimes be controlled in the analysis by identifying factors that are related to subject selection and controlling for them as confounders. For example, if white-collar workers are more likely to be selected for (or participate in) a study than manual workers (and white-collar work is negatively or positively related to the exposure of interest), then this bias can be partially controlled by collecting information on social class and controlling for social class in the analysis as a confounder.

Information bias

Information bias involves misclassification of the study participants with respect to disease or exposure status. Thus, the concept of information bias refers to those people actually included in the study, whereas selection bias refers to the selection of the study participants from the source population, and confounding generally refers to noncomparability of subgroups within the source population.

Nondifferential information bias. Nondifferential information bias occurs when the likelihood of misclassification of exposure is the same for asthmatics and non-asthmatics (or when the likelihood of misclassification of asthma is the same for exposed and nonexposed persons). Nondifferential misclassification of exposure generally (but not always) biases the relative risk estimate toward the null value of 1.0 (Copeland et al, 1977; Dosemeci et al, 1990). Hence, nondifferential information bias tends to produce "false negative" findings and is of particular concern in studies that find a negligible association between exposure and disease. One important condition is needed to ensure that exposure misclassification procedures bias toward the null, however: the exposure classification errors must be independent of other errors. Without this condition, nondifferential exposure misclassification can produce bias in any direction (Chavance et al, 1992; Kristensen, 1992).

Example 3.8

There are considerable problems of measuring asthma prevalence in population surveys (see Chapter 4), and it often occurs that some asthmatics will be wrongly classified as non-asthmatic, and vice versa. Table 3.6 illustrates this situation with hypothetical data from a study of asthma prevalence in childhood. Suppose the true
prevalence rates are 40% in the exposed group, and 20% in the nonexposed group; the
prevalence ratio is thus 2.0, and the prevalence odds ratio is 2.7. Suppose that 20% of
asthmatics are incorrectly classified as non-asthmatics (i.e., a sensitivity of 0.80), and
that 10% of non-asthmatics are incorrectly classified as asthmatics (i.e., a specificity
of 0.90). As a result, the observed prevalences will be 38% and 24%, respectively
(Table 3.6); the observed prevalence ratio will be 1.6 (instead of the true value of 2.0),
and the observed prevalence odds ratio will be 1.9 (instead of the true value of 2.7).
Because of nondifferential misclassification, prevalence in the exposed group has
been biased downward, and prevalence in the nonexposed group has been biased
upward. The net effect is to bias the prevalence ratio toward the null value of 1.0 (the
relationship between sensitivity, specificity, and the extent of the nondifferential information bias in prevalence studies is discussed in more detail in Chapter 4).

Differential information bias. Differential information bias occurs when the
likelihood of misclassification of exposure is different in asthmatics and non-
asthmatics (or the likelihood of misclassification of asthma is different in
exposed and nonexposed persons). This can bias the observed effect estimate
in either direction, either toward or away from the null value. For example, in
a prevalence case-control study, the recall of exposures (such as passive smoking) in non-asthmatics might be different from that of asthmatics. In this
situation, differential information bias would occur, and it could bias the
odds ratio toward or away from the null, depending on whether asthmatics
were more or less likely to recall previous exposures than non-asthmatics.

Example 3.9

Example 3.8 considered a hypothetical situation in which information bias was
nondifferential—that is, the misclassification of asthma was not related to exposure.

Table 3.6. Hypothetical data from a prevalence study in which 20% of asthmatics and
10% of non-asthmatics are incorrectly classified

	Actual		Observed	
	Exposed	Nonexposed	Exposed	Nonexposed
Asthmatics	40	20	32 + 6 = 38	16 + 8 = 24
Non-asthmatics	60	80	54 + 8 = 62	72 + 4 = 76
Total	100	100	100	100
Prevalence ratio	2.0		1.6	
Prevalence odds ratio	2.7		1.9	

However, in international asthma prevalence comparisons, the "exposures" being compared involve residence in a particular country or region, and the classification, or misclassification, of asthma may well vary among countries, particularly if different languages are involved. In this situation, information bias will be differential. This is illustrated by the study of Osterman et al (1991), which compared responses to French and English versions of the American Thoracic Society respiratory questionnaire in a bilingual working population. French-speaking workers reported significantly less wheeze with colds (OR = 0.60) and wheeze apart from colds (OR = 0.55) than the English-speaking group, although the occurrence of "wheeze on most days or nights" was similar for both groups. For 66 bilingual workers who completed both French and English questionnaires at a time interval of about 2 months, highly consistent results were found for socioeconomic data, smoking habits, cough, phlegm, breathlessness, and chronic bronchitis, but not for wheeze with or apart from colds. The authors concluded that these results reflected the difficulties in translating the concept of "wheeze" from English to French.

Information bias can drastically affect the validity of a study. It is often helpful to ensure that the misclassification is nondifferential by ensuring that exposure information is collected in an identical manner in asthmatics and non-asthmatics (or that disease information is collected in an identical manner in the exposed and nonexposed groups). In this situation, if it is independent of other errors, misclassification tends to produce false-negative findings and is thus of greatest concern in studies that have not found an important effect of exposure; it is of much less concern in studies with positive findings because these findings are likely to have been even more strongly positive if misclassification had not occurred.

It is sometimes said that the aim of data collection is not to collect perfect information, but to collect information in a similar manner from the groups being compared, even if this means ignoring more detailed exposure information if this is not available for both groups. However, more valid results can sometimes be obtained by collecting information that is as detailed and accurate as possible, even if that information is not collected in a similar manner in the groups being compared (Greenland and Robins, 1985b).

Effect Modification

Effect modification occurs when the measure of exposure effect depends on the level of another factor in the source population (Miettinen, 1974b). The terms *statistical interaction* and *effect-measure modification* are also used. Effect modification is distinct from confounding (and selection and information bias) in that it does not represent a bias (which should be removed or controlled), but rather a real difference in the measure of exposure effect in various subgroups (which may be of considerable interest). For example, in a cohort study of passive smoking and asthma in children, the rate ratio for passive smoking might be different in different age groups, or in males and females.

The clearest example of effect modification is when a factor is hazardous in one group and has no effect or is actually protective in another group (see Example 3.10). More generally, the risk might be elevated in both groups, but the size of the effect measure may vary. In this situation, effect modification should be interpreted with considerable care because the presence of effect modification usually depends on the measure of effect one uses. In fact, all secondary risk factors modify either the rate ratio or the rate difference, as uniformity over one measure implies nonuniformity over the other. Similarly, all such factors modify at least one of the risk ratio, risk difference, or odds ratio.

Example 3.10

Stoddard and Miller (1995) conducted a prevalence survey of wheezing respiratory illness in 7578 children and youths less than 18 years of age in the United States. Children whose mothers smoked at the time of the survey were more likely than children of nonsmoking mothers to experience wheezing respiratory illness (odds ratio = 1.36). However, the odds ratio varied by age of the child: in children aged 0 to 2 years, maternal smoking doubled the risk of wheezing respiratory illness, whereas it had little effect on the risk of wheezing respiratory illness in those aged 13 to 17 years (Table 3.7). Thus, the effect of maternal smoking on childhood wheezing respiratory illness depended on (was modified by) the age of the child.

If the assessment of the joint effect of two factors is a fundamental goal of the study, then this can be done by calculating stratum-specific effect estimates, as in Example 3.10. It is less clear how to proceed if effect modification is occurring but assessment of joint effects is not an analytical goal. Some authors (e.g., Kleinbaum et al, 1982) argue that it is often not appropriate in this situation to calculate an overall estimate of effect summarized

Table 3.7. Childhood wheezing respiratory illness (asthma or wheezing) in relation to maternal smoking

Child's age (years)	Odds ratio	95% CI
0–2	1.90	1.23–2.94
3–5	1.53	0.99–2.37
6–12	1.35	1.01–1.81
13–17	1.07	0.76–1.49
Total	1.36	1.14–1.62

Source: Stoddard and Miller (1995).

Table 3.8. Relationship between epidemic asthma and airborne exposure to soybean (measured as the area of residence or daily walking expressed in kilometers), according to atopy (number of positive skin reactions) and tobacco smoking

Airborne soybean exposure	Skin test	Nonsmokers				Smokers			
		Cases (*n*)	Controls (*n*)	Odds ratio	95% CI	Cases (*n*)	Controls (*n*)	Odds ratio	95% CI
<4	0	4	10	1.0		8	13	1.5	0.3–8.5
≥4	0	10	18	1.4	0.3–6.5	13	11	2.9	0.6–15.5
<4	1+	29	30	2.4	0.6–5.2	18	14	3.2	0.7–15.6
≥4	1+	33	29	2.8	0.7–12.2	44	14	7.9	1.8–36.0

Source: Sunyer et al (1992).

across levels of the effect modifier. However, it is common to ignore this stipulation if the difference in effect estimates is not too great (Pearce, 1989). In fact, the methods of standardization described above have been specifically developed for this situation (Rothman and Greenland, 1997).

Example 3.11

Table 3.8 shows the stratum-specific estimates from the study of Sunyer et al (1992) of 169 cases of "epidemic asthma" emergency room admissions at four large urban hospitals in Barcelona, and 172 controls selected from emergency room admissions at the same hospitals during "non-epidemic" periods. The authors had previously found a causal relationship between the epidemics of emergency room admissions and the airborne soybean dust released from a harbor silo where soybeans were being unloaded. Table 3.8 shows the stratum-specific estimates for the separate effects of airborne soybean exposure, atopy (number of positive skin reactions), and tobacco smoking. It shows that these were all independent risk factors for epidemic asthma, and that they modified each other's effects on a multiplicative scale; for example, in those with negative skin tests, the odds ratio for soybean exposure was 1.4 in non-smokers, but nearly twofold in smokers (2.9 vs 1.5) and the combination of soybean exposure and smoking carried a nearly threefold risk. The authors concluded that the findings suggest a multifactorial process for epidemic asthma, in which atopy and tobacco smoking played an important synergistic role.

Summary

The greatest concern in epidemiological studies usually relates to confounding because exposure has not been randomly allocated, and the groups under study may therefore be noncomparable with respect to their baseline disease risk. However, to be a significant confounder, a factor must be strongly predictive of disease and strongly associated with exposure. Thus, although confounding is constantly a source of concern, the strength of confounding is often considerably less than might be expected; it should be appreciated, however, that this appearance may be illusory, for non-differential misclassification of a confounder (which is common) will usually make the confounding appear smaller than it really is.

The problem of information bias (misclassification of exposure or disease) is of particular concern in asthma epidemiology studies because of the difficulties in defining and measuring asthma, and the difficulties in obtaining exposure information in the etiologically relevant time period. However, provided that information has been collected in a standardized manner, then misclassification will be nondifferential, and any bias it produces will usually be toward the null value. In this situation, misclassification—if it is independent of other errors—tends to produce false-negative findings and is thus of greatest concern in studies that have not found an important effect of exposure; it is of much less concern in studies with positive findings because these findings are likely to have been even more strongly positive if misclassification had not occurred. Again, one should appreciate the limitations of these observations: it may be difficult to be sure that the exposure and disease misclassification is nondifferential, and nondifferential misclassification of a confounder can lead to bias away from the null if the confounder produces confounding toward the null.

References

Anderson HR, Pottier AC, Strachan DP (1992). Asthma from birth to age 23: incidence and relation to prior and concurrent disease. Thorax 47: 537–42.

Axelson O (1978). Aspects on confounding in occupational health epidemiology. Scand J Work Environ Health 4: 85–9.

Breslow NE, Day NE (1980). Statistical Methods in Cancer Research. Vol I: The Analysis of Case-Control Studies. Lyon, France: IARC.

Breslow NE, Day NE (1987). Statistical Methods in Cancer Research. Vol II: The Analysis of Cohort Studies. Lyon, France: IARC.

Chavance M, Dellatolas G, Lellouch J (1992). Correlated nondifferential misclassifications of disease and exposure: application to a cross-sectional study of the relationship between handedness and immune disorders. Int J Epidemiol 21: 537–46.

Checkoway HA, Pearce NE, Crawford-Brown DJ (1989). Research Methods in Occupational Epidemiology. New York: Oxford University Press.

Clayton D, Hills M (1993). Statistical Models in Epidemiology. Oxford: Oxford Scientific Publications.

Copeland KT, Checkoway H, McMichael AJ, et al (1977). Bias due to misclassification in the estimation of relative risk. Am J Epidemiol 105: 488–95.

Crane J, Lewis S, Slater T, et al (1994). The self-reported prevalence of asthma symptoms amongst adult New Zealanders. N Z Med J 107: 417–21.

Dean J, Dean A, Burton A, Dicker R (1990). Epi Info. Version 5.01. Atlanta, GA: CDC.

Dosemeci M, Wacholder S, Lubin JH (1990). Does nondifferential misclassification of exposure always bias a true effect toward the null value? Am J Epidemiol 132: 746–8.

Drane J (1991). Imputing nonresponses to mail-back questionnaires. Am J Epidemiol 134: 908–12.

Goodman SN, Berlin JA (1994). The use of predicted confidence intervals when planning experiments and the misuse of power when interpreting results. Ann Intern Med 121: 200–6.

Greenland S (1980). The effect of misclassification in the presence of covariates. Am J Epidemiol 112: 564–9.

Greenland S (1983). Tests for interaction in epidemiologic studies: a review and a study of power. Stat Med 2: 243–51.

Greenland S (1988a). On sample-size and power calculations for studies using confidence intervals. Am J Epidemiol 128: 231–7.

Greenland S (1988b). Statistical uncertainty due to misclassification: implications for validation substudies. J Clin Epidemiol 41: 1167–74.

Greenland S, Neutra R (1981). An analysis of detection bias and proposed corrections in the study of estrogens and endometrial cancer. J Chron Dis 34: 433–8.

Greenland S, Robins JM (1985a). Estimation of a common effect parameter from sparse follow-up data. Biometrics 41: 55–68.

Greenland S, Robins JM (1985b). Confounding and misclassification. Am J Epidemiol 122: 495–506.

Greenland S, Robins JM (1986). Identifiability, exchangeability and epidemiological confounding. Int J Epidemiol 15: 412–8.

Hosmer D, Lemeshow S (1989). Applied Logistic Regression. New York: Wiley.

Kleinbaum DG, Kupper LL, Morgenstern H (1982). Epidemiologic Research: Principles and Quantitative Methods. Belmont, CA: Lifetime Learning Publications.

Kleinbaum DG, Kupper LL, Muller K (1988). Applied Regression Analysis and Other Multivariable Methods. 2nd ed. Belmont, CA: Wadsworth.

Kristensen P (1992). Bias from nondifferential but dependent misclassification of exposure and outcome. Epidemiology 13: 210–5.

Mantel N, Haenszel W (1959). Statistical aspects of the analysis of data from retrospective studies of disease. J Natl Cancer Inst 22: 719–48.

Miettinen OS (1974a). Standardization of risk ratios. Am J Epidemiol 96: 383–8.

Miettinen OS (1974b). Confounding and effect modification. Am J Epidemiol 100: 350–3.

Miettinen OS (1985). Theoretical Epidemiology. New York: Wiley and Sons.

Olivetti JF, Kercsmar CM, Redline S. Pre- and perinatal risk factors for asthma in inner city African-American children. Am J Epidemiol 143: 570–7.

Osterman JW, Armstrong BG, Ledoux E, et al (1991). Comparison of French and English versions of the American Thoracic Society Respiratory Questionnaire in a bilingual working population. Int J Epidemiol 20: 138–43.

Pearce NE (1989). Analytic implications of epidemiological concepts of interaction. Int J Epidemiol 18: 976–80.

Pearce NE (1992). Time-related confounders and intermediate variables in epidemiologic studies. Epidemiology 3: 279–81.

Pearce NE, Checkoway HA, Dement JM (1988). Exponential models for analyses of time-related factors: illustrated with asbestos textile worker mortality data. J Occup Med 30: 517–22.

Robins J (1987). A graphical approach to the identification and estimation of causal parameters in mortality studies with sustained exposure periods. J Chron Dis 40 (suppl 2): 139S–161S.

Robins J (1989). The control of confounding by intermediate variables. Stat Med 8: 679–701.

Robins JM, Breslow NE, Greenland S (1986). Estimation of the Mantel-Haenszel variance consistent with both sparse-data and large-strata limiting models. Biometrics 42: 311–23.

Robins JM, Blevins D, Ritter G, et al (1992). G-estimation of the effect of prophylaxis therapy for pneumocystic carinii pneumonia on the survival of AIDS patients. Epidemiology 3: 319–36.

Rothman KJ, Greenland S (1997). Modern Epidemiology. 2nd ed. Philadelphia: Lippincott.

Schlesselman JJ (1982). Case-control Studies: Design, Conduct, Analysis. New York: Oxford University Press.

Segi M (1960). Cancer mortality for selected sites in 24 countries (1950–1957). Sendai, Japan: Department of Public Health, Tohoku University School of Medicine.

Siemiatycki J, Wacholder S, Dewar R, et al (1988). Smoking and degree of occupational exposure: are internal analyses in cohort studies likely to be confounded by smoking status? Am J Ind Med 13: 59–69.

Smith AH, Bates M (1992). Confidence limit analyses should replace power calculations in the interpretation of epidemiologic studies. Epidemiology 3: 449–52.

Stoddard JJ, Miller T (1995). Impact of parental smoking on the prevalence of wheezing respiratory illness in children. Am J Epidemiol 141: 96–102.

Sunyer J, Antó JM, Sabriá J, et al (1992). Risk factors of soybean epidemic asthma: the role of smoking and atopy. Am Rev Respir Dis 145: 1098–1102.

Walker AM (1982). Anamorphic analysis: sampling and estimation for covariate effects when both exposure and disease are known. Biometrics 38: 1025–32.

Walter SD (1977). Determination of significant relative risks and optimal sampling procedures in prospective and retrospective studies of various sizes. Am J Epidemiol 105: 387–97.

Weinberg CR (1993). Toward a clearer definition of confounding. Am J Epidemiol 137: 1–8.

White JE (1982). A two-stage design for the study of the relationship between a rare exposure and a rare disease. Am J Epidemiol 115: 119–28.

Part II
ASTHMA MORBIDITY

4

Measuring Asthma Prevalence

Most asthma prevalence studies must, by necessity, focus on factors that are related to, or symptomatic of, asthma but that can be readily assessed on a particular day. The main options in this regard are symptoms and physiological measures. The choice of specific techniques should be motivated by the need to use simple and practical methods in order to obtain valid data on large numbers of people, with high response rates, in a manner that is comparable across the social groups, regions, or countries being compared. Thus, symptom-based questionnaires remain the cornerstone of asthma prevalence surveys, although these are often supplemented by bronchial responsiveness testing or other physiological measures.

Introduction

The need for prevalence studies

The prevalence and causes of asthma and related conditions can be studied at many different levels including populations, individuals, organs, tissues, or cells. All of these approaches are potentially useful, and individual researchers will focus on different "levels of analysis" depending on their training, areas of interest, and availability of funding (Pearce, 1996). In the past however, the major contribution of epidemiology to the study of chronic diseases has been the focus on the population level, including analyses of patterns of disease prevalence and incidence across demographic groups and geographic areas and across time ("person, place, and time"). In particular, many of the epidemiological hypotheses concerning the causes of chronic disease have stemmed, at least in part, from geographical comparisons (Reid, 1975).

Example 4.1

Von Mutius et al (1992) compared the prevalence of asthma among children in Munich (western Germany) and Leipzig (eastern Germany), where environmental

Table 4.1. Lifetime prevalence of respiratory disorders among 9- to 11-year-old children in Leipzig and Munich

	Leipzig		Munich		Odds ratio	95% CI
	n	Percent	n	Percent		
Diagnosed asthma	72	7.3%	435	9.3%	0.8	0.6–1.0
Wheeze	191	20.0%	786	17.0%	1.2	1.0–1.5
Attacks of shortness of breath	73	7.3%	416	8.7%	0.8	0.6–1.1
Nocturnal cough	34	3.4%	166	3.4%	1.0	0.7–1.4
Cough after exercise or during foggy or cold weather	182	18.6%	560	11.7%	1.7	1.4–2.0

Source: Von Mutius et al (1992).

exposures, particularly air concentrations of sulfur dioxide and particulate matter, and living conditions have differed over the past 45 years. Questionnaires were completed by the parents of 7445 children in Munich and 1429 children in Leipzig. No significant differences were found in the lifetime prevalence of asthma or wheezing between children in Leipzig and Munich (Table 4.1), but if anything the prevalence tended to be lower in Leipzig. The authors concluded that the findings supported other evidence that long-term exposure to sulfur dioxide and particulate matter, even at high levels, does not have a major effect on the population prevalence of asthma.

For example, many of the recent discoveries on the causes of cancer (including dietary factors and colon cancer, hepatitis B and liver cancer, aflatoxins and liver cancer, human papilloma virus [HPV] and cervical cancer) have their origins, directly or indirectly, in the systematic international comparisons of cancer incidence conducted in the 1950s and 1960s (e.g., Doll et al, 1966). These revealed that there were major international differences in cancer incidence, particularly between industrialized countries and the developing world. These international patterns suggested hypotheses concerning the possible causes of these patterns, which were investigated in more depth in further studies. In some instances these hypotheses were consistent with biological knowledge at the time and may have been advanced at some stage even if the international comparisons had not been made. However, in other instances, the epidemiological hypotheses that were suggested were new and striking (otherwise they would have been proposed and tested at an earlier date) and might not have been proposed, or might not have been investigated further, if the international comparisons had not been made. The same logic applies to epidemiological studies involving comparisons within populations in Western countries. For example, of the 30 to 40 known occupational causes of cancer (Neutra, 1990), almost all of them were apparently first "discovered" in case reports and epidemiological studies (Pearce, 1994); none of them were first discovered in the laboratory, and in some instances (e.g., arsenic benzene) it took many years of laboratory research to replicate the epidemiological findings and to establish the etiologic mechanisms involved.

It is notable that the striking international differences in cancer incidence may not have been apparent if the cancer incidence analyses had been confined to Western countries, as the differences in cancer incidence (and in the lifestyle-related risk factors that cause the incidence patterns) in many instances would not have been sufficiently great. More generally, Rose (1985, 1992) has noted that whole populations, or regions of the world, may be exposed to risk factors for disease (e.g., high levels of exposure to dietary fat), and the associations of these factors with disease may only be readily apparent when comparisons are made between populations, or regions of the world, rather than within populations.

Is asthma prevalence increasing?

A further reason for conducting standardized international prevalence studies is the current concern that the prevalence of asthma may be increasing (Burr, 1987; Anderson, 1989; Weitzman et al, 1992; Anderson et al, 1994; Balfe et al, 1996; Woolcock and Peat, 1997). This is based on studies that have determined the prevalence of asthma symptoms, using the same methodology in the same community at different times. These studies have reported that asthma prevalence has increased in recent decades with the magnitude of the increase in some cases being substantial. Although methodological differences in these studies make it difficult to compare the magnitude of the differences in asthma prevalence between countries, the trend of increasing prevalence among populations in countries of widely differing lifestyles and ethnic groups is generally consistent. In a number of these studies the prevalence of other atopic disorders has also increased in parallel.

Table 4.2 summarizes 23 studies of changes in asthma prevalence over time. The studies used a wide variety of questions for assessing asthma prevalence, but in each instance the same questions have been used in a second "repeat" study in the same population at a later time. Thus, the findings for different populations are not comparable, as different questions were used, but the findings within a particular population can be compared over time. The studies found marked increases in asthma prevalence in virtually all countries considered. For example, Hsieh and Tsai (1992) examined the prevalence of allergic disorders in schoolchildren aged 7 to 15 years in Taipei, Taiwan, and found that the prevalence of childhood asthma increased from 1.3% in 1974 to 5.1% in 1985 and 5.8% in 1991. There were similar two- to threefold increases in the prevalence of allergic rhinitis, eczema, and urticaria, but these occurred at a later stage. The reduction in

Table 4.2. Changes in asthma prevalence in children and young adults

Country	Period	Asthma prevalence 1st study	2nd study	Reference
Australia	1964–1990	19.1%	46.0%	Robertson et al (1991)
	1982–1992	12.9%	19.3%	Peat et al (1994)
Canada	1980–1983	3.8%	6.5%	Infante-Rivard et al (1987)
England	1956–1975	1.8%	6.3%	Morrison Smith (1976)
	1966–1990	18.3%	21.8%	Whincup et al (1993)
	1973–1986	2.4%	3.6%	Burney et al (1990)
Finland	1961–1986	0.1%	1.8%	Haahtela et al (1990)
France	1968–1982	3.3%	5.4%	Perdrizet et al (1987)
Israel	1986–1990	7.9%	9.6%	Auerbach et al (1993)
Italy	1983–1993	2.9%	4.4%	Ciprandi et al (1996)
Japan	1982–1992	3.3%	4.6%	Nishima (1993)
Netherlands	1977–1992	19%	31%	Tirimanna et al (1996)
New Zealand	1969–1982	7.1%	13.5%	Mitchell (1983)
	1975–1989	26.2%	34.0%	Shaw et al (1990)
	1981–1990	22.8%	30.8%	Kljakovic (1991)
Papua New Guinea	1973–1984	0.0%	0.6%	Dowse et al (1985)
Scotland	1964–1989	10.4%	19.8%	Ninan and Russell (1992)
Sweden	1971–1981	1.9%	2.8%	Alberg (1989)
Tahiti	1979–1984	11.5%	14.3%	Liard et al (1988)
Taiwan	1974–1985	1.3%	5.1%	Hsieh et al (1988)
USA	1971–1976	4.8%	7.6%	Gergen et al (1988)
	1981–1988	3.1%	4.3%	Weitzman et al (1992)
Wales	1973–1988	4.0%	9.0%	Burr et al (1989)

air pollution during this period suggested that air pollution was not the main cause of the trends in asthma prevalence.

Example 4.2

Haahtela et al (1990) analyzed the medical examination reports of approximately 900,000 conscripts to the Finnish defense forces during 1966–89, and a proportional but unknown number examined in 1926–61. During 1926–61 the prevalence of asthma recorded at call-up examinations was in the range of 0.02 to 0.08%. However, asthma prevalence increased from 0.29% in 1966 to 1.79% in 1989 (Fig. 4.1). The authors concluded that the increase was unlikely to be due to improved diagnostic methods, and that much of the increase was likely to be real. This conclusion was strengthened by a concomitant rise (from 0.12% in 1966 to 0.75% in 1989) in exemptions and discharges due to asthma.

International prevalence comparisons

Thus, in many respects, the epidemiology of asthma is currently in a situation similar to that of cancer epidemiology in the 1950s and 1960s when international and regional prevalence comparisons were undertaken as a

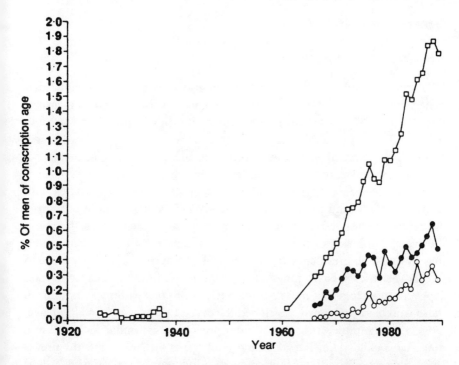

Figure 4.1. Prevalence of asthma in Finnish young men during 1926–89 expressed as percentage of male candidates for military conscription with diagnosis of asthma at or before call-up medical examination (□), percentage of men exempted at call up for military service by virtue of disabling asthma (●), and percentage of conscripts discharged during course of military service because of asthma (○). (Source: Haahtela et al, 1990.)

first step in ascertaining the causes of different forms of cancer (e.g. Doll et al, 1966). In considering methods of measuring asthma prevalence, we therefore focus on the issues involved in geographical comparisons (although asthma prevalence studies can also be conducted within a single center, as a prelude to prevalence case-control studies examining various risk factors for asthma (see Chapter 6)). Until recently, although hundreds of asthma prevalence studies had been conducted in various parts of the world, these studies had not adopted a standardized approach and there had been very few international or regional comparisons of asthma prevalence that had used identical techniques in different countries or centers. However, an international survey of asthma prevalence in adults has recently been conducted (Burney et al, 1994; ECRHS, 1996), and an International Study of Asthma and Allergies in Childhood (ISAAC) is also under way (Pearce et al, 1993; Asher et al, 1995). The methodologies used in these two major studies have become the standards for asthma prevalence comparisons, and we will therefore refer to them in reviewing the various methods for measuring asthma prevalence.

General Considerations

Prevalence, incidence, and duration

Ideally, we would wish to compare international patterns of asthma incidence. In practice, however, asthma incidence is very difficult to measure, both because of the intensive long-term monitoring required and because of the difficulty of establishing the date of onset of the condition (Gregg, 1983). Therefore, most studies involve prevalence rather than incidence. Techniques similar to those described in this chapter can be used in incidence studies (e.g., Larsson, 1995), except that incidence studies with intensive monitoring may enable a diagnosis of asthma to be more firmly established. Asthma prevalence reflects both the incidence of asthma and the average duration of the condition (see Chapter 2). Thus, a population may have a high prevalence of asthma either because of a high exposure to factors (genetic or environmental) that induce asthma or because of high exposure to factors that incite, exacerbate, or prolong asthma symptoms in those who have previously developed the disease (Dolovich and Hargreave, 1981). For example, asthma symptom prevalence is similar in Maori and non-Maori children in New Zealand (Robson et al, 1993), but the prevalence is greater in adult Maori than in adult non-Maori (Fig. 4.2) and does not decrease with age, whereas prevalence decreases with age in non-Maori (Crane et al, 1994). The reasons for this are unclear, but one possible explanation is that asthma symptoms are being prolonged or exacerbated in Maori because of environmental exposures (e.g., environmental tobacco smoke) or inappropriate management (e.g., underprescribing of inhaled corticosteroids).

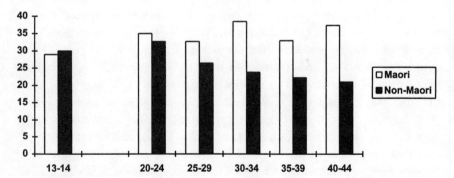

Figure 4.2. Asthma prevalence by age in Maori and non-Maori New Zealanders. (Source: Adapted from Crane et al, 1994; Robson et al, 1993.)

Definitions of asthma

Because clinicians, physiologists, and pathologists cannot agree on how to define asthma, it is not surprising that epidemiologists also have problems with this issue. As discussed in Chapter 1, the definition of asthma has become more complex as our understanding of its pathophysiology has increased. However, despite this increased complexity, the basic characteristic features of reversible airflow obstruction and bronchial hyperresponsiveness by which one recognizes or diagnoses the disease have changed little over recent years. These clinical features were the basis of the WHO (1975) definition:

> . . . a chronic condition characterised by recurrent bronchospasm resulting from a tendency to develop reversible narrowing of the airway lumina in response to stimuli of a level or intensity not inducing such narrowing in most individuals.

Although these features receive lesser prominence 20 years later, as the importance of airways inflammation is appropriately recognized, they still form the basis of the recent WHO/NHLBI definition (Anonymous, 1994) of asthma as:

> . . . a chronic inflammatory disorder of the airways in which many cells play a role, in particular mast cells, eosinophils and T lymphocytes. In susceptible individuals this inflammation causes recurrent episodes of wheezing, breathlessness, chest tightness and cough, particularly at night and/or in the early morning. These symptoms are usually associated with widespread but variable airflow limitation and is at least partly reversible either spontaneously or with treatment. The inflammation also causes an associated increase in airway responsiveness to a variety of stimuli.

A fundamental problem is that even when a single definition is accepted, the diagnosis of asthma involves an overall assessment of the patient's medical history, physical examination, and laboratory test results, and there are no universally accepted rules for combining the information from these various sources. A related problem is that biomedical definitions of disease are usually based on unifying pathophysiologic mechanisms, whereas the term asthma encompasses a disparate group of disease processes that produce similar clinical effects (i.e., variable airflow obstruction) (Josephs et al, 1990). In this sense, at least for purposes of epidemiological studies, asthma could be regarded as a "condition" or "syndrome" rather than a disease (Gergen and Weiss, 1995), and it is currently most useful to define asthma in terms of the phenomena involved without making any etiologic implications (Gross, 1980). Thus, although asthma can be conceptualized either in terms of symptoms such as wheezing, or in terms of the underlying bronchial inflammation, the essential feature of asthma (at least in clinical and epidemiological terms) is variable airflow obstruction that can be reversed by treatment or is self-limiting (Gregg, 1983).

Diagnosed asthma

This poses several problems with the use of "diagnosed asthma" in asthma prevalence studies because the diagnosis of "variable airflow obstruction" usually requires several medical consultations over an extended period. It is therefore not surprising that several studies have found the prevalence of physician-diagnosed asthma to be substantially lower than the prevalence of asthma symptoms (e.g., Baumann et al, 1992; Burr et al, 1994; Dales et al, 1994; Lee et al, 1983; Pearce et al, 1993). For example, Ehrlich et al (1995), in a survey of schoolchildren in Cape Town, found that among children with more than 12 attacks of wheezing in the previous 12 months, only 60% were reported as asthmatic and only 55% as receiving regular treatment.

These problems with "diagnosed asthma" as a measure not only affect prevalence estimates but also affect time trends (Hill et al, 1989) and geographical and social patterns of asthma prevalence. For example, some studies (e.g., Peckham and Butler, 1978) have found diagnosed asthma to be more common in upper social class children, possibly because of greater access to health care and therefore greater likelihood of being labeled as asthmatic (see also Chapter 6). The same concerns apply, perhaps to a greater extent, in surveys of use of asthma medication or health services. Although such information may be of value in morbidity studies (see Chapter 5) it is of very limited use in asthma prevalence studies.

Example 4.3

Lee et al (1983) conducted a prevalence survey of all 7-year-old children in North Tyneside in 1979. Questionnaires were completed by parents. A total of 11% of children were reported to have had episodes of wheeze since school entry: 9.3% were reported to have had episodic wheeze during the previous year, and 1.8% were reported to have had similar symptoms since starting school but not during the previous year. Only 1.2% of children in the survey had previously been diagnosed as having asthma. However, all of those children with current symptoms who were followed up subsequently responded to one or more of the drugs used in the management of asthma. The authors concluded that all these wheezy children had symptoms of asthma and that they should all have been both diagnosed and treated.

These issues are of particular concern in geographical prevalence comparisons because there are major international and regional differences in access to health care and labeling of asthma. Thus, some international comparisons have found differences in diagnosed asthma to be much greater than differences in reported asthma symptoms (e.g., Pearce et al, 1993); these differences in diagnosed asthma may partially reflect differences in access to health services and diagnostic practice rather than genuine differences in asthma prevalence. For example, Dodge and Burrows (1980) suggest that "the epidemiology of asthma is a reflection of the diagnostic habits of physicians in the locale, as well as an indicator of the frequency of a specific syndrome."

Such problems of differences in diagnostic practice could be minimized by using a standardized protocol for asthma diagnosis in prevalence studies. However, this is rarely a realistic option because it requires repeated contacts between the study participants and physicians, and this is not possible or affordable in large-scale epidemiological studies. One exception occurs when comprehensive medical examinations are performed routinely on a well-defined population, such as that described by Haahtela et al (1990) (see also Example 4.3). Although self-reported histories of physician-diagnosed asthma have been found to be relatively valid (Burr et al, 1975), this relates to diagnosed asthma rather than true asthma prevalence.

Validation

Thus, most epidemiological studies must, by necessity, focus on factors that are related to, or symptomatic of, asthma but that can be readily assessed on a particular day. The main options in this regard are symptoms or physiological measurements (Burney and Chinn, 1987).

A key difficulty in choosing between the various possible measures of asthma prevalence is the problem of validation when there is no practical "gold standard" for asthma. As noted above, the real gold standard is to give all study participants a series of physician examinations in order to diagnose all cases of clinical asthma, but this is rarely practical in epidemiological studies. Most commonly, validation has been performed against bronchial hyperresponsiveness (BHR) (Samet, 1987). BHR is not specific to asthma (see below), but BHR testing does at least provide a reliable marker of one physiologic characteristic associated with asthma (Burney et al, 1989a, 1989b) and remains the principal validation instrument for asthma prevalence surveys.

Such validations usually involve classifying study participants as having or not having BHR, and comparing this classification to the results using the instrument to be validated. For example, for a particular question (e.g., wheezing) the response to the question (yes or no) will be compared with the results of the BHR testing (yes or no). The *sensitivity* of the questions

Table 4.3. Sensitivity and specificity

		"Gold Standard"	
		Yes	No
Instrument	Yes	a	1 − b
	No	1 − a	b

(for BHR) is then the proportion of those classified as positive on the basis of the question (Table 4.3). The *specificity* is the proportion of those classified as negative for BHR who were classified as negative on the basis of the question. *Youden's index* is the sum of the sensitivity and specificity minus 1, and provides an overall measure of the validity of the question. In fact (Burney et al, 1989b), if:

a = sensitivity
b = specificity
P = the true proportion of positive responses (according to the gold standard)

then the observed proportion of positive responses to the question is:

$$a P + (1 - b)(1 - P) = P(a + b - 1) + (1 - b)$$

Therefore, if two populations are being compared, and their true prevalences (according to the gold standard) are P_1 and P_2, respectively, then the observed difference in prevalence between the two centers is:

$$(P_1 - P_2)(a + b - 1)$$

The expression $(a + b - 1)$ is Youden's index. When this is equal to 1 (which occurs only when the sensitivity and specificity are both 1) then the observed difference in prevalence will be exactly equal to the true difference in prevalence. More commonly, Youden's index will be less than 1 and the observed prevalence difference will be reduced accordingly; for example, if Youden's index is 0.75, then the observed prevalence difference will be 0.75 times the true prevalence difference. If the question has a sensitivity and specificity no better than chance (e.g. both equal to 0.5) then Youden's Index is zero and the expected value of the observed prevalence difference is zero. Youden's index therefore provides the most appropriate measure of the validity of a particular question or technique in prevalence comparisons.

Example 4.4

Example 3.8 (Chapter 3) considered hypothetical data from a study of asthma prevalence in childhood (see Table 3.6). The true prevalence rates were 40% in the exposed group and 20% in the nonexposed group; the true prevalence difference was thus 20%. If 20% of asthmatics are incorrectly classified as non-asthmatics (i.e., a sensitivity of 0.80), and 10% of non-asthmatics are incorrectly classified as asthmatics (i.e., a specificity of 0.90), then the observed prevalence will be 38% and 24%, respectively (Table 3.6); the observed prevalence difference will then be 14% (instead of the true value of 20%). The net effect is to bias the prevalence difference toward the null value of zero. The extent of the bias is related to Youden's index: this is $0.80 + 0.90 - 1.0 = 0.7$, and the observed prevalence difference of 14% is 0.7 times the true value of 20%.

It should be stressed that a perfect measure of asthma prevalence for use in epidemiological surveys does not exist. Epidemiological surveys of asthma prevalence need not (and cannot) produce perfect data, and the method that has the greatest validity within a particular population may not be most appropriate for regional or international comparisons. The objective is to produce data that are of comparable accuracy across the various groups, regions, or countries being compared—that is, it is important to ensure that any misclassification of the disease is nondifferential. In this situation, although some individuals may be misclassified, the study findings will reflect the true overall pattern of asthma prevalence (although the size of the prevalence differences between populations may be attenuated). Thus, when choosing possible approaches to comparing asthma prevalence in different populations, the emphasis must be on the comparability across populations of the information, rather than the absolute accuracy of the information in every individual study participant.

Response rates

It is also important that prevalence studies have good response rates. Response rates may be poor if participation in the study is time-consuming, involves travel, is potentially unpleasant (e.g., BHR testing), or is inconvenient in some other way. Nonresponse will not seriously bias the survey findings if the reasons for nonresponse are unrelated to asthma symptoms. However, it might be expected that people with asthma symptoms might be more likely to participate in such a study than people without asthma symptoms (even if the term "asthma" is not used in the invitation to participate). In this situation, a low response rate may seriously bias both the prevalence estimate and the comparison of asthma prevalence between different groups or centers. The best solution to this problem is to avoid it by achieving a high response rate. This is an important consideration in the choice of survey instrument because the most valid instrument will not give the most valid results if it produces low response rates. If, despite strenuous efforts, a survey has a low response rate, either overall or for some subgroups, then an attempt may be made to "adjust" the study findings for nonresponse, by attempting to estimate the prevalence of symptoms in the group of non-responders (Example 3.7 in Chapter 3 illustrates this approach).

Symptoms

Questionnaires on asthma symptoms are the cornerstone of large-scale epidemiological surveys of asthma prevalence (Anderson, 1989). These have the advantage of being inexpensive and simple to administer to large numbers of participants on a single day, and they will discriminate those with variable airflow obstruction that causes noticeable symptoms. The key issue is that questionnaires should obtain information in a standardized manner on symptoms that are directly related to "variable airflow obstruction." This definition of asthma implies a condition in which symptoms occur from time to time, rather than the presence or absence of symptoms on a particular day. Thus, operational definitions of asthma involve specification of the time period during which symptoms may have occurred. In particular, "current symptoms" are usually defined as symptoms at any time in the previous 12 months. Although there has been concern that repeated questioning of subjects could increase awareness of respiratory symptoms, a recent comparison of findings from an intensive longitudinal study and a prevalence study within similar populations found very similar symptom prevalences, suggesting that repeated questioning of the longitudinal study population had not biased prevalence rates (Sears et al, 1997).

Written questionnaires

Standard written questionnaires have been the principal instrument for measuring asthma symptom prevalence in community surveys, and in homogeneous populations these have been standardized, validated, and shown to be reproducible (Burney et al, 1989a). A number of symptoms, including wheezing, chest tightness, breathlessness, and coughing with or without sputum, are recognized by physicians as indicative of asthma. Of these the most important symptom for the identification of asthma in epidemiological studies is wheezing (Gergen et al, 1988; Lee et al, 1983), and most questionnaires have focused on this. However, symptoms such as wheeze may be absent despite variable airflow obstruction (asthma), and symptoms may also occur in the absence of asthma (Weiss et al, 1980). For example, a study in New Mexico (Samet et al, 1982; Samet, 1987) found that wheezing (apart from colds) occurred in 74.1% of current doctor-diagnosed asthmatics, but also occurred in 17.6% of smokers and 9.7% of nonsmokers without diagnosed asthma. Thus, wheezing is not synonymous with diagnosed asthma; in some instances, wheezing may indicate asthma that has not been diagnosed, but it may also indicate other diseases (particularly chronic bronchitis and emphysema in persons aged 45 years or more) or may be unrelated to other symptoms or disease; conversely, diagnosed asthmatics may not experience or recognize wheeze as a symptom. Nevertheless, wheezing remains the symptom that is most characteristic of asthma, particularly in persons aged 5 to 34 years, in whom asthma is less likely to be confused with bronchitis or emphysema. Furthermore, self-reported wheezing has reasonable sensitivity and specificity for other prevalence measures such as BHR (Burney et al, 1989a,b; Shaw et al, 1992a,b, 1995). Thus, most asthma symptom prevalence questionnaires focus on "current wheezing" (defined as wheezing at any time in the previous 12 months), but they usually also include additional questions on the frequency of wheezing and the circumstances in which wheezing occurs (wheezing while at rest, wheezing after exercise, waking with wheezing), as well as questions on related symptoms (e.g., waking with cough and severe episodes of breathlessness).

A large number of such questions have been used in epidemiological surveys in the last decade; Figure 4.3 shows questions related to wheezing and attacks of wheezing in the American Thoracic Society Questionnaire for adults (Samet, 1987). However, it is only in the past few years that standardized questionnaires have become available for prevalence studies in adults (Burney et al, 1994) and in children (Asher et al, 1995).

10A. Does your chest ever sound wheezing or whistling?
    1.   When you have a cold?
    2.   Occasionally apart from colds?
    3.   Most days or nights?

10B. (If yes to 1, 2 or 3 in 10A) For how many years has this been present?

11A. Have you ever had an attack of wheezing that has made you feel short of breath?

11B. (If yes to 11A) How old were you when you had your first such attack?

11C. Have you had two or more such episodes?

11D. Have you ever required medicine or treatment for the(se) attacks?

Figure 4.3 Questions related to wheezing and attacks of wheezing in the American Thoracic Society Questionnaire for adults (ATS-DLD-78). Source: Samet (1987).

The European Community Respiratory Health Survey (ECRHS) questionnaire

Figure 4.4 shows the phase I screening questionnaire for European Community Respiratory Health Survey (ECRHS) in adults (Burney et al, 1994). This is based on the International Union Against Tuberculosis and Lung Disease (IUATLD) bronchial symptoms questionnaire. It was initially developed in English in the 1980s (Burney and Chinn, 1987), and has now been translated into many languages, using translation and back-translation. The questionnaire was sent by post and self-administered. The questions primarily relate to asthma symptoms and medication use during the previous 12 months.

Example 4.5

Burney et al (1989a) conducted a validation of the IUATLD questionnaire in four European centers: Helsinki (n = 42), Berlin (n = 42), Paris (n = 51), and Nottingham (n = 40). The questionnaire was translated into Finnish, German, and French and the translations checked by back-translation into English. Table 4.4 shows the

---

**TO ANSWER THE QUESTIONS PLEASE CHOOSE THE APPROPRIATE BOX.
IF YOU ARE UNSURE OF THE ANSWER PLEASE CHOOSE 'NO.'**
  1. Have you had a wheezing or whistling in your chest at any time in the last *12 months?*
IF 'NO' GO TO QUESTION 2, IF 'YES'
      1.1   Have you been at all breathless when the wheeze noise was present?
      1.2   Have you had this wheezing or whistling when you did not have a cold?
  2. Have you woken up with a feeling of tightness in your chest at any time in the last *12 months?*
  3. Have you been woken by an attack of shortness of breath at any time in the last *12 months?*
  4. Have you been woken by an attack of coughing at any time in the last *12 months?*
  5. Have you had an attack of asthma in the last *12 months?*
  6. Are you currently taking any medicine (including inhalers, aerosols or tablets) for asthma?
  7. Do you have any nasal allergies including hay fever?
  8. What is your *date of birth?*
  9. What is *today's date?*
  10. Are you male or female?

Figure 4.4. Phase I screening questionnaire for the European Community Respiratory Health Survey (ECRHS).

Table 4.4. Sensitivity (Sens) and specificity (Spec) for BHR of selected questions from the IUATLD bronchial symptoms questionnaire

Question	Helsinki			Berlin			Paris			Nottingham		
	Sens	Spec	Youden	Sens	Spec	Youden	Sens	Spec	Youden	Sens	Spec	Youden
Wheeze	0.95	0.74	0.69	0.59	0.80	0.39	0.73	0.65	0.38	0.89	0.62	0.51
Morning tightness	0.74	0.87	0.61	0.33	0.93	0.26	0.53	0.72	0.25	0.79	0.57	0.36
Attacks of shortness of breath	0.58	0.78	0.36	0.11	0.80	-0.09	0.73	0.68	0.41	0.74	0.67	0.41
Waking with shortness of breath	0.47	0.83	0.31	0.37	0.80	0.17	0.69	0.77	0.46	0.74	0.97	0.71
Phlegm	0.63	0.74	0.37	0.26	0.87	0.13	0.50	0.62	0.12	0.74	0.79	0.23
Asthma ever	0.73	0.91	0.65	0.33	0.93	0.26	0.80	0.74	0.54	0.53	1.00	0.53
Asthma last 12 months	0.68	0.91	0.59	0.26	0.93	0.19	0.50	0.76	0.26	0.47	1.00	0.47

Source: Burney et al (1989a).

findings for sensitivity, specificity, and Youden's index when validated against BHR. In most of the centers, the best value of Youden's index was obtained with the general question on wheeze during the past 12 months. Most other questions had poorer sensitivity and better specificity, but the overall value of Youden's index was lower. In general, Youden's index was lower in Germany than in the other countries studied. Although the reason for this difference is not clear, it may relate to the difficulty of translating "wheezing" into German, for which word there is no colloquial term. In this study, for the translation into German, a phrase (rather than a single word) was used that did not bear an immediate resemblance to the original question relating to "wheeze."

The International Study of Asthma and Allergies in Childhood (ISAAC) questionnaire

A similar questionnaire (Fig. 4.5) has now been developed for the International Study on Asthma and Allergies in Childhood (ISAAC). The ISAAC

---

1. Have you *ever* had wheezing or whistling in the chest at any time in the past?
    Yes [ ]   No [ ]
    IF YOU ANSWERED "NO" PLEASE SKIP TO QUESTION 6
2. Have you had wheezing or whistling in the chest *in the last 12 months?*
    Yes [ ]   No [ ]
    IF YOU ANSWERED "NO" PLEASE SKIP TO QUESTION 6
3. How many attacks of wheezing have you had *in the last 12 months?*
    None [ ]   1 to 3 [ ]   4 to 12 [ ]   More than 12 [ ]
4. *In the last 12 months,* how often, on average, has your sleep been disturbed due to wheezing?
    Never woken with wheezing [ ]
    Less than one night per week [ ]
    One or more nights per week [ ]
5. *In the last 12 months,* has wheezing ever been severe enough to limit your speech to only one or two words at a time between breaths?
    Yes [ ]   No [ ]
6. Have you *ever* had asthma?
    Yes [ ]   No [ ]
7. *In the last 12 months,* has your chest sounded wheezy during or after exercise?
    Yes [ ]   No [ ]
8. *In the last 12 months,* have you had a dry cough at night, apart from a cough associated with a cold or a chest infection?
    Yes [ ]   No [ ]

Figure 4.5. ISAAC Phase I asthma symptom questionnaire.

Table 4.5. Sensitivity, specificity, and Youden's index for the ISAAC written and video questionnaires in 12- to 15-year-olds in Wellington

Question	Sensitivity	Specificity	Youden's index	95% CI
WRITTEN QUESTIONNAIRE				
1. Wheezing	0.65 (17/26)	0.62 (38/61)	0.27	0.05–0.49
2. Wheezing with exercise	0.58 (15/26)	0.72 (44/61)	0.30	0.08–0.52
3. Nocturnal wheezing	0.54 (14/26)	0.84 (51/61)	0.38	0.16–0.60
4. Nocturnal cough	0.38 (10/26)	0.75 (46/61)	0.13	−0.08–0.35
5. Severe wheezing	0.50 (13/26)	0.85 (52/61)	0.35	0.13–0.57
VIDEO QUESTIONNAIRE				
1. Wheezing	0.70 (46/66)	0.76 (96/127)	0.46	0.33–0.59
2. Wheezing with exercise	0.68 (45/66)	0.66 (84/127)	0.34	0.20–0.48
3. Nocturnal wheezing	0.47 (31/66)	0.90 (114/127)	0.37	0.24–0.40
4. Nocturnal cough	0.61 (40/66)	0.65 (82/127)	0.26	0.12–0.40
5. Severe wheezing	0.52 (34/66)	0.89 (113/127)	0.38	0.25–0.51

Source: Shaw et al (1995).

questionnaire is based on several similar questionnaires that had previously been used in studies of children in Australia, England, and New Zealand (e.g., Mitchell et al, 1990; Anderson et al, 1983; Robertson et al, 1991). Once again, the questions primarily relate to asthma symptoms during the previous 12 months.

Example 4.6

Table 4.5 shows the findings of a validation study of the ISAAC written questionnaire in samples of New Zealand high school students aged 12 to 15 years (Shaw et al, 1995). The study involved self-completion of the questionnaire by the students. Similar values of Youden's index were obtained for the various questions employed. The values of Youden's index were less, but not significantly so, than those obtained using similar questions in adults (see Table 4.4).

Translation of written questionnaires

One of the major problems with the use of written questionnaires in international comparisons is their translation into the different languages of the communities studied. As discussed above, this problem has been experienced with the translation into German of the IUATLD questionnaire (Burney et al, 1989a), for there is no colloquial term for "wheezing" in the German language. Similar problems have been recognized in a recent study in a French-speaking population (Osterman et al, 1991), and in studies that have been undertaken of asthma prevalence in remote Pacific atoll communities (Crane et al, 1989). For example, in the Tokelau Islands the indigenous language contains no single word for "wheezing," and the word normally used encompasses a wide range of respiratory symptoms including breathlessness and coughing. To ensure that data regarding the frequency and severity of symptoms are comparable in international comparisons of asthma prevalence, it is important that the questionnaire be translated in a manner that ensures that the terms describing symptoms correspond as closely as possible to the international recommended questions.

Example 4.7

Weiland et al (1993) studied how children and adolescents with asthma, as well as their parents, describe their symptoms for the purpose of translating the term "wheeze" for use in the ISAAC written symptom questionnaire. Children aged 7 to 15 years and their parents were asked to rate different descriptions of breathing and sounds of breathing during asthma attacks. The descriptions were those that had been used in existing questionnaires as well as those deemed appropriate to ask, and those that appeared unsuitable were used as control items. Description evaluation and cluster analysis showed the best-valued descriptions. In describing the sounds of asthmatic breathing, the item "pfeifend aus brustkorb" (whistling from the chest) was rated the best term. The order of the rating of terms was relatively independent of the sex of the child and whether the child or caregiver answered the question, indicating that in Germany at least it is possible to develop a questionnaire that can be answered by parents and children in a consistent manner. In contrast the study showed that the use of language by the patients does not correlate closely with the use by doctors.

As a result of the study described in Example 4.7, Weiland (1994) developed guidelines for the translation of the ISAAC study questionnaires. These recommended that:

1. The questionnaires be translated by one or more persons who are bilingual and familiar with the area in which the questionnaire will be used.
2. In order to find the most appropriate translation for difficult terms, for example, "wheezing" or "whistling in the chest," the following are proposed:
   a. Ask local doctors about local words to describe these terms.
   b. Ask children with asthma and parents of children with asthma how they would describe the breathing during an asthma episode.
   c. Show the asthma video (see below) and ask children with asthma and parents of children with asthma how they would describe the breathing of the children and adolescents in the video.
   d. Submit a list of possible descriptors to children with asthma and par-

ents of children with asthma and ask them to indicate (e.g., using a rating system) which description(s) they favor best.

3. The most appropriate translation should be agreed upon among a group of national experts on the basis of 2(a)–2(d). The national questionnaires should allow for differences in the wording of questionnaires according to the local use of language.
4. The questionnaires should be translated back into English by an independent translator. Modifications should be made if necessary.
5. The questionnaires should be tested in populations representative of the study populations. Modifications should be made if necessary.
6. Steps 2 to 5 are repeated if necessary.

The ISAAC video questionnaire

In response to the problems of validity associated with the use of standard written questionnaires in studies of populations speaking different languages, and from different cultural backgrounds, a video questionnaire involving the audiovisual presentation of clinical signs and symptoms of asthma has also been developed (Shaw et al, 1992a,b). This video questionnaire attempts to minimize these difficulties of comparability of information in large surveys among diverse populations (the accompanying questionnaire is shown in Fig. 4.6). In particular, the video questionnaire was developed to avoid problems of translation and comprehension of terms such as "wheeze" or "whistling in the chest," and their use in culturally heterogeneous populations (Burr, 1992). A pilot video questionnaire (AVQ1.0) was tested in 1989 (Shaw et al, 1992a), and a second version (AVQ2.0) was developed in 1990 (Shaw et al, 1992b). The questionnaire involves five sequences of clinical asthma symptoms in young persons: wheezing at rest; wheezing after exercise; waking with wheezing; waking with cough; a severe asthma attack. After each sequence, participants are asked whether their breathing had ever been like that of the person in the video; if so, they are asked whether this had occurred in the past year, and whether this had occurred one or more times a month (Fig. 4.6). The term asthma or wheezing is not mentioned at any stage in the video questionnaire. In a validation exercise, the video questionnaire was found to be as sensitive and specific for predicting bronchial hyperresponsiveness (BHR) as the ISAAC written questionnaire (see Table 4.5 in example 4.6). The first ISAAC version of the video (AVQ2.0) was produced in New Zealand using Caucasian asthmatics, but this was subsequently replaced by an international version of the video, featuring asthmatics from various continents and ethnic groups (AVQ3.0). Two sequences are common to both versions of the video, thereby permitting comparability between the two versions. Chan et al (1997) validated the international version of the video

- *The first scene is of a young person at rest.*

(First scene comes on here)

- *Question 1.* Has your breathing been like this at any time in your life?
  If Yes, has this happened in the last year?
  If Yes, has this happened at least once a month?

- *The second scene is of two young people after exercise.*
  One is in a dark shirt, and one is in a light shirt.

(Second scene comes on here)

- *Question 2.* Has your breathing been like the boy's in the dark shirt following exercise at any time in your life?
  If Yes, has this happened in the last year?
  If Yes, has this happened at least once a month?

- *The third scene is of a young person waking at night.*

(Third scene comes on here)

- *Question 3.* Have you been woken at night like this at any time in your life?
  If Yes, has this happened in the last year?
  If Yes, has this happened at least once a month?

- *The fourth scene is also of a young person waking at night.*

(Fourth scene comes on here)

- *Question 4.* Have you been woken at night like this at any time in your life?
  If Yes, has this happened in the last year?
  If Yes, has this happened at least once a month?

- *The final scene is of another person at rest.*

(Fifth scene comes on here)

- *Question 5.* Has your breathing been like this at any time in your life?
  If Yes, has this happened in the last year?
  If Yes, has this happened at least once a month?

Figure 4.6. ISAAC Phase I asthma video questionnaire.

questionnaire and found it to be at least as effective as the ISAAC written questionnaire in predicting BHR.

Physiological Measures

The problems of validity, repeatability and translation of questionnaires have led to attempts to find more "objective" physiological measures for use in prevalence studies. These measures carry with them their own set of limitations with regard to both their "objectivity" (i.e., they are not un-equivocally measures of asthma prevalence) and their practicality in large population-based surveys. Nevertheless, they form a useful complement to symptom questionnaires.

Lung function

Diminished lung function, as well as being used as an outcome measure in prevalence studies, is also a risk factor for the development of wheezing and/ or asthma (Martinez et al, 1988). Lung function measurements include forced expiratory volume in one second (FEV_1), forced vital capacity (FVC), and peak expiratory flow rate (PEFR). These are all forced expiratory maneuvers undertaken following a maximum inspiratory maneuver. While maximum inspiratory and expiratory maneuvers may lead to small transient changes in airway caliber, the simplicity, standardization, and reproducibility of such maximal expiratory maneuvers (particularly FEV_1 and FVC although PEFR has many practical advantages in field studies) make them the lung function measurements of choice in epidemiological studies (Quanjer et al, 1993), and standardized guidelines are available (American Thoracic Society, 1987; Quanjer et al, 1997).

However, such measures may have limited use in prevalence studies because the airflow obstruction in asthma is reversible over short periods of time and may not be present on the day of assessment (Josephs et al, 1990). Indeed, one of the characteristic features of reversible airflow obstruction in asthma is its diurnal variation, in that the degree of airflow obstruction is greatest at night or on wakening, and least during the day when lung function measurement is likely to be undertaken (Lebowitz et al, 1997). Thus, a significant proportion of asthmatics may have lung function within normal limits on any one day and may not exhibit the recognized 15% improvement in FEV_1 or PEF values after inhaled bronchodilator that is required for a physiological diagnosis of asthma to be made. A better alternative is to undertake repeat measurements of lung function before and after inhaling bronchodilator, at different times of day over a period of time (e.g., 2 weeks); however, this inevitably requires greater resources. It is this variation and reversibility of changes in lung function that typifies asthma, and this cannot be captured in a one-off prevalence survey on a particular day. Similarly, a one-off clinical examination with auscultation of the chest to identify the proportion of subjects with wheeze is also of limited value.

Example 4.8

Kelly et al (1988) studied an age-matched group of 247 subjects who had had asthma as children and 39 controls; both groups were studied with lung function

Table 4.6. FEV$_1$/VC (and 95% CI) by age and asthma severity

Age	Control	Class S*	Class T†	Class U‡	Class V§
7	90.3	89.4	88.5	85.4	85.5
	(88.6–92.0)	(88.1–90.7)	(86.5–90.5)	(82.9–87.8)	(82.9–88.0)
10	88.5	86.8	85.4	86.1	82.0
	(86.3–90.6)	(85.1–88.5)	(83.4–87.5)	(84.4–87.8)	(78.9–85.1)
14	87.2	86.5	82.0	85.2	79.2
	(85.1–89.2)	(85.2–87.8)	(78.7–85.3)	(83.2–87.3)	(75.5–83.0)
21	83.6	83.5	80.6	82.1	75.6
	(81.3–85.9)	(81.8–85.3)	(77.7–83.5)	(80.0–84.1)	(71.5–79.6)
28	82.1	81.3	77.3	77.3	67.4
	(79.9–84.2)	(80.0–82.7)	(74.7–79.9)	(75.0–79.6)	(64.3–70.5)

*Not wheezed for 3 or more years.
†Wheezed in previous 3 years, but not in previous 3 months.
‡Wheezed in previous 3 months, but less than once a week.
§Wheezed more than once a week in previous 3 months.
Source: Adapted from Kelly et al (1988).

testing at ages 7, 10, 14, 21, and 28 years. Those with the most severe asthma at age 28 showed the steepest decline in their FEV$_1$/VC from the age of 10 years than those with less severe asthma and those with no asthma (Table 4.6). The authors concluded that airways obstruction becomes more common as wheezing frequency increases. On the other hand, they found no evidence of a decline in lung function related to bronchial hyperreactivity (BHR). These findings are consistent with other evidence of reduced lung growth throughout childhood and adolescence in those with persistent asthma symptoms (Buist and Vollmer, 1987).

Bronchial responsiveness

Measurements of bronchial responsiveness in epidemiological studies of obstructive respiratory disease have been increasingly used in the past decade, and standard procedures are now well established (Rijcken and Schouten, 1993). Bronchial hyperresponsiveness (BHR) testing was originally developed in a clinical setting and has conventionally been defined in terms of the dose of agonist producing a 20% fall in FEV$_1$ (Abramson et al, 1990), although more recently analysis of breath sounds has been proposed as an alternative method (Gavriely, 1996). Although BHR is often defined in terms of a dichotomy (e.g., subjects are defined as having BHR if they experience a 20% fall in FEV$_1$ at a dose of agonist below a specified level), it can also be regarded as a continuous measure using the dose-response slope (O'Connor et al, 1987; Muñoz and Sunyer, 1996).

BHR tests are neither wholly sensitive nor specific for asthma. For example, Josephs et al (1989) found that within a group of asthmatics, levels of BHR are related to the average severity of the asthma, but that levels of BHR in individuals were not consistently related to concurrent asthma severity. BHR usually, but not always, precedes the development of asthma

(Hopp et al, 1990; Carey et al, 1996) but also occurs in chronic bronchitis and in tobacco smokers (Burney et al, 1987). BHR has been reported in 6 to 8% of children without symptoms, and was absent in one third of those with recurrent wheezing (Josephs et al, 1990). Similarly, BHR occurs in 3% of normal adults and more frequently in relatives of atopic or asthmatic patients (Josephs et al, 1990). BHR also persists in patients with a past history of asthma, although usually at lower levels than in patients with current disease (Townley et al, 1971).

Perhaps the fundamental problem is that BHR may (by definition) represent the potential to respond to stimuli, rather than the response itself. Thus, persons with nonspecific BHR may have a greater tendency to experience asthma symptoms if they are exposed to the relevant stimulus, but whether they do actually experience asthma symptoms will depend on whether exposure occurs, and at what level. Thus, the severity of airflow obstruction may be determined by the interaction of nonspecific reactivity and the strength of a provoking bronchoconstrictor stimulus (Josephs et al, 1990; Cockroft et al, 1979). Furthermore, BHR is only one mechanism contributing to the clinical expression of variable airflow obstruction and may contribute to a greater or lesser extent in different individuals and within the same individual at different times (Josephs et al, 1990). Thus, although BHR is clearly related to asthma, and may be involved in many of the pathways by which variable airflow obstruction may occur, variable airflow obstruction may occur independently of BHR, and vice versa (Sears et al, 1986). They are separate phenomena that both involve inflammation of the airways (Chung, 1986), and that are both worthy of study in their own right.

Example 4.9

Backer et al (1991) studied 495 randomly selected children and adolescents aged 7 to 16 years in Copenhagen. All participants were interviewed and completed a questionnaire about asthmatic symptoms; 28 were then classified as asthmatic, and 467 as non-asthmatic. Both groups then underwent histamine challenge tests. Table 4.7 shows the sensitivity, specificity, value of Youden's index, and positive and negative predictive value for BHR as a predictor of asthma, using three different cutoff points and two different concentrations of histamine. When stricter criteria were used for defining BHR, the sensitivity of the test for asthma increased, but the specificity decreased. The authors concluded that BHR testing has a low positive predictive value for asthma, and that it has at most a supplementary role in population studies.

Methods of testing for BHR. A number of factors can affect the results of challenge tests, including the selection of patients, criteria for carrying out the

Table 4.7. Sensitivity, specificity, Youden's index, and positive and negative predictive value of BHR testing for asthma, using three different cutoff points (for the % fall in FEV_1) and two different concentrations of histamine

Percentage fall in FEV_1	Sensitivity	Specificity	Youden's index	Positive predictive value	Negative predictive value
CUTOFF AT 2.4 MG/ML					
PC_6	1.00	0.74	0.74	19%	100%
PC_{12}	0.75	0.93	0.68	40%	98%
PC_{20}	0.57	0.98	0.55	59%	97%
CUTOFF AT 8.0 MG/ML					
PC_6	1.00	0.46	0.46	10%	100%
PC_{12}	1.00	0.73	0.73	18%	100%
PC_{20}	1.00	0.89	0.89	35%	100%

Source: Adapted from Backer et al (1991).

challenge test, technical factors, the provoking agent used, the dosing schedule, the lung function tests that are carried out, and the analysis of the data (Weeke et al, 1987). Protocols for challenge procedures therefore require detailed inclusion and exclusion criteria. For example in the European Community Respiratory Health Study (ECRHS) subjects were excluded if they had heart disease currently requiring medication, had epilepsy, or were pregnant or breast-feeding. Medication that might interfere with the test also must be considered; inhaled short-acting beta$_2$ agonists or anti-muscarinics are usually withheld for 4 to 6 hours prior to testing; oral beta$_2$ agonists or oral theophyllines are usually withheld for 8 hours, and for slow-release preparations more than 24 hours may be required. Other drugs such as beta adrenergic blockers may also influence test results.

The measurement of BHR in children has been confounded by problems of changing lung size and difficulty controlling for this variable. BHR is common in healthy infants (Le Souef et al, 1989), and declines with age in children (Hopp et al, 1985). One possibility is that BHR in children may be a reflection of increased dose to the airway in relation to size. The situation is further complicated by patterns of breathing that can influence aerosol deposition and vary considerably with age in children. Le Souef (1993) has argued that in the absence of suitable techniques for correcting for lung size, comparisons of BHR between children of different sizes are precluded. Nevertheless, bronchial challenge testing can be readily performed in children aged 5 years or more, and in adolescents (Hopp et al, 1986).

A wide variety of methodologies, bronchoconstrictors (including physiological and nonphysiological agents) and physical methods have been used to induce bronchoconstriction in susceptible individuals. These include exercise, isocapnic hyperventilation, cold/dry air, hypo- and hypertonic aerosols, pharmacological agents, allergens, occupational sensitizers, and a variety of experimental challenge agents (Sterk et al, 1993).

For each of these methods, standardization and reproducibility are obviously important. In the case of aerosol generation, calibration and quality control procedures need to be incorporated into any study protocol. Increasing concentrations of the agonists are used to provide a series of known concentrations or doses delivered to the airways over a period of approximately 30 minutes. The amount of agonist required to produce bronchoconstriction is considered in terms of a cumulative dose or concentration. Practical protocols usually incorporate two dosing regimens to provide a rapid rise in agonist dose for those without symptoms or with normal baseline spirometry and slower incremental dosing for those with abnormal spirometry or with a history of airways obstruction. Protocols specify baseline conditions under which a challenge should not be undertaken; these are usually defined in terms of a reduced FEV_1/FVC ratio. The challenge test usually commences with a diluent or normal saline challenge, and change in FEV_1 following each agonist dose is calculated from this post-diluent value. The procedure usually terminates when a 20% fall in FEV_1 has been achieved or the highest dose or concentration in the protocol has been delivered. Spirometry is normally undertaken with subjects sitting rather than standing, and nose clips are used to prevent nasal exhalation during forced expiratory maneuvers.

In large-scale surveys, challenges with histamine and methacholine have been the most widely used methods and have been best standardized and validated, with methacholine having less systemic and local side effects at higher doses than histamine. These agents are usually considered interchangeable with good correlation in responsiveness in a group of subjects (Juniper et al, 1981), although not necessarily in individuals (Josephs et al, 1990). Results are expressed either as a dose in micromols causing a 10% or 20% fall in FEV_1 (PD_{10} and PD_{20}) from baseline, or in the case of tidal breathing methods, the concentration required to cause a fall of 10% or 20% (PC_{10} or PC_{20}).

These doses are usually calculated by plotting the cumulative dose of bronchoconstrictor delivered to the airways on a log scale against the percentage fall in FEV_1 with extrapolation of the dose-response curve if required. More recently some investigators have suggested the use of the dose-response slope rather than the PD_{20} or PC_{20}, essentially providing a measure of the percentage decline in FEV_1 per mol of methacholine or histamine administered (O'Connor et al, 1987). This technique has the advantage of providing information on a much larger proportion of the population under study rather than simply categorizing individuals as responsive or nonresponsive. In the laboratory setting—under optimal conditions and with patients whose respiratory status is stable—the 95% confidence interval for single measurements of PD_{20} or PC_{20} is less than one twofold dose or concentration difference; in the community setting, where clinical stability and inter-technician variability is less easily controlled, the 95% confidence interval may increase to two to three twofold dose differences (Sterk et al, 1993).

Three principal methods of reproducible aerosol generation have been employed in testing for BHR using histamine or methacholine: (1) powered nebulizers (Chai et al, 1975); (2) handheld nebulizers (Yan et al, 1983); and (3) tidal breathing from a jet nebulizer (Cockroft et al, 1977). There is good correlation between these methods (Josephs et al, 1990). Woolcock et al have used the Yan technique (Yan et al, 1983) for measuring nonspecific BHR in an extensive program of asthma epidemiological studies predominantly among children (Peat et al, 1989, 1992, 1994; Salome et al, 1987; Woolcock et al, 1987). It employs small glass or plastic handheld and hand-operated nebulizers (De Vilbiss 40 glass nebulizers) to deliver discrete doses of histamine or methacholine. The method was developed for field use (Woolcock et al, 1983), and has the considerable advantage of being easily portable and does not require an electricity supply for a nebulizer. In the European Community Respiratory Health Survey (ECRHS), Burney et al (1994) have used a dosimeter method in the laboratory, with Mefar MB3 dosimeters, Biomed Spirometers, and standard methacholine solutions. There is good agreement between the ECRHS and Yan methods (Toelle et al, 1994).

Example 4.10

Hopp et al (1986) tested bronchial hyperresponsiveness in 400 subjects aged 5 to 21 years in Omaha. The methacholine challenge results were expressed as the area under the dose-response curve determined by the integration of the best-fit parabola. This was categorized into 4 response ranges: high (strongly positive), medium, low (weakly positive) and negative. All 55 asthmatics reacted to methacholine, with 82% having strongly positive responses. However, 52% of nonasthmatics and 47% of nonallergic subjects also reacted to methacholine. The challenge test results were also affected by age, and family history of asthma. The authors concluded that methacholine challenge studies in pediatric patients must be interpreted with age, personal atopic status, and family asthma history in mind.

Recently concerns have been raised in a number of countries by health and regulatory authorities over the use of methacholine and histamine from laboratory sources that have not been approved for human use. Difficulty in obtaining supplies or gaining the appropriate authority to use these agents has led to a renewed interest in alternative methods for assessing airway hyperresponsiveness in field studies. For example, a school-based study in southwestern Germany using methacholine raised considerable concern and press coverage, resulting in a very low response rate (Frischer et al, 1991; Nicolai et al, 1993).

Exercise challenge using a variety of standardized exercise protocols and often peak flow measurements rather than FEV_1 has been used extensively in epidemiological studies, particularly among children (e.g., Busquets et al, 1996). Free running is preferred in field studies but in the laboratory a bicycle ergometer has the advantage of providing a workload independent of weight (Sterk et al, 1993). Burr et al (1989) have used a 6-minute indoor running stimulus with measurement of the peak expiratory flow rates (PEFR) before and after exercise. Haby et al (1993) have recently developed a standardized protocol for field use with spirometry and a free-running stimulus. Two problems arise for exercise challenge in epidemiological studies: between subject standardization of ventilation with resulting difference in the magnitude of the exercise stimulus; and the impact of varying absolute water content on the response (Anderson, 1985). Continuous measurement of heart rate together with a measure of the total distance covered allows an indirect estimate of ventilation to be made (Haby et al, 1993) and thus an estimate of the size of the individual stimulus. Restriction of studies to times when the ambient water content is below 10 mg H_2O/L minimizes the loss of sensitivity to exercise (Anderson, 1985).

More recently *hypertonic saline* challenge has been trialled for use in epidemiological studies and has been specified as an alternative to methacholine challenge testing in Phase II of the ISAAC study (Strachan, 1995) (see Example 4.11).

Cold air challenge has also been used to measure airway hyperresponsiveness in epidemiological studies, although the relative complexity of the equipment required has been a significant limiting factor. Nicolai et al (1993) report that cold air has a lower sensitivity than does histamine (31% versus 52%) and a similar specificity (about 90%).

Finally, challenge with *distilled water* has also been used in population studies (Frischer et al, 1992).

Example 4.11

Riedler et al (1994) evaluated the sensitivity and specificity of a 4.5% hypertonic saline challenge, and a free-running exercise challenge, in 393 schoolchildren in Melbourne who completed the Phase I ISAAC asthma symptom questionnaire.

Table 4.8. BHR, lung function, self-reported symptom frequency, diagnosed asthma, and medication use in 352 children aged 7 to 12 years

	Normal	BHR only	Wheeze only	BHR and wheeze
BRONCHIAL RESPONSIVENESS				
$PD_{20}FEV_1$	—	2.4	—	0.9
Dose-response slope (DRS)	3.6	12.0	3.9	23.4
Abnormal DRS (%)	0	50.0	0	84.9
LUNG FUNCTION				
Mean airflow meter variability	12.6	19.0	16.5	31.7
FEV_1 (% predicted)	86.9	89.0	88.7	85.9
SYMPTOMS				
Symptoms recorded (%)	26.9	34.4	55.8	61.3
Symptoms limiting activity (%)	6.4	9.4	14.0	27.4
Night cough (%)	18.7	25.0	34.9	60.0
ASTHMA				
Diagnosed asthma (%)	10.5	31.3	74.4	88.7
Medications (%)	2.3	6.2	20.9	47.2
Total number	171	43	32	106

Source: Adapted from Toelle et al (1992).

Hypertonic saline challenge tests were based on the protocol of Smith and Anderson (1990). A 6-minute free-running exercise test was based on a protocol developed by Haby et al (1993); this involved a 6-minute run on a flat oval at a medium jog to keep the heart rate above 180 bpm after running for 2 minutes. The sensitivity and specificity of the hypertonic saline challenge for "current wheeze" were 47% and 92%, respectively (Youden's index 0.45), and the corresponding figures for the exercise challenge were 46% and 88% (Youden's index 0.34). The authors concluded that hypertonic saline challenge had sensitivity and specificity similar to that of standardized exercise challenge and pharmacologic challenges and a higher sensitivity than cold air hyperventilation and distilled water.

Combining BHR testing with symptoms. It has been suggested that a combination of recent symptoms and abnormal BHR may be the most useful epidemiological definition of asthma currently available (Woolcock, 1987; Toelle et al, 1992). This has some attractive features because neither wheezing nor BHR alone provides definitive data on asthma prevalence. Toelle et al (1992) studied 352 children aged 7 to 12 years in New South Wales and found that children with both current wheeze (in the previous 12 months) and BHR showed greater BHR, symptoms, diagnosed asthma, and asthma medication use than either marker alone (Table 4.8). The combination of current wheeze and BHR (which Toelle et al defined as "current asthma") therefore denotes a group with relatively high asthma prevalence. However, the interpretation of the findings for the "wheeze only" and "BHR only" groups is not so clear (Table 4.8). Toelle et al argued that the group with

"BHR only" was intermediate between the "normal" group and the group with both characteristics, whereas the group with "wheeze only" was more similar to the normal group. However, this pattern is only evident with the measures related to BHR, which is to be expected because the groups are defined in terms of their results for BHR testing. For asthma symptoms, diagnosed asthma, and asthma medications, the "wheeze only" group showed greater severity than the "BHR only" group and for measures of lung function there was little difference between the two groups. In a recent New Zealand study (D'Souza et al, unpublished) the pattern was similar, but there was if anything an even greater tendency for the "wheeze only" group to be more consistently severe than the "BHR only" group. These findings are consistent with other data showing that symptom questionnaires have greater sensitivity and specificity for physician-diagnosed asthma than does BHR testing or a combination of symptoms and BHR (see Example 4.12).

Example 4.12

Jenkins et al (1996) studied 361 children who were given the ISAAC written questionnaire and 93 adults who were given a similar written questionnaire; 168 children and 91 adults completed bronchial challenge with hypertonic saline. All study participants were interviewed by a pediatric respiratory physician who was blinded to the results of the symptom questionnaires and BHR testing. A physician diagnosis of "current asthma" was defined as a history of wheeze suggestive of a clinical diagnosis of asthma within the past 12 months. Table 4.9 shows that the symptom questionnaire gave a higher value of Youden's index than the BHR testing or a combination of symptoms and BHR. The authors noted that comparisons of BHR prevalence may give considerable underestimates of differences in asthma prevalence; for example, in adults the value of Youden's index was 0.29, indicating that the observed prevalence difference between populations would be less than one third of the true difference.

Table 4.9. Sensitivity, specificity, and Youden's index of symptom questionnaire and BHR for physician-diagnosed asthma

	Sensitivity (95% CI)	Specificity (95% CI)	Youden's index (95% CI)
ADULTS			
Symptoms	0.80 (0.58–0.93)	0.97 (0.90–0.99)	0.76 (0.54–0.90)
BHR	0.39 (0.21–0.61)	0.90 (0.80–0.96)	0.29 (0.09–0.51)
BHR+symptoms	0.37 (0.20–0.59)	0.99 (0.95–1.00)	0.36 (0.18–0.58)
CHILDREN			
Symptoms	0.85 (0.73–0.93)	0.81 (0.76–0.86)	0.66 (0.53–0.76)
BHR	0.54 (0.40–0.67)	0.89 (0.83–0.94)	0.43 (0.29–0.57)
BHR+symptoms	0.47 (0.35–0.60)	0.94 (0.90–0.97)	0.41 (0.28–0.55)

Source: Adapted from Jenkins et al (1996).

Strategies for Measuring Asthma Prevalence

BHR testing is time-consuming and generally yields lower response rates than simple questionnaire surveys. Therefore, it is generally impractical for routine use in large epidemiological surveys. Similar considerations apply to lung function testing and to testing for various risk factors for asthma such as serum IgE, skin-prick tests to common allergens, and indoor allergen exposures (see Chapter 6). Therefore, researchers have begun to develop more efficient strategies in which large surveys are complemented by BHR testing in subsamples of participants. The essential problem is that epidemiological surveys of asthma prevalence require large numbers and high response rates in order to obtain valid information. For example, asthma prevalence surveys typically require a minimum of 1000 persons, and ideally 3000 persons, with a response rate of greater than 90%, in order to estimate asthma prevalence and severity with reasonable precision (Asher et al, 1995). Thus, the key problem is to gain information on the largest possible number of people in random samples collected in a comparable manner across social groups, regions, and countries.

This is quite different from the clinical situation where the aim is to gain the maximum possible information on a single patient. Such clinical considerations have often led to asthma prevalence surveys involving a high number of sophisticated, expensive, and often invasive, tests on a small number of people. Such methods may gain good information on the small number of study subjects, but they are of little value in prevalence comparisons because of their small numbers, and low response rates (as well as the usual problems of possible noncomparability of methods).

For these reasons, comparisons of asthma prevalence are increasingly being based on a simple comparison of symptom prevalence in a questionnaire survey in a large number of people (phase I), followed by more intensive testing of physiologic measures related to asthma (BHR, lung function) and risk factors for asthma (skin-prick testing, serum IgE, indoor allergens, and other exposures) in a subsample (phase II). This approach is being used in the international survey of asthma prevalence in adults (Burney et al, 1994), and in the International Study of Asthma and Allergies in Childhood (Asher et al, 1995).

The European Community Respiratory Health Survey (ECRHS)

The European Community Respiratory Health Survey (Burney et al, 1994) had as objectives:

1. To determine the variation in the prevalence of asthma, asthma-like symptoms, and bronchial lability in Europe

2. To estimate variation in exposure to known or suspected risk factors for asthma; to measure their association with asthma; and to further assess the extent to which they may explain variations in prevalence across Europe
3. To estimate the variation in treatment practice for asthma in the European Community.

In each center a representative sample of 3000 adults, aged 20 to 44 years, completed a phase I screening questionnaire (Fig. 4.4) seeking information on asthma symptoms and medication use. Individuals answering "yes" to waking with an attack of shortness of breath (question 3), an attack of asthma (question 5), or current asthma medications (question 6) were defined as asthmatic.

A random subsample of 600 subjects and an additional sample of up to 150 "asthmatic" individuals were then studied in more detail in phase II, with measurements of skin-prick test to common allergens, serum total and specific IgE, bronchial responsiveness to inhaled methacholine and urine electrolytes, as well as an additional questionnaire on asthma symptoms and medical history, occupation and social status, smoking, the home environment, and the use of medications and medical services.

The phase I results (ECRHS, 1996) include data from 48 centers in 22 countries, predominantly in western Europe, with only nine centers from six countries (Algeria, Iceland, India, New Zealand, Australia, USA) being from outside of Europe. Nevertheless, the study found a wide variation in asthma symptom prevalence. Prevalence was generally higher in the British Isles, Republic of Ireland, New Zealand, Australia, and the United States (i.e., in English-speaking countries), and lower in centers in the Baltic, Algeria and India, with most continental European centers being intermediate. The Phase II results were just beginning to be published (Sunyer et al, 1996) at time of preparation of this book.

The International Study of Asthma and Allergies in Childhood (ISAAC)

The International Study of Asthma and Allergies in Childhood (ISAAC) (Asher et al, 1995) had as objectives:

1. To describe the prevalence and severity of asthma, rhinitis, and eczema in children living in different centers, and to make comparisons within and between countries
2. To obtain baseline measures for assessment of future trends in the prevalence and severity of these diseases
3. To provide a framework for further etiologic research into lifestyle, environmental, genetic, and medical care factors affecting these diseases.

The ISAAC study has a similar study design to that of the ECRHS. However, the emphasis is on obtaining the maximum possible participation

Table 4.10. ECRHS and ISAAC phase I study designs

	ISAAC 6–7 years	ISAAC 13–14 years	ECRHS 20–44 years
Sample size	3000	3000	3000
Information source	Parents	Self-reported	Self-reported
Wheezing questionnaire	Strongly recommended	Compulsory	Compulsory
Video wheezing questionnaire	Not used	Strongly recommended	Not used
Rhinitis questionnaire	Strongly recommended	Compulsory	Not used
Eczema questionnaire	Strongly recommended	Compulsory	Not used

across the world in order to obtain a global overview of asthma prevalence in children. For this reason, the phase I questionnaire modules have been designed to be simple and to require minimal resources to administer. Furthermore, in order to maximize participation from centers around the world, phase I and phase II have been separated and need not be performed in the same groups of children (in fact, phase II is optional).

The characteristics of phase I of the ISAAC study are summarized and compared with those of the ECRHS in Table 4.10. The population of interest is schoolchildren aged 6 to 7 years and 13 to 14 years within specified geographical areas. The older age group was chosen to reflect the period when morbidity from asthma is common and to enable the use of self-completed questionnaires (Figs. 4.5 and 4.6). The younger age group was chosen to give a reflection of the early childhood years, and involves parent completion of questionnaires.

The phase I results were not published at the time of preparation of this book. However, the preliminary results, covering approximately 120 centers in 50 countries and involving more than 620,000 children, showed striking international differences in asthma symptom prevalence, with particularly high prevalences in English-speaking countries (using both the written and video questionnaires), and low prevalence in eastern Europe and most developing countries (Pearce et al, 1993, 1996; Asher et al, 1996).

Further studies

International comparisons are only the first step in investigating the determinants of asthma incidence and prevalence. The next step is to conduct prevalence case-control studies and cohort studies to investigate which risk factors could account for the prevalence patterns that have been observed. As noted in Chapter 2, prevalence case-control studies involve identifying cases of "wheeze" or "asthma" in a prevalence study, together with a sample of controls who report not having any recent asthma symptoms (e.g., within the past year). Both groups are then assessed with respect to their exposure to various possible risk factors for asthma. Of course, in some instances it may not be advisable to conduct a case-control study in a single center because everyone in a particular center may be exposed to a risk factor (e.g., cold weather) and there may therefore be no appropriate "nonexposed" comparison subgroup. However, for many other factors, there may be exposed and nonexposed subgroups (e.g., smokers and nonsmokers), or at least subgroups with varying levels of exposure to a particular factor (e.g., house dust mites) within the same population. In this situation, it is possible to build nested case-control studies into the data collection for a population-based prevalence study.

Summary

In summary, most asthma prevalence studies focus on factors that are related to, or symptomatic of, asthma but that can be readily assessed on a particular day. The main options in this regard are symptoms, lung function, or bronchial responsiveness testing. The choice of techniques should be motivated by the need to use simple techniques to obtain valid data on large numbers of people, with high response rates, in a manner that is comparable across the social groups, regions, or countries being compared. Thus, questionnaires remain the cornerstone of asthma prevalence surveys, although these can be supplemented by bronchial responsiveness testing in subgroups of the study population. Such studies are the first stage in the research process, and lead on to nested case-control studies or cohort studies, which measure the exposure to possible asthma risk factors in cases of "asthma" and symptom-free controls, in order to ascertain the possible causes of the prevalence patterns that have been observed. The measurement of such risk factors is discussed further in Chapter 6.

References

Abramson MJ, Saunders NA, Hensley M (1990). Analysis of bronchial reactivity in epidemiological studies. Thorax 45: 924–9.

Alberg N (1989). Asthma and allergic rhinitis in Swedish conscripts. Clin Exp Allergy 19: 59–63.

Anderson HR (1989). Is the prevalence of asthma changing? Arch Dis Child 64: 172–5.

Anderson HR, Bailey PA, Cooper JS, et al (1983). Morbidity and school absence caused by asthma and wheezing illness. Arch Dis Child 58: 777–84.

Anderson HR, Butland BK, Strachan DP (1994). Trends in prevalence and severity of childhood asthma. BMJ 308: 1600–4.

Anderson S (1985). Airway cooling as the stimulus to exercise induced asthma—a reevaluation. Eur J Respir Dis 67: 20–30.

Anonymous (1994). Global Strategy for Asthma Management and Prevention. NHLBI/WHO Workshop Report. Global Initiatives for Asthma. Washington, DC: NHLBI.

Asher I, Keil U, Anderson HR, et al (1995). International Study of Asthma and Allergies in Childhood (ISAAC): rationale and methods. Eur Respir J 8: 483–91.

Asher I, and the ISAAC Steering Committee (1996). ISAAC Phase I—Worldwide variation in the prevalence of wheezing and asthma in children. Eur Respir J 9: 410s (abstract).

American Thoracic Society (ATS) (1987). Standardization of spirometry—1987 update. Am Rev Respir Dis 136: 1285–98.

Asher MI, Pattemore PK, Harrison AC, et al (1988). International comparison of the prevalence of asthma symptoms and bronchial hyperresponsiveness. Am Rev Respir Dis 138: 524–9.

Auerbach I, Springer C, Godfrey S (1993). Total population survey of the frequency and severity of asthma in 17 year old boys in an urban area in Israel. Thorax 48: 139–41.

Backer V, Groth S, Dirksen A, et al (1991). Sensitivity and specificity of the histamine challenge test for the diagnosis of asthma in an unselected sample of children and adolescents. Eur Respir J 4: 1093–1100.

Balfe D, Crane J, Beasley R, Pearce N (1996). The worldwide increase in the prevalence of asthma in children and young adults. Continuing Med Education J 14: 433–42.

Baumann A, Hunt J, Young L, et al (1992). Asthma under-recognition and under-treatment in an Australian community. Aust N Z J Med 22: 36–40.

Buist AS, Vollmer WM (1987). Prospective investigations in asthma: what have we learned from longitudinal studies about lung growth and senescence in asthma? Chest 91: 119S–136S.

Burney P, Chinn S (1987). Developing a new questionnaire for measuring the prevalence and distribution of asthma. Chest 91: 79S–83S.

Burney PGJ, Laitinen LA, Perdrizet S, et al (1989a). Validity and repeatability of the IUATLD (1984) bronchial symptoms questionnaire: an international comparison. Eur Respir J 2: 940–5.

Burney PGJ, Britton JR, Chinn S, et al (1987). Descriptive epidemiology of bronchial reactivity in an adult population: results from a community study. Thorax 42: 38–44.

Burney PGJ, Anderson HR, Burrows B, et al (1989). Epidemiology. In: Holgate S, Howell JBL, Burney PGJ, et al (eds). The Role of Inflammatory Processes in Airway Responsiveness. Oxford: Blackwell Scientific.

Burney PG, Chinn S, Rona RJ (1990). Has the prevalence of asthma increased in children? Evidence from the national study of health and growth 1973–1986. BMJ 300: 1306–10.

Burney PGJ, Luczynska C, Chinn S, Jarvis D (1994). The European Community Respiratory Health Survey. Eur Respir J 7: 954–60.

Burr ML (1987). Is asthma increasing? J Epidemiol Community Health 41: 185–9.

Burr ML (1992). Diagnosing asthma by questionnaire in epidemiological surveys. Clin Exp Allergy 22: 509–10.

Burr ML, St. Leger AS, Bevan C, Menett TG (1975). A community survey of asthmatic characteristics. Thorax 30: 663–8.

Burr ML, Butland BK, King S, et al (1989). Changes in asthma prevalence: two surveys 15 years apart. Arch Dis Child 64: 1452–6.

Burr ML, Limb ES, Andrae S, et al (1994). Childhood asthma in four countries: a comparative survey. Int J Epidemiol 23: 341–7.

Busquets RM, Antó JM, Sunyer J, et al (1996). Prevalence of asthma-related symptoms and bronchial responsiveness to exercise in children aged 13–14 years in Barcelona, Spain. Eur Respir J 9: 2094–8.

Carey VJ, Weiss ST, Tager IB, et al (1996). Airways responsiveness, wheeze onset, and recurrent asthma episodes in young adolescents: The East Boston Childhood Respiratory Disease Cohort. Am J Respir Crit Care Med 153: 356–61.

Chai H, Farr RS, Froelich LA, et al (1975). Standardization of bronchial inhalation challenge procedures. J Allergy Clin Immunol 56: 323–7.

Chan JKW, Leung R, Ho SS, Lai CKW (1997). Validation of an international video questionnaire for measuring asthma prevalence. Aust N Z J Med 27: 232 (abstract).

Chung KF (1986). Role of inflammation in the hyperreactivity of the airways in asthma. Thorax 41: 657–62.

Cockroft D, Killian D, Mellon J, Hargreaves F (1977). Bronchial reactivity to inhaled histamine: a method and clinical survey. Clin Allergy 7: 235–43.

Cockroft DW, Ruffin RE, Frith PA, et al (1979). Determinants of allergen-induced asthma: dose of allergen, circulating IgE antibody concentration and bronchial responsiveness to inhaled histamine. Am Rev Respir Dis 120: 1053–8.

Crane J, O'Donnell TV, Prior IAM, et al (1989). Symptoms of asthma, methacholine airway responsiveness and atopy in migrant Tokelauan children. N Z Med J 102: 36–8.

Crane J, Lewis S, Slater T, et al (1994). The self-reported prevalence of asthma symptoms amongst adult New Zealanders. N Z Med J 107: 417–21.

Dales RE, Raizenne M, El-Saadanny S, et al (1994). Prevalence of childhood asthma across Canada. Int J Epidemiol 23: 775–81.

Dodge RB, Burrows B (1980). The prevalence and incidence of asthma and asthma-like symptoms in a general population sample. Am Rev Respir Dis 122: 57–75.

Doll R, Payne P, Waterhouse J (eds) (1966). Cancer Incidence in Five Continents. Vol I. Berlin: Springer-Verlag.

Dolovich J, Hargreave FE (1981). The asthma syndrome: inciters, inducers and host characteristics. Thorax 36: 641–4.

Dowse GK, Turner KJ, Stewart GA, et al (1985). The association between Dermatophagoides mites and the increasing prevalence of asthma in village communities within the Papua New Guinea highlands. J Allergy Clin Immunol 75: 75–83.

Ehrlich RI, Du Toit D, Jordaan E, et al (1995). Prevalence and reliability of asthma symptoms in primary school children in Cape Town. Int J Epidemiol 24: 1138–46.

European Community Respiratory Health Survey (ECRHS) (1996). Variations in the prevalence of respiratory symptoms, self-reported asthma attacks, and use of asthma medication in the European Community Respiratory Health Survey (ECRHS). Eur Respir J 9: 687–95.

Frischer T, Kühr HR, Meinert R, et al (1991). Prävalenz Allergischer Manifestationen im Schulkindalter in Südbaden. Münch Med Wschr 133: 671–4.

Frischer T, Studnicka M, Neumann M, Götz M (1992). Determinants of airway response to challenge with distilled water in a population sample of children aged 7 to 10 years old. Chest 102: 764–70.

Gavriely N (1996). Analysis of breath sounds in bronchial provocation tests. Am J Respir Crit Care Med 153: 1469–71.

Gergen PJ, Mullally DI, Evans R (1988). National survey of prevalence of asthma among children in the United States, 1976 to 1980. Paediatrics 81: 1–7.

Gergen PJ, Weiss KB (1995). Epidemiology of asthma. In: Busse W, Holgate S (eds). Asthma and Rhinitis. Oxford: Blackwell Scientific, pp 15–31.

Gregg I (1983). Epidemiological aspects. In: Clark TJK, Godfrey S (eds). Asthma. London: Chapman Hall.

Gross NJ (1980). What is this thing called love? or, defining asthma. Am Rev Respir Dis 121: 203–4.

Haahtela T, Lindholm H, Bjorksten F, et al (1990). Prevalence of asthma in Finnish young men. BMJ 301: 266–8.

Haby M, Anderson S, Peat J, et al (1993). An exercise challenge protocol for epidemiological studies of asthma in children: comparison with histamine challenge. Eur Respir J 7: 43–9.

Hill R, Williams J, Tattersfield A, Britton J (1989). Change in use of asthma as a diagnostic label for wheezing illness in schoolchildren. BMJ 299: 898.

Hopp R, Bewtra A, Nair N, Townley R (1985). The effect of age on methacholine response. J Allergy Clin Immunol 76: 908–13.

Hopp RJ, Bewtra AK, Nair NM, et al (1986). Methacholine challenge studies in a selected pediatric population. Am Rev Respir Dis 134: 994–8.

Hopp RJ, Townley RG, Biven RE, et al (1990). The presence of airway reactivity before the development of asthma. Am Rev Respir Dis 141: 2–8.

Hsieh K-H, Shen J-J (1988). Prevalence of childhood asthma in Taipei, Taiwan and other Asian Pacific countries. J Asthma 25: 73–82.

Hsieh K-H, Tsai Y-T (1992). Increasing prevalence of childhood allergic disease in Taipei, Taiwan, and the outcome. In: Miyamoto T, Okuda M (eds). Progress in allergy and clinical immunology. Vol 2: Proceedings of the 14th International Congress of Allergology and Clinical Immunology. Gottingen: Hogrefe & Huber, pp 223–5.

Infante-Rivard C, Sukia SE, Roberge D, Baumgarten M (1987). The changing frequency of childhood asthma. J Asthma 24: 283–8.

Jenkins MA, Clarke JR, Carlin JB, et al (1996). Validation of questionnaire and bronchial hyperresponsiveness against respiratory physician assessment in the diagnosis of asthma. Int J Epidemiol 25: 609–16.

Josephs LK, Gregg I, Mullee MA, Holgate ST (1989). Nonspecific bronchial reactivity and its relationship to the clinical expression of asthma. Am Rev Respir Dis 140: 350–7.

Josephs LK, Gregg I, Holgate ST (1990). Does non-specific bronchial responsiveness indicate the severity of asthma? Eur Respir J 3: 220–7.

Juniper EF, Frith PA, Hargreave FE (1981). Airway responsiveness to histamine and methacholine: relationship to minimum treatment to control symptoms of asthma. Thorax 36: 575–9.

Kelly WJW, Hudson I, Raven J, et al (1988). Childhood asthma and adult lung function. Am Rev Respir Dis 138: 26–30.

Kljakovic M (1991). The change in prevalence of wheeze in seven year old children over 19 years. N Z Med J 104: 378–80.

Larsson L (1995). Incidence of asthma in Swedish teenagers: relation to sex and smoking habits. Thorax 50: 260–4.

Lee DA, Winslow NR, Speight ANP, Hey EN (1983). Prevalence and spectrum of asthma in childhood. BMJ 286: 1256–8.

Lebowitz MD, Krzyzanowski M, Quackenboss JJ, O'Rourke MK. (1997). Diurnal variation of PEF and its use in epidemiological studies. Eur Respir J 10(suppl 24): 495–565.

Le Souef PN (1993). Can measurements of airway responsiveness be standardized in children? Eur Respir J 6: 1085–7.

Le Souef P, Geelhoed G, Turner D, et al (1989). Response of normal infants to inhaled histamine. Am Rev Respir Dis 139: 62–6.

Liard R, Chansin R, Neukirch F, et al (1988). Prevalence of asthma among teenagers attending school in Tahiti. J Epidemiol Community Health 42: 149–51.

Martinez FD, Morgan WJ, Wright AL, et al (1988). Diminished lung function as a predisposing factor for wheezing respiratory illness in infants. N Engl J Med 319: 1112–7.

Mitchell EA (1983). Increasing prevalence of asthma in children. N Z Med J 96: 463–4.

Mitchell EA, Anderson RA, Freeling P, White P (1990). Why are hospital admission rates for childhood asthma higher in New Zealand than in the United Kingdom? Thorax 1990; 45: 176–82.

Morrison Smith J (1976). The prevalence of asthma and wheezing in children. Br J Dis Chest 70: 73–7.

Muñoz A, Sunyer J (1996). Comparison of semiparametric and parametric survival models for the analysis of bronchial hyperresponsiveness. Am J Respir Crit Care Med 154: S234–9.

Neutra RM (1990). Counterpoint from a cluster buster. Am J Epidemiol 132: 1–8.

Nicolai T, Von Mutius E, Reitmeir P, Wjst M (1993). Reactivity to cold-air hyperventilation in normal and asthmatic children in a survey of 5,697 schoolchildren in Southern Bavaria. Am Rev Respir Dis 147: 565–72.

Ninan TK, Russell G (1992). Respiratory symptoms and atopy in Aberdeen schoolchildren: evidence from two surveys 25 years apart. BMJ 304: 873–5.

Nishima S (1993). A study of the prevalence of bronchial asthma in school children in western districts of Japan: comparison between the studies in 1982 and in 1992 with the same methods and same districts. Arerugi 42: 192–204.

O'Connor G, Sparrow D, Taylor D, et al (1987). Analysis of dose-response curves to methacholine. An approach suitable for population studies. Am Rev Respir Dis 136: 1412–7.

Osterman JW, Armstrong BG, Ledoux E, et al (1991). Comparison of French and English versions of the American Thoracic Society Respiratory Questionnaire in a bilingual working population. Int J Epidemiol 20: 138–43.

Pearce N (1994). Disease clusters and high-risk occupations. People and Work. Research Reports 1. Proceedings of the International Symposium on New Epidemics in Occupational Health. Helsinki: Finnish Institute of Occupational Health, pp 214–20.

Pearce N (1996). Traditional epidemiology, modern epidemiology, and public health. Am J Public Health 86: 678–83.

Pearce NE, Weiland S, Keil U, et al (1993). Self-reported prevalence of asthma symptoms in children in Australia, England, Germany and New Zealand: an international comparison using the ISAAC written and video questionnaires. Eur Respir J 6: 1455–61.

Pearce N, and the ISAAC Steering Committee (1996). ISAAC—The International Study of Asthma and Allergies in Childhood: background and methods. Eur Respir J 9: 410s (abstract).

Peat JK, Salome CM, Sedgwick CS, et al (1989). A prospective study of bronchial hyperresponsiveness and respiratory symptoms in a population of Australian schoolchildren. Clin Exper Allergy 19: 299–306.

Peat JK, Haby M, Spijker J, et al (1992). Prevalence of asthma in adults in Busselton, Western Australia. BMJ 305: 1326–9.

Peat JK, van den Berg RH, Green WF, et al (1994). Changing prevalence of asthma in Australian children. BMJ 308: 1591–6.

Peckham C, Butler N (1978). A national study of asthma in childhood. J Epidemiol Community Health 32: 79–85.

Perdrizet S, Neukirch F, Cooreman J, Liard R (1987). Prevalence of asthma in adolescents in various parts of France and its relationship to respiratory allergic manifestations. Chest 91: 104S–106S.

Quanjer P, Tammeling GJ, Cotes JE, et al (1993). Lung volumes and forced ventilatory flows. Eur Respir J 6 (suppl 16): 4–39.

Quanjer PH, Lebowitz MD, Gregg I, et al (1997). Peak expiratory flow: conclusions and recommendations of a working party of the European Respiratory Society. Eur Respir J 10(suppl 24): 2s–8s.

Reid DD (1975). International studies in epidemiology. Am J Epidemiol 102: 469–76.

Riedler J, Reade T, Dalton M, et al (1994). Hypertonic saline challenge in an epidemiologic survey of asthma in children. Am J Respir Crit Care Med 150: 1632–9.

Rijcken B, Schouten JP (1993). Measuring bronchial hyperresponsiveness in epidemiology. Eur Respir J 6: 617–8.

Robertson C, Heycock E, Bishop J, et al (1991). Prevalence of asthma in Melbourne schoolchildren: changes over 26 years. BMJ 302: 1116–8.

Robson B, Woodman K, Burgess C, et al (1993). Prevalence of asthma symptoms among adolescents in the Wellington region, by area and ethnicity. N Z Med J 106: 239–41.

Rose G (1985). Sick individuals and sick populations. Int J Epidemiol 14: 32–3.

Rose G (1992). The Strategy of Preventive Medicine. Oxford: Oxford University Press.

Salome CM, Peat JK, Britton WJ, Woolcock AJ (1987). Bronchial hyperresponsiveness in two populations of Australian schoolchildren. I. Relation to respiratory symptoms and diagnosed asthma. Clin Allergy 17: 271–81.

Samet JM (1987). Epidemiologic approaches for the identification of asthma. Chest 91: 74S–78S.

Samet JM, Schrag SD, Howard CA, et al (1982). Respiratory disease in a New Mexico population sample of Hispanic and non-Hispanic whites. Am Rev Respir Dis 125: 152–7.

Sears MR. Jones DT, Holdaway MD, et al (1986). Prevalence of bronchial reactivity to inhaled methacholine in New Zealand children. Thorax 41: 283–9.

Sears MR, Lewis S, Herbison GP, et al (1997). Comparison of reported prevalences of recent asthma in longitudinal and cross-sectional studies. Eur Respir J 10: 51–4.

Shaw RA, Crane J, O'Donnell TV, et al (1990). Increasing asthma prevalence in a rural New Zealand adolescent population: 1975–89. Arch Dis Child 63: 1319–23.

Shaw RA, Crane J, O'Donnell TV, et al (1992a). The use of a videotaped questionnaire for studying asthma prevalence: a pilot study amongst New Zealand adolescents. Aust N Z J Med 157: 311–4.

Shaw RA, Crane J, Pearce NE, et al (1992b). Validation of a video questionnaire for assessing asthma prevalence. Clin Exp Allergy 22: 562–9.

Shaw R, Woodman K, Ayson M, et al (1995). Measuring the prevalence of bronchial hyperresponsiveness in children. Int J Epidemiol 24: 597–602.

Smith CM, Anderson SD (1990). Inhalation challenge using hypertonic saline in asthmatic subjects: a comparison with response to hyperpnoea, methacholine and water. Eur Respir J 3: 144–51.

Sterk PJ, Fabbri LM, Quanjer PhM, et al (1993). Airway responsiveness: standardized challenge testing with pharmacological physical and sensitizing stimuli. Eur Respir J 6 (suppl 16): 53–83.

Strachan DP (1995). International Study of Asthma and Allergies in Childhood (ISAAC). Phase II modules. London: St George's Hospital Medical School.

Sunyer JM, Antó J, Castellsaque JB, et al (1996). Total serum IgE is associated with asthma independently of specific IgE levels. Eur Respir J 9: 1880–4.

Tirimanna PR, van Schayk CP, den Otter JJ, et al (1996). Prevalence of asthma and COPD in general practice in 1992: has it changed since 1977? Brit J Gen Practice 46: 277–81.

Toelle BG, Peat JK, Salome CM, et al (1992). Toward a definition of asthma for epidemiology. Am Rev Respir Dis 146: 633–7.

Toelle BG, Peat JK, Salome CM, et al (1994). Comparison of two epidemiological protocols for measuring airway responsiveness and allergic sensitivity in adults. Eur Respir J 7: 1798–1804.

Townley RG, Ryo UY, Kang B (1971). Bronchial sensitivity to methacholine in asthmatic subjects free of symptoms for one to twenty-one years. J Allergy 47: 91–2.

Von Mutius E, Fritzsch C, Weiland SK, et al (1992). Prevalence of asthma and allergic disorders among children in united Germany: a descriptive comparison. BMJ 305: 1395–9.

Weeke B, Madsen F, Frolund L (1987). Reproducibility of challenge tests at different times. Chest 91: 83S–88S.

Weiland S (1994). Guidelines for the translation of questionnaires. ISAAC Newsletter. March, 1994. ISAAC Document 041, p 2.

Weiland SK, Kugler J, von Mutius E, et al (1993). Die Sprach Asthmakranaker Kinder. Monatsschr Kinderheilkd 141: 878–82.

Weiss ST, Tager IB, Speizer FE, Rosner B (1980). Persistent wheeze: its relation to respiratory illness, cigarette smoking, and level of pulmonary function in a population sample of children. Am Rev Respir Dis 122: 697–707.

Weitzman M, Gortmaker SL, Sobol AM, et al (1992). Recent trends in the prevalence and severity of childhood asthma. JAMA 268: 2673–7.

Whincup PH, Cook DP, Strachan DP, Papacosta O (1993). Time trends in respiratory symptoms in childhood over a 24 year period. Arch Dis Child 68: 729–34.

Woolcock AJ (1987). Epidemiologic methods for measuring prevalence of asthma. Chest 91: 89S–92S.

Woolcock AJ, Peat JK (1997). Evidence for the increase in asthma worldwide. 1997

The rising trends in asthma. Ciba Foundation Symposium 206. Chichester: Wiley, pp 122–39.

Woolcock AJ, Dowse GK, Temple K, et al (1983). The prevalence of asthma in the South-Fore people of Papua New Guinea. A method for field studies of bronchial reactivity. Eur J Respir Dis 64: 571–81.

Woolcock AJ, Peat JK, Salome CM, et al (1987). Prevalence of bronchial hyperresponsiveness and asthma in a rural adult population. Thorax 42: 361–8.

World Health Organisation (WHO) (1975). Epidemiology of chronic non-specific respiratory diseases. Bull WHO 52: 251–9.

Yan K, Salome C, Woolcock AJ (1983). Rapid method for measuring bronchial responsiveness. Thorax 38: 760–5.

5

Measuring Asthma Morbidity

Morbidity studies are usually conducted to assess the effects of a hazardous exposure or the effects of an intervention believed to be beneficial. The general approach is to measure asthma severity or control at the start of the study, and then to measure changes in asthma severity or control over time. Measures of asthma mobidity fall into five major groups: symptoms, physiological measures, health service and medication usage, quality of life and knowledge of asthma, and composite measures. In this chapter we review these various approaches to measuring asthma morbidity, and we argue that symptoms and physiological measures, although imperfect, are generally the most appropriate and valid outcome measures in morbidity studies.

Introduction

Whereas prevalence studies usually involve a general population sample (as the denominator) with asthma as the outcome under study (i.e., the numerator), morbidity studies involve studying an asthmatic population (as the denominator) and examining changes in "asthma severity" over time. The concept of "asthma severity" can relate to overall asthma severity (chronic severity) or the severity of an acute attack (acute severity). Furthermore, Cockroft and Swystun (1996) argue that asthma severity is usually defined in terms of factors such as symptoms, medication requirements, and physiologic abnormalities, but most of these criteria relate to a lack of asthma control and/or the severity of a particular attack of exacerbation, whereas the underlying severity may be reflected by the minimal medication required to achieve adequate control. Severe exacerbations can also be divided into those with sudden onset and those with slow onset (Picado, 1996). We use the term "morbidity studies" to encompass all studies in which the denominator is an asthmatic population and the intention is to assess changes in the level of morbidity (asthma severity, asthma control, quality of life, knowledge of asthma) over time. Similarly, the term "asthma severity" is used here to indicate both markers of (lack of) asthma control and markers of the underyling disease severity.

The most common reasons for measuring asthma morbidity are to study the effects of an exposure believed to be hazardous (e.g., air pollution) or to study the effects of an intervention believed to be beneficial (e.g., a new asthma drug, or a program of allergen avoidance). The study of hazardous exposures cannot be randomized (for practical and ethical reasons) and requires an epidemiological (nonrandomized) approach, whereas the study of the effects of an intervention can involve either randomized or non-randomized studies. If having a nonexposed group (or nonintervention group) is impractical or unethical, then the study may just involve one group with each asthmatic serving as his or her own control in a "before and after" comparison (e.g., D'Souza et al, 1994, 1996), or in the case of a variable exposure (e.g., air pollution), time series comparisons can be made (within the same individuals) of levels of morbidity on high exposure and low exposure days.

Example 5.1

Ignacio-Garcia nad Gonzalez-Santos (1995) conducted a controlled trial of a self-managment plan incorporating home monitoring of peak expiratory flow rate (PEFR). Thirty-five patients managed themselves, using peak flow readings as the basis for the therapeutic plan coupled with educational intervention, whereas 35 control patients used symptoms and spirometric data for following physicians' treatment plans. After a 6-month study period, the patients in the experimental group showed significant improvements in asthma morbidity parameters (Table 5.1) as

Table 5.1. Comparison of experimental and control groups' changes in morbidity parameters (mean ± SE) 6 months before and 6 months after intervention

Morbidity parameters	Control group				Experimental group			
	Before		After		Before		After	
Days lost from work	25.4	±5.1	20.0	±4.9	22.2	±6.2	4.9	±1.1
Acute asthma exacerbations	4.4	±0.5	3.1	±0.3	3.8	±0.4	2.3	±0.3
Days on antibiotic therapy	27.7	±3.8	22.5	±3.0	26.8	±3.5	15.7	±1.9
Physician consultations	7.2	±0.9	4.5	±0.7	5.8	±0.9	1.5	±0.2
Emergency room admissions	2.1	±0.4	1.9	±0. 5	1.9	±0.2	0.7	±0.1
Nocturnal wakening			37.9	±6.1			16.5	±2.5
Number of hospital admissions	4		5		4		0	

* Mean ± SEM.
Source: Ignacio-Garcia and Gonzalez-Santos (1995).

well as improvements in lung function and reductions in use of asthma medication. The authors concluded that the personal use of PEFR measurements in association with the self-management plan leads to an improvement in the patient's condition.

A number of different outcome measures can be used in morbidity studies (Bailey et al, 1994), and these fall into five major groups: symptoms, physiological measures, health service and medication usage, quality of life and knowledge of asthma, and composite measures. These various outcome measures are reviewed in the following sections.

Symptoms

The most straightforward method for assessing morbidity is to use symptom questionnaires similar to those used in prevalence studies, and to examine changes over time. However, morbidity studies usually require more information on the intensity, duration, and frequency of symptoms than is required for prevalence studies. Many different detailed questionnaires are in current use, but a recent review (O'Connor and Weiss, 1994) concluded that there was no clear evidence to suggest that a particular questionnaire was preferred as the standard.

Questionnaires on symptom frequency and severity generally have similar advantages and disadvantages as those of questionnaires on symptom prevalence used in prevalence studies, but one advantage in morbidity studies is that the population under study comprises asthmatics who should already be familiar with terms such as wheezing, although increased recognition or labeling of such terms over the study period may still be a source of bias.

The key difficulty in using symptom questionnaires is the problem of recall, particularly because recall of symptoms may be affected by participation in a study. One solution is the use of daily asthma symptom diaries; this may considerably add to the cost of a study because of the need to monitor the participants and to ensure that the diaries are being completed adequately, but it will provide information that is less affected by problems of recall. However, it may still be affected by problems of recognition and reporting of current symptoms. The reporting of symptoms can be improved by techniques such as the use of visual analogue scales (Adams et al, 1985; Horn and Cochrane, 1989).

Another problem with studying symptoms such as breathlessness, wheezing, and chest tightness is that they may be a poor guide to the severity of airflow obstruction in asthma. This is illustrated by studies that have shown that a significant proportion of adults with chronic asthma may have minimal symptoms despite marked airflow obstruction as measured by the reduction in the FEV_1 from predicted to normal values (Rubinfeld and Pain, 1976). Patients with the most severe asthma have the worst perception of the degree of airflow obstruction, suggesting that in these patients symptoms may not accurately reflect exacerbations of asthma (Burdon et al, 1982).

The problems of recognition and recall of symptoms mean that it is usually preferable to study the frequency of clearly identified symptom "events" rather than more general symptoms such as wheeze. One possible outcome event is the occurrence of an "attack" of wheezing, but this measure is problematic because many asthmatics do not consider that they suffer from attacks, and the labeling of an episode of wheezing as an attack is subjective. These problems have led to an approach based on symptom events that are relatively common and reasonably clearly defined. The main options are nocturnal waking with wheezing or coughing, and days lost from work or school due to being "out of action" because of asthma (D'Souza, 1994). Symptoms experienced during the night and day are usually recorded separately because of the marked diurnal variation in airflow obstruction that characterizes asthma. This is particularly important in unstable asthma, in which increasingly frequent and severe nocturnal asthma may develop, despite little change in daytime symptoms and lung function.

Example 5.2

Barnes et al (1993) conducted a double-blind randomized parallel group study comparing the efficacy of 1 mg per day of fluticasone propionate (a new topically active inhaled corticosteroid) to that of 2 mg per day of beclomethasone dipropionate in severe adult asthma. Patients noted the severity of their asthma symptoms by day and night using 4-point rating scales. Symptoms during the day were rated as follows:

0 = none

1 = wheezing or shortness of breath on strenuous exercise/hurrying, otherwise asthma not unduly troublesome

2 = wheezing or shortness of breath most of the day, normal activities difficult

3 = unable to carry out normal activities because of shortness of breath.

Symptoms during the night were rated as:

0 = none

1 = symptoms caused waking once or early waking

2 = woken 2 or 3 times by cough/wheeze/breathlessness/asthma

3 = awake most of the night with cough/wheeze/breathlessness/asthma.

At the end of the 6-week treatment period, patients in both groups reported fewer asthma symptoms by day and at night, with no significant differences between treatments.

In some instances (e.g., air pollution studies) all of the individuals in the study may be exposed on a particular day, but the level of exposure may change markedly from day to day. Such studies involve a "time series" comparison of exposed and nonexposed days with each asthmatic serving as his or her own control. Once again, measures of symptom prevalence can be used to assess variations in asthma morbidity over time, except that in this situation it is important that symptoms be measured on each specific day, rather than being averaged over an extended period.

Example 5.3

Romieu et al (1996) conducted a time series study of the effects of air pollution on the respiratory health of 71 children with mild asthma living in the northern part of Mexico City. Parents and children were instructed to complete daily diaries about respiratory symptoms and medication use. Parents were asked to bring the children to the clinic at the end of each week for a clinical examination and a new diary was issued. Daily air pollution data were obtained from the government's air monitoring station located in the northern part of the city. Table 5.2 shows the odds ratios for various respiratory symptoms and various air pollutants. For example, the table shows that an increase in the PM_{10} level of 20 $\mu g/m^3$ was associated with a small increased risk for cough on the same day (OR=1.10, 95% CI 1.06–1.15), the next day (OR=1.08, 1.04–1.12) and the increased risk was still present 2 days later (OR=1.08, 95% CI 1.02–1.12). The authors concluded that children with mild asthma are affected by the high ambient levels of particulate matter and ozone observed in the northern part of Mexico City.

Table 5.2. Association of respiratory symptoms and ambient air pollution, Mexico City, 1991–1992

Pollutants	Cough Odds ratio 95% CI	Phlegm Odds ratio 95% CI	Wheezing Odds ratio 95% CI
PM_{10}, 20 $\mu g/m^3$	1.10 1.06–1.15	1.08 1.00–1.17	1.04 0.96–1.12
PM_{10}, lag 1 day	1.08 1.04–1.12	1.04 0.98–1.12	1.06 0.96–1.15
PM_{10}, lag 2 days	1.08 1.02–1.12	1.02 0.96–1.10	1.02 0.96–1.12
PM_{10}, 7 day moving average	1.10 1.04–1.19	1.06 0.96–1.17	1.06 0.94–1.21
Ozone, 50 ppb	1.11 1.05–1.18	1.06 0.96–1.19	1.03 0.91–1.16
Ozone, lag 1 day	1.12 1.06–1.19	1.05 0.95–1.16	1.02 0.89–1.18
Ozone, lag 2 days	1.06 0.99–1.14	1.04 0.94–1.15	1.02 0.90–1.12

Note: All analyses adjusted for minimum temperature.
Source: Adapted from Romieu et al (1996).

Physiological Measures

Lung function

As in prevalence studies, symptom questionnaires may be supplemented by physiological measurements of lung function, including forced vital capacity (FVC), forced expiratory volume in one second (FEV_1), and peak expiratory flow rate (PEFR). As noted in Chapter 4, these are not good measures in cross-sectional studies, because asthma essentially involves reversible airways obstruction and the change in lung function from day to day is much more important than the absolute level of lung function recorded on a particular day. However, lung function measurements are more useful in longitudinal studies because repeated measurements can be used to study changes in lung function over the period of the study.

The measurement of peak flow rates is particularly valuable in this regard because this can be readily done by study participants and entered into a daily diary. This is simple and inexpensive and provides perhaps the most practicable approach to collecting daily lung function data over an extended period. When the morning PEFR is subtracted from the evening PEFR, the diurnal variation in PEFR can be calculated, and excessive PEFR variability measured in this way is related to bronchial hyperresponsiveness (Neukirch et al, 1992). An alternative method of calculating PEFR variability is the highest post-bronchodilator value (usually in the afternoon) minus the lowest pre-bronchodilator value (usually in the morning). This method demonstrates a considerably higher correlation coefficient with BHR than when calculating the amplitude from pre-bronchodilator values only, and adds another component to the assessment of disease severity, that is, the degree of reversibility to a beta agonist (Ryan et al, 1982). PEFR appears to be less sensitive than FEV_1 in detecting airways obstruction, but PEFR will detect significant changes in airways resistance (Paggiaro et al, 1997) and has many practical advantages in epidemiologic studies.

The measurement of FEV_1 and FVC is more complex and is usually performed by the investigators rather than the participants themselves. Therefore, such measurements cannot usually be made on a daily basis. Other lung function tests, such as absolute lung volumes and airways resistance, are expensive and technically demanding (Enright et al, 1994) and are not practical for most asthma epidemiology studies. Lung function changes with age, increasing during childhood and decreasing during most of adulthood; the extent of the change with age differs by person, place, and time, and there may be significant period and cohort effects (mostly related to period of birth), making it important to control for these differences in long-term longitudinal studies (Lebowitz, 1996).

Example 5.4

Haahtela et al (1991) compared the inhaled corticosteroid budesonide with the beta agonist terbutaline in the long-term treatment of asthma. During the 2-year study period, patients recorded their PEFR before they took their medication in the morning and evening, together with daily recordings of use of supplemental medication and symptoms scores. FEV_1 was assessed on nine occasions. In the budesonide group there were significant increases in the morning and evening PEFR values. The average increase over the pretreatment value in PEFR in the morning for budesonide (33 L/min) was significantly greater than that for terbutaline (5 L/min). The increase in FEV_1 in the steroid group was also significantly greater than that in the beta agonist group.

Bronchial responsiveness

The problems of using tests of bronchial responsiveness in prevalance studies have already been discussed in Chapter 4. Similar considerations apply in studies of asthma morbidity, but the problems may be of even more concern because morbidity studies usually involve following individuals over time and there is no simple relationship between current asthma severity and current levels of BHR in individuals (Josephs et al, 1990). Within a group of asthmatics, levels of BHR are related to the average severity of the asthma, but the association is not so clear at the individual level. For example, Rubinfeld and Pain (1976) studied 11 adult asthmatics over an 18-month period and found no correlation between BHR and the severity of asthma as defined by the frequency or severity of wheeze, sleep disturbance, impairment of activities, absence from work, or treatment needs.

Other studies have found more consistent correlations at the group level (e.g., Beaupre and Malo, 1981; Britton et al, 1988; Geubelle et al, 1971), but the association was not so clear at the individual level. For example, Josephs et al (1990) studied 20 patients over a period of 12 to 18 months and found that overall levels of responsiveness were highest in the group that were considered to have clinically severe asthma, but there were only six subjects in whom changes in BHR appeared to reflect simultaneous trends in symptoms or peak flow rates. Thus, in studies of asthma morbidity, changes in bronchial hyperresponsiveness may be valuable for measuring changes in asthma severity in a group of asthmatics but may not be suitable for monitoring changes in asthma severity in individual asthmatics.

Example 5.5

Kerstjens et al (1992) compared three inhalation regimens in which a beta-2-agonist (terbutaline, 2000 μg daily) was combined with a corticosteroid (beclomethasone,

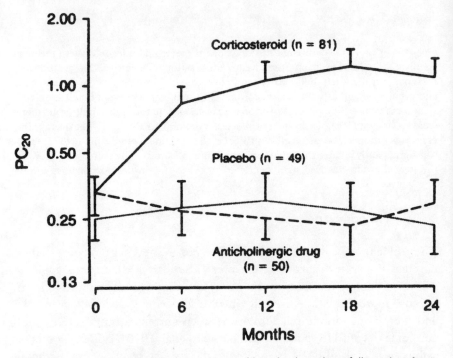

Figure 5.1. Geometric mean PC_{20} in response to histamine in patients followed up for at least 24 months. (Source: Kerstjens et al, 1992, Copyright 1992, Massachusetts Medical Society. All rights reserved.)

800 mg daily), an anticholinergic bronchodilator (ipratropium bromide, 160 μg daily), or placebo. The study involved 274 patients aged 18 to 60 years with airways hyperresponsiveness and obstruction, who were followed for $2\frac{1}{2}$ years. Withdrawal from the study was less common in the corticosteroid group (12 of 91 patients) than in the anticholinergic drug group (45 of 92 patients) or the placebo group (44 of 91 patients). Figure 5.1 shows the geometric mean PC_{20} in response to histamine in patients followed for at least 24 months. The PC_{20} increased by two doubling concentrations in the corticosteroid group but did not change in the other groups. Other markers of asthma morbidity also improved significantly in the corticosteroid group. The authors concluded that the addition of an inhaled corticosteroid—but not an inhaled anticholinergic agent—to maintenance treatment with a beta-2- agonist (terbutaline) substantially reduced morbidity, bronchial hyperresponsiveness, and airways obstruction in patients with a spectrum of obstructive airways disease.

One of the problems in assessing bronchial hyperresponsiveness relates to the choice of the bronchoconstrictor agonist. This is illustrated by the recent demonstration that in asthmatic children, responsiveness to the bronchocon-strictor agonist AMP correlates better with the clinical expression of their disease than the more traditional test of BHR with histamine or metha-choline (Avital et al, 1995). Furthermore, in both children and adults, the therapeutic response to inhaled corticosteroids is more closely associated with a reduction in airway responsiveness to AMP than it is to methacholine. These findings suggest that BHR testing to agents that more directly reflect the underlying inflammatory process in asthma may be a more appropriate method of assessing severity in clinical asthma.

Health Service and Medication Usage

Measures of health service usage (including hospitalizations) have some advantages as outcome measures in epidemiologic studies because they represent a well-defined outcome and are usually available at national and local levels and can be uniformly coded throughout the world (Vollmer et al, 1994). However, a key issue in studies using health service and medication usage as outcome measures is that increased contact with the health services is often an intended or unintended effect of participation in a study. In fact, even modest changes in patterns of self-referral and physician referral can greatly influence hospital admission rates (Anderson, 1989). Thus, in intervention studies, measures of contact with the health services may just be surrogates for compliance with the intervention and may not be valid measures of the real clinical effects of the intervention. For example, it might be hoped that the introduction of a self-management plan might eventually lead to better asthma control and a fall in doctor visits and hospital admission rates. However, such plans usually involve the early detection of worsening asthma and the seeking of medical help at an early stage of disease deterioration. Thus, a self-management plan might be expected to initially lead to an increase in doctor visits and hospital admissions, even if usage of health services and medication fell in the long term. For example, Shields et al (1990) report a randomized trial of a patient education program in which emergency room visits were actually more frequent in the intervention group. Even in a study in which the intervention does not inherently involve changes in medication or use of health services, this may be an indirect consequence of increased patient contact at clinics during the course of the study. An additional problem in "before and after" studies is that hospital admission rates can also be affected by more general changes in the organization and delivery of acute asthma care (Vollmer et al, 1993), or by more general trends in hospitalization rates (e.g., Gergen and Weiss, 1990).

Nevertheless, information on health service and medication usage may be important in determining why an intervention did or did not work, and there are some situations in which health service and medication usage may be valid outcome measures in themselves. In particular, in time series studies in which asthma symptoms are assessed on a daily basis and associated with environmental exposures, any tendency for increased contact with the health services might be assumed to apply equally through the study period, and to be unlikely to be correlated with environmental exposure levels. For example, emergency room visits are reasonably common and may be a useful marker in studies of the effects of time-limited climate change (Vollmer et al, 1994).

Example 5.6

The identification of soybean dust as a causative factor of the community outbreaks of asthma in Barcelona was primarily based on the temporal association between emergency room admissions with asthma and the unloading of soybean from ships in the harbor (Antó et al, 1989). An "unusual asthma day" was defined as a day on which the number of emergency room visits for asthma were so high that the probability that such a number or a higher one would occur by chance (assuming that in fact soybean dust exposure had no effect on asthma emergency room visits) was 0.025 or less. An asthma "epidemic day" was defined as an unusual asthma day on which the cases were clustered on an hourly basis. An "hourly cluster" was defined as the occurrence in one 4-hour period of so many emergency room visits for asthma that the probability that such a high number of visits was the result of chance was 0.05 or less. Table 5.3 shows the association between asthma epidemic days and various products that were unloaded in the harbor during 1985–1986. All 13 asthma epidemic days coincided with the unloading of soybeans at the nearby port,

Table 5.3. Association between asthma epidemic days and various products that were unloaded in the harbor of Barcelona over a 730-day period

	Unloading		No unloading			
Product	Total days	Asthma days	Total days	Asthma days	Risk ratio	95% CI
Soybeans	262	13	468	0	UH*	7.2–UH*
Wheat	30	3	700	10	7.0	2.3–21.0
Cement	503	12	227	1	5.4	0.9–32.0
Potassium chloride	511	11	219	2	2.4	0.6–10.0
Petroleum	56	2	674	11	2.2	0.5–9.4
Phosphates	217	6	513	7	2.0	0.7–5.8
Gas	229	6	500	7	1.9	0.7–5.4
Coal	200	4	530	9	1.2	0.4–3.8
Fuel oil	153	3	577	10	1.1	0.3–4.1
Cotton	406	7	324	6	0.9	0.3–2.7
Coffee	305	5	425	8	0.9	0.3–2.6
Minerals	276	4	454	9	0.7	0.2–2.3
Gasoline	182	2	548	11	0.6	0.1–2.4
Chemicals	548	8	182	5	0.5	0.2–1.6
Corn	136	1	594	12	0.4	0.1–2.5
Butane	141	1	589	12	0.4	0.1–2.4

*UH: unquantifiably high.
Source: Antó et al (1989).

whereas no epidemic days occurred when soybean unloading did not take place. The authors concluded that the outbreaks were caused by the inhalation of soybean dust released during the unloading of soybeans at the city harbor.

A further advantage that outcome measures such as hospital admissions or emergency room attendances have over twice-daily recording of symptoms and lung function is that they do not rely on patient recall and reporting and the necessary information is available through medical records. For example, Gottlieb et al (1995) report a small area analysis of asthma hospitalization rates in Boston in which hospitalization rates were highest in poor nonwhite neighborhoods and were negatively correlated with the ratio of inhaled anti-inflammatory to beta-agonist medication use. They concluded that underuse of inhaled anti-inflammatory medication could be contributing to the excess hospitalization.

The requirement for inhaled beta agonist therapy may be a useful marker of asthma severity if patients are instructed to use this drug treatment as required for the relief of symptoms. In particular, a markedly increased use of beta agonist therapy is an important marker of severe asthma, predictive of an adverse outcome such as requirement for hospital admission (Windom et al, 1990). The frequency of use of beta agonist drugs can be recorded either in a daily diary or on a computer chip that is subsequently downloaded for analysis. Other medications that are also useful as markers of severe attacks of asthma are the requirement for nebulized bronchodilator and courses of oral steroids. While such medication usage may be influenced by interventions that modify management, they are good markers of frequency and severity of attacks of asthma in studies of causative factors and pharmacological agents. For example, Van Ganse et al (1995) report a case-control study of asthma medications and disease exacerbations in which "cases" of disease exacerbation comprised asthmatics who used oral corticosteroids intermittently; controls were asthmatics who did not use oral corticosteroids. They then determined other asthma medication use in cases and controls and reported that the use of oral xanthines and inhaled fenoterol, but not inhaled salbutamol, corticosteroids, cromoglycate or ipratropium bromide, was associated with an increased probability of exacerbations.

Example 5.7

Tinkelman et al (1993) compared the benefits and adverse reactions of theophylline and beclomethasone (BDP) in the long-term control of asthma in 195 children aged

Table 5.4. Supplemental bronchodilator medication use (%) in a trial of aerosol beclomethasone dipropionate compared with theophylline

Month	n	Beclomethasone None	Moderate	High	n	Theophylline None	Moderate	High
Baseline	98	4.1%	78.6%	17.4%	91	9.9%	74.7%	15.4%
1	99	14.1%	80.8%	5.1%	90	14.4%	75.6%	10.0%
2	94	20.2%	74.5%	5.3%	88	22.7%	62.5%	14.8%
3	88	36.4%	58.0%	5.7%	80	26.3%	60.0%	13.8%
4	80	33.8%	62.5%	3.8%	78	23.1%	69.2%	7.7%
5	78	44.9%	52.6%	2.6%	77	26.0%	63.6%	10.4%
6	81	38.3%	58.0%	3.7%	73	24.7%	64.4%	11.0%
7	79	40.5%	54.4%	5.1%	72	27.8%	62.5%	9.7%
8	76	39.5%	55.3%	5.3%	67	29.9%	59.7%	10.5%
9	74	31.1%	63.5%	5.4%	66	27.3%	60.6%	12.1%
10	70	44.3%	51.4%	4.3%	67	23.9%	61.2%	14.9%
11	73	38.4%	57.5%	4.1%	68	33.8%	51.5%	14.7%
12	73	38.4%	56.2%	5.5%	64	34.4%	51.6%	14.1%

Source: Tinkelman et al (1993).

6 to 16 years who were randomized to treatment with either BDP (84 μg four times a day) or sustained-release theophylline administered twice daily in doses adjusted for optimum control of symptoms. Each patient kept a diary on daily asthma symptoms, peak flow rates, doses of study medications, supplemental bronchodilator use, absence from work or school due to asthma, and doctor or emergency department visits or hospitalizations for asthma. For each month, supplemental brochodilator use was defined as follows:

- none = none used
- moderate = mean puffs of aerosol bronchodilator greater than zero up to (and including) six per day and/or oral bronchodilator use on 1% to 75% of days
- high = mean puffs greater than six per day or oral bronchodilator use on more than 75% of days.

Beclomethasone resulted in comparable symptom control with less bronchodilator use than did theophylline (Table 5.4).

Information on medication usage and contact with the health services may also be useful when information can be obtained for the period prior to the start of the study and for the period following the formal end of the study. Such information may be useful in terms of assessing the long-term effects of the intervention. Ideally, it should be validated against medical records (e.g., hospital admission records). Although various scoring systems are available, this approach is fraught with difficulties because of changes in the philosophy of asthma therapy over time. Thus, it is important to obtain separate information on bronchodilator use and anti-inflammatory use (Busse et al, 1994).

Example 5.8

In the controlled study of Mayo et al (1990), the effect of an outpatient asthma management program was investigated in a high risk group of disadvantaged asthmatic patients. There were 104 adult asthmatic patients who had previously required multiple hospitalizations for asthma, who were randomly assigned to receive either their previous outpatient care or an intensive outpatient treatment program. The main factors used to determine efficacy of the program were readmission rates and hospital days. Comparison of treated with untreated patients indicated that the program resulted in a threefold reduction in readmission rate and a twofold reduction in hospital day use rate. The authors concluded that by using a vigorous medical regimen and intensive educational program, it was possible to decrease severe asthma morbidity among a group of adult asthmatics who had previously required repeated readmissions for acute asthma attacks.

Finally, information on health service and medication usage may provide valid outcome measures in a randomized trial, particularly if the trial is double-blind and the changes in these behaviors are not an integral part of the intervention.

Quality of Life and Knowledge of Asthma

Quality of Life

It has been proposed that in a chronic disease such as asthma, there are four basic objectives of therapy (Jones et al, 1994): reduced mortality, modification of the natural history of the disease, fewer acute episodes, and a reduction in the impact of the disease on daily life. Quality of life measures are designed to quantify the latter (Jones et al, 1994). Although the other asthma morbidity measures discussed in this chapter (symptoms, physiological measures, medication and health services usage) are invaluable in assessing whether asthma severity has improved or deteriorated, they provide only part of the picture of asthma morbidity, and they do not tell us whether patients actually function better in their daily lives. For example, physiological measures do not fully reflect all the disease processes that occur in asthma, and it can be difficult to determine whether a small improvement in airways function translates into a clinically worthwhile improvement (Jones, 1995). Quality of life questionnaires can help to fill this knowledge gap; for example, one study (Rutten-Van Mölken et al, 1995) found that a clinically significant improvement in health was obtained if therapy produced a 33 L/min improvement in morning peak flow or a 9% predicted improvement in FEV_1 (Jones, 1995). In additional, quality of life questionnaires may provide further validation of other measures of asthma morbidity, as well as facilitating global consideration of a variety of morbidity measures.

General quality of life questionnaires

A number of general quality of life questionnaires are available and have been used in respiratory disease studies.

The Quality of Wellbeing Index (QWB). Richards and Hemstreet (1994) discuss the Quality of Wellbeing (QWB) measure (Kaplan et al, 1984), which is based on summing scores for level of mobility, level of physical activity, level of social activity, and "symptom complex." The only symptom complex directly relevant to asthma is "cough, wheezing, or shortness of breath." The scores are based on a scale of 0.0 to 1.0, but there is no procedure for combining the various utilities into an overall score; rather the overall score is based on the worst score for any specific symptom. Thus, if one symptom complex is relieved, then the score for "symptom complex" becomes the next "most undesirable" symptom complex. Richards and Hemstreet (1994) illustrate this with data derived from Kaplan and Atkins (1989), and this is shown in Table 5.5: all study participants showed an improvement if their asthma symptoms were treated and relieved, but the improvement in the score depended on whether other symptoms (unrelated to asthma) remained unrelieved. In some instances (e.g., for people with arthritis), the relief of asthma symptoms reduced their overall QWB score.

The Sickness Impact Profile (SIP). The Sickness Impact Profile (SIP) is a generic quality of life measure developed by Bergner et al (1981). It measures health-related dysfunction in 12 domains: ambulation, mobility, body care and movement, social interaction, emotional behavior, alertness behavior, communication, work, eating, sleep and rest, household management, and recreation and pastimes (Williams and Bury, 1989). It asks patients to consider their situation on the day they complete the questionnaire. The SIP provides summary scores for physical, psychosocial, and overall behavioral dysfunction as well as separate scores for the 12 domains.

Table 5.5. Impact of relief of asthma symptoms on quality of well-being (QWB) scores when other symptom complexes are present

Other symptom complex	QWB with asthma symptoms		Improvement in QWB
	Present	Absent	
None	0.743	1.000	0.257
Wears eyeglasses	0.743	0.899	0.156
Takes some medication	0.743	0.856	0.113
Is overweight	0.743	0.812	0.069
Has pain or stiffness in joints	0.743	0.701	−0.042

Source: Richards and Hemstreet (1994), derived from Kaplan and Atkins (1989).

The Medical Outcomes Study Short Form (SF-36). The SF-36 (Ware, 1993) includes scales to measure physical functioning, role functioning, bodily pain, mental health, and general health perceptions. The SF-36 scales have been widely used in clinical research in a wide variety of populations to assess overall health status. Relevant sections include the Physical and Emotional Role Functioning scales, which measure the extent to which physical health (or emotional problems) interfere with work or other daily activities; the Mental Health Scale, which includes depression and anxiety; and the General Health Perceptions Scale (Katz et al, 1997). Dyer and Sinclair (1997) found that mean SF-36 scores were significantly worse in hospitalized asthmatics than in non-asthmatic hospital controls, particularly for components of physical function, physical role limitation, energy, health change, and general health perception.

Limitations of general quality of life questionnaires. Although general quality of life questionnaires have sometimes been successfully applied in asthma studies, asthma-specific questionnaires are usually considered to be of more value because they focus on areas of function that are of particular relevance to asthma, and they are therefore more responsive to small but important changes (Juniper et al, 1993). Furthermore, most general measures of quality of life tend to produce scores that are severely skewed with a small subgroup of people having very poor scores, whereas in asthma the distributions are reasonably similar to those of the general population and measures developed primarily for life-threatening disease are unlikely to be relevant, because life-threatening asthma is uncommon. In the next section, we consider five asthma-specific quality of life questionnaires.

Asthma-specific quality of life questionnaires

The Asthma Quality of Life Questionnaire (AQLQ). The Asthma Quality of Life Questionnaire (Juniper et al, 1992) was developed specifically for use in clinical trials in asthma. The aim was to develop a questionnaire that was capable of measuring change in quality of life over time within individuals (Kirshner and Guyatt, 1985) and that would (Juniper et al, 1993):

- Include both physical and emotional health
- Reflect areas of function that are important to adult patients with asthma
- Be reproducible when the clinical state is stable
- Be responsive to changes that are important to the patient even if the changes are small
- Be valid—i.e., actually measure quality of life in asthma

Impairment of quality of life was evaluated from structured interviews in which patients were asked to identify the parts of their daily lives affected by asthma (Juniper et al, 1992). Areas of impairment included asthma symptoms, responses to environmental stimuli, the need to avoid these stimuli, limitation of activities, and emotional dysfunction. The items of quality of life impairment were very similar across strata of severity, age, and sex; a single questionnaire was therefore developed for all adult patients with asthma. The questionnaire has 32 items in four domains: activity limitation (11 items), symptoms (12 items), emotional function (5 items), and environmental stimuli (4 items). Patients rate the impairment they have experienced during the previous 14 days, responding to each item on a 7-point scale (1 = maximum impairment, 7 = no impairment). The minimal important difference for both quality of life and individual domains has been estimated as a change in score of 0.5 per item (Juniper et al, 1994).

The questionnaire was designed as an evaluative rather than as a discriminative instrument—that is, it was primarily designed to capture small within-subject changes over time (such as would occur in an intervention or clinical trial) rather than to distinguish between patients in a one-off cross-sectional survey. However, the questionnaire appears to be also reliable and valid for discriminative purposes (Juniper et al, 1993).

Example 5.9

Juniper et al (1995) compared the effects of salmeterol (50 μg daily), salbutamol (200 μg four times a day), and placebo on asthma-specific quality of life in a 12-week multicenter, double-blind, randomized, placebo-controlled crossover trial with each trial medication taken for 4 weeks. The participants were 140 adults with mild to moderate asthma enrolled from 14 respiratory clinics across Canada. The outcome measures included the Asthma Quality of Life Questionnaire (Juniper et al, 1992), which was administered at the end of each treatment period. Table 5.6 shows the differences in mean quality of life scores. The scores, both overall and for the individual domains, were better with salmeterol than with placebo ($p < 0.0001$)

Table 5.6. Differences in quality of life (QOL) scores between treatments

	Differences in scores ($n=140$)					
	Salmeterol minus placebo		Salmeterol minus salbutamol		Salbutamol minus placebo	
Domain	Mean	95% CI	Mean	95% CI	Mean	95% CI
Symptoms	0.7	0.5–0.8	0.5	0.3–0.7	0.2	0.0–0.3
Emotions	0.7	0.4–0.9	0.5	0.3–0.7	0.2	−0.1–0.4
Activity limitation	0.4	0.3–0.6	0.3	0.2–0.5	0.1	0.0–0.3
Environment	0.5	0.3–0.6	0.3	0.1–0.4	0.2	0.0–0.3
Overall QOL	0.6	0.4–0.7	0.4	0.3–0.6	0.2	0.0–0.3

Source: Adapted from Juniper et al (1995).

or salbutamol (p<0.001); the differences were considered by the authors to be clinically important.

The St George's Respiratory Questionnaire. The St George's Respiratory Questionnaire (SGRQ) is another asthma-specific quality of life questionnaire (Jones et al, 1991). It comprises 76 weighted responses to a range of questions divided into three sections: (1) symptoms (distress caused by specific respiratory symptoms), (2) activity (physical activities that cause or are limited by breathlessness), and (3) impact (social and psychological effects of the disease). A total score is derived from all items. Each item in the questionnaire has an empirically derived weight based on a study of 140 patients, in six countries, with a wide range of ages and severity of asthma. The questionnaire has been shown to be both repeatable and sensitive (Jones et al, 1992).

Example 5.10

Jones et al (1994) used the SGRQ together with the Sickness Impact Profile and Hospital Anxiety and Depression Scale in a year-long multicenter double-blind placebo-controlled group comparative study to measure the effect of the anti-inflammatory drug nedocromil sodium on the quality of life in asthmatic subjects. The impacts component of the SGRQ was significantly improved in patients receiving nedocromil sodium, in association with a reduction in symptoms and requirement for inhaled bronchodilator use. This particular component of the SGRQ draws together the effects of the disease on social function and emotional well-being, and has been shown to correlate predominantly with severity of disability, exercise tolerance, and level of anxiety. The improvement in the SGRQ score in the nedocromil sodium–treated patients was about double that considered to be clinically significant. The questionnaire appeared to be used similarly in different countries despite differences in language and culture.

The Sydney Asthma Quality of Life Questionnaire. Marks et al (1992) have developed another asthma quality of life questionnaire for use in studies in adults. Items for inclusion on an initial questionnaire were derived from a focus group of people with asthma, from a literature review, and from asthma educators and other asthma health professionals. After pilot testing, the questionnaire, which contained 69 items, was tested on 284 adults with asthma and a principal components analysis was used to identify 20 items that were considered to relate to quality of life. These were used in the final questionnaire with 5-point responses. The questionnaire is self-administered and patients are asked to consider the impact of asthma over the preceding 4 weeks. The *Total* scale score is calculated from addition of the 20 item scores, and four subscale scores are derived from subsets of the items: *Breathlessness* and physical restrictions; *Mood* disturbance; *Social* disruption; and *Concerns* for health. The questionnaire has been shown to be capable of detecting differences between improved and stable patients (Marks et al, 1993).

The Living With Asthma Questionnaire (LWAQ). The Living With Asthma Questionnaire (Hyland et al, 1991a,b) was developed through focus groups and a series of validation studies. It comprises 68 statements covering 11 domains: social/leisure, sport, holidays, sleep, work/other activities, colds, mobility, effects on others, medication usage, sex, and dysphoric states and attitudes. These have been grouped into two main constructs: health knowledge (49 items) and health appraisal (19 items). The questionnaire contains both positive and negative statements, and patients are asked to indicate for each statement whether it is untrue, slightly true, very true, or not applicable. For negative statements, these responses are scored as 0, 1, 2, and 0 respectively; for positive statements, they are scored as 2, 1, 0, 0. Results can be expressed as an overall score, scores for the two main constructs, and scores for the 11 domains; in each instance, scores are based on averaging across all valid statements (excluding the statements that were "not applicable" or "not answered"). Thus, the overall score and the subscores range from 0 to 2 with a lower score indicating a better quality of life. The questionnaire has been shown to be valid and reliable (Hyland et al 1991a, 1991b) and there is some evidence that it may be responsive to change (Rutten-Van Mölken et al, 1995).

Example 5.11

Rutten-Van Mölken et al (1995) compared the performance of four instruments in evaluating the effects of salmeterol on asthma quality of life. In a double-blind parallel group study, 120 patients with moderate asthma, aged 18 to 70 years, received either inhaled salmeterol 50 μg b.i.d. or inhaled salbutamol 400 μg b.i.d. Quality of life was measured at 6 weeks' follow-up using (1) the Asthma Quality of Life Questionnaire (AQLQ), (2) the Living With Asthma Questionnaire (LWAQ), (3) the Sickness Impact Profile (SIP), and (4) the Rating Scale (RS) and Standard Gamble (SG) utilities. The Rating Scale ranges from "perfect health" equal to 100 to "death" equal to 0. Table 5.7 shows the mean differences (across all patients) between the salmeterol period and the salbutamol period, the standard deviations (SD) of the mean differences, and the ratio of the mean difference to the standard deviation. The latter ratio is used to permit a comparison of the effect sizes of different instruments that use different scales and have different ranges of variations. Although all the instruments showed a difference in favor of salmeterol, only the AQLQ and RS utility showed significantly greater improvement on salmeterol than on salbutamol. The study also found (not shown in table) that the AQLQ showed the best correlations with symptom scores, the patient's overall assessment of efficacy, and changes in lung function.

Table 5.7. Effect sizes in the salmeterol group as measured by each of four quality of life instruments

Instrument	Within-subject salmeterol effect	Pooled within-subject SD of change	Effect size*
AQLQ	0.492	0.600	0.820
Activities	0.573	0.666	0.860
Symptoms	0.581	0.803	0.723
Environment	0.438	0.797	0.550
Emotions	0.176	0.583	0.302
LWAQ	0.118	0.170	0.694
Health knowledge	0.130	0.208	0.625
Health appraisal	0.064	0.192	0.333
SIP	1.585	4.956	0.320
Physical	0.827	3.950	0.209
Psychosocial	2.815	6.648	0.423
Utilities			
Rating Scale	7.345	10.381	0.708
Standard Gamble	0.008	0.161	0.050

Source: Rutten-Van Mölken et al (1995).
* Within-subject salmeterol effect divided by pooled within- subject SD of change.

The Perceived Control of Asthma Questionnaire (PCAQ). The Perceived Control of Asthma Questionnaire (PCAQ) (Katz et al, 1997) comprises 11 questions focusing on the individual's perceived ability to effectively deal with asthma and its exacerbations. Figure 5.2 shows the 11 questions, each of which is scored from 1 to 5 (four "negative" questions are reverse scored), yielding an overall score in the range of 11 to 55. Katz et al (1997)

---

1. Managing asthma is largely my own responsibility
2. I can reduce asthma by staying calm and relaxed
3. Too often, my asthma seems to just hit me out of the blue*
4. If I do all the right things, I can successfully manage my asthma
5. I can do a lot of things myself to cope with my asthma
6. When I manage my personal life well, my asthma does not affect me as much
7. I have considerable ability to control my asthma
8. I would feel helpless if I couldn't rely on other people for help when I'm not feeling well from asthma*
9. No matter what I do, or how hard I try, I just can't seem to get relief from my asthma*
10. I am coping effectively with my asthma
11. It seems as though fate and other factors beyond my control affect my asthma*

---

* Negatively scored.

Figure 5.2. Questions in the Perceived Control of Asthma Questionnaire (PCAQ). (Source: Katz et al, 1997).

found that the questionnaire showed internal consistency and excellent construct validity, correlating strongly with asthma severity, quality of life, and SF-36 measures.

Knowledge of asthma

Intervention trials involving asthma education may be intended to improve knowledge and self-management of asthma, and there are a variety of outcome measures that may be used in such studies. However, positive changes in knowledge of asthma may not necessarily lead to a beneficial effect, and such changes have not been very successful to date in predicting changes in behavior (Clark and Starr-Schneidkraut, 1994; Blessing-Moore, 1996). The reasons for this are complex, but it should be noted that such patterns have been observed in many other areas of health education. For example, knowledge of the hazards of tobacco smoking may not lead to significant changes in smoking prevalence, which is more strongly influenced by other health problems, poverty, low self-esteem, and peer-group behavior (Graham, 1989; Power et al, 1991). Nevertheless, although many asthma education programs have had mixed results (e.g., Hilton et al, 1986), and participants in such programs may not be representative of all asthmatics (Yoon et al, 1991), the overall evidence suggests that asthma education can lead to improved outcomes and can be cost-effective (Partridge, 1995), provided that the programs focus on self-management skills and address special cultural and educational issues rather than adopting a "one size fits all" approach (Pomare et al, 1992; Blessing-Moore, 1996). In the current context, the key issue is that increased knowledge of asthma may not result in behavior change, or improvements in asthma morbidity. However, evaluating changes in knowledge of asthma is one important component in evaluating why an intervention did or did not lead to changes in behavior or improvements in other morbidity measures.

Example 5.12

Yoon et al (1993) conducted a randomized controlled trial of an asthma education program in 76 adult patients admitted to hospital for asthma. The intervention group (n = 37), received education soon after the first visit, whereas the control group (n = 39) waited until the third visit (about 12 months). A self-administered questionnaire (Yoon et al, 1991) was used at baseline and at 10 months. Table 5.8 shows that both groups showed improvements in most of the questionnaire measures, but the intervention group showed a significantly greater improvement in some measures of asthma knowledge and self-management skills. There was no consistent difference between the groups in various physiological measures, but there was only one readmission in the intervention group compared with seven in the control group during the 10-

Table 5.8. Mean scores from questionnaires at baseline and 10 months after education in intervention and control groups

	Maximal or possible score	Intervention group		Control group		P-value for difference
		Baseline	10 months	Baseline	10 months	
Action plan	10	2.89	4.79	3.32	3.03	<0.001
Differentiate mild from severe attack	10	2.18	4.07	2.68	2.85	0.005
Asthma severity	1–8	4.65	2.78	4.35	2.81	0.85
Symptom score	3–12	7.81	5.43	7.03	5.67	0.54
Psychosocial disturbance	12	7.21	4.00	6.75	3.96	0.87
Knowledge of asthma	4	2.89	3.09	3.22	2.80	0.07
Asthma health beliefs	5	1.32	2.46	1.68	1.28	<0.001
Knowledge of asthma drugs	14		9.25		7.57	<0.05

Source: Yoon et al (1993).

month follow-up period. The authors concluded that despite minimal effect on measures of airway function, substantial changes in illness behavior and use of health care facilities were achieved by the brief asthma education program.

Composite Measures

Finally, composite measures may be used in order to summarize all of the information on symptoms, lung function, health service and medication usage, and quality of life in each participant. Of course, each of these measures may themselves be composite scores. For example, it is possible to obtain a summation of different asthma symptoms into a single symptom index. One approach is to ask study participants to themselves give an overall score of the severity of their asthma in a given period; the alternative approach is to collect information on multiple, specific symptoms and to then combine this information into an overall symptom score (O'Connor and Weiss, 1994). More complex approaches may combine symptom scores with information on health service and medication usage and other asthma morbidity information. One observation that supports the use of composite scores is that changes in peak flow, PC_{20}, FEV_1, and symptom scores vary in their time course response to treatment, suggesting that they provide different information. As a result it has been recommended that these markers should be used in combination rather than in isolation (Kerstjens et al, 1992).

It is possible to combine information in a qualitative rather than a quantitative fashion. For example, Sears et al (1990) made a subjective composite use of information on morbidity based on daily diaries, recording nocturnal cough and wheeze, number of puffs of known bronchodilator used overnight and during the day, morning peak flow rate, daytime symptoms, and all medication taken. The investigators examined the diaries of each participant to determine the treatment period during which asthma was better controlled, and the use of "composite" information of this type may permit a more comprehensive overall evaluation of asthma severity. However, the qualitative nature of such assessments does not permit an estimation of the magnitude of the effect under study (Nelson et al, 1991).

On the other hand, quantitative composite measures may be problematic in that a single overall "asthma score" may mask important patterns in particular measures. However, they may have the advantage of including a more inclusive picture of the patient's experience than is obtained with a single narrowly focused measure (Marks et al, 1993). Such composite measures may be able to show an improvement in quality of life or knowledge about asthma even when the actual improvement in morbidity is small (Hyland et al, 1991b). This situation is particularly relevant in the evaluation of asthma education programs because these often produce little improvement in morbidity (Sibbald, 1989) but may have other benefits in terms of increased knowledge, confidence, or quality of life. Composite measures may also be used to combine information on symptoms and health service and medication usage (see Example 5.13).

Example 5.13

Lahdensuo et al (1996) conducted a randomized trial of guided self-management and traditional treatment of asthma over one year. Patients were randomized to receive traditional treatment (n=59) or guided self-management (n=56) based on daily morning peak expiratory flow (PEF) measurements. Table 5.9 shows that there were significantly fewer incidents (unscheduled outpatient visits, days off work, courses of antibiotics, courses of prednisolone) per patient in the self-management group than in the traditional treatment group over a 1-year period. Figure 5.3 combines the information from these various outcome measures and shows that the cumulative percentage of patients not having had any incident caused by asthma was consistently higher in the self-management group than in the tradi-

Table 5.9. Mean number of incidents (and SD) per patient caused by asthma in self-management and traditional treatment groups during one year

	Self-management (n=56)	Traditional treatment (n=59)	P-value
Unscheduled outpatient visits	0.5 (0.4)	1.0 (0.4)	0.04
Days off work	2.8 (0.6)	4.8 (0.3)	0.02
Courses of antibiotics	0.4 (0.4)	0.9 (0.4)	0.009
Courses of prednisolone	0.4 (0.4)	1.0 (0.5)	0.006
Total (any incident caused by asthma)	0.6 (0.4)	2.1 (0.8)	<0.0001

Source: Lahdensuo et al (1996).

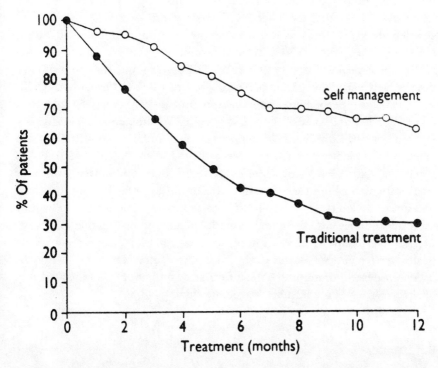

Figure 5.3. Cumulative percentage of patients not having any incident caused by asthma in self-management and traditional treatment groups. (Source: Lahdensuo et al, 1996, BMJ Publishing Group.)

tional treatment group ($P<0.0001$). The authors also used components of the St George's Respiratory Questionnaire to evaluate quality of life and found a higher mean quality of life score (16.6 versus 8.4) at 12 months in the self-management group (not shown in table).

Summary

Whereas prevalence studies usually involve a general population sample (as the denominator) with asthma as the outcome under study (the numerator), morbidity studies involve studying an asthmatic population (as the denominator) with the intention of ascertaining which factors affect the level of asthma severity or control within this population. Measures of asthma morbidity fall into five major groups: symptoms, physiological measures, health service and medication usage, quality of life and knowledge of asthma, and composite measures. As in prevalence studies, symptoms are the cornerstone of studies of asthma morbidity but questionnaires on asthma symptom severity in morbidity studies usually require more information on the intensity, duration, and frequency of symptoms than is required for prevalence studies. As in prevalence studies, symptom questionnaires may be supplemented by physiological measurements of lung function, including forced vital capacity (FVC), forced expiratory volume in one second (FEV_1), and peak expiratory flow rate (PEFR). The measurement of peak flow rates is particularly valuable in this regard because this can be readily done by study participants and entered into a daily diary. Measures of health service and medication usage are more problematic because increased contact with the health services is often an intended or unintended effect of participation in a study. Nevertheless, there are still a number of situations, particularly time series studies and some randomized controlled trials, in which health service and medication usage may be valid outcome measures. A variety of quality of life scores are available for use in asthma morbidity studies, and these may provide valuable complementary information to that obtained from symptom reporting, physiological measures, and health service and medication usage. Finally, composite measures may be used in order to summarize all the information on symptoms, lung function, health service and medication usage, and quality of life.

References

Adams L, Chronos N, Lane R, Guz A (1985). The measurement of breathlessness induced in normal subjects: validity of two scaling techniques. Clin Sci 69: 7–16.

Anderson HR (1989). Is the prevalence of asthma changing? Arch Dis Child 64: 172–5.

Antó JM, Sunyer J, Rodriguez-Roisin R, et al (1989). Community outbreaks of asthma associated with inhalation of soybean dust. N Engl J Med 320: 1097–1102.

Avital A, Springer C, Bar-Yishay E, Godfrey S (1995). Adenosine, methacholine, and exercise challenges in children with asthma of paediatric chronic obstructive pulmonary disease. Thorax 50: 511–6.

Bailey WC, Wilson SR, Weiss KB, et al (1994). Measures for use in asthma clinical research. Overview of the NIH Workshop. Am J Respir Crit Care Med 149: S1–S8.

Barnes NC, Marone G, Maria GU, et al (1993). A comparison of fluticasone propionate, 1 mg daily, with beclomethasone dipropionate, 2 mg daily, in the treatment of severe asthma. Eur Respir J 6: 877–84.

Beaupre A, Malo JL (1981). Histamine dose-response curves in asthma: relevant of the distinction between PC_{20} and reactivity in characterising clinical state. Thorax 36: 731–6.

Bergner M, Bobbitt RA, Carter WB, et al (1981). The Sickness Impact Profile: development and final revision of a health status measure. Med Care 19: 787–805.

Blessing-Moore J (1996). Does asthma education change behaviour? Chest 109: 9–11.

Britton JR, Burney PGJ, Chinn S, et al (1988). The relation between airway reactivity and change in respiratory symptoms and medication in a community study. Am Rev Respir Dis 138: 530–4.

Burdon JGW, Juniper EF, Killian KJ, et al (1982). Perception of breathlessness in asthma. Am Rev Respir Dis 126: 825–8.

Busse WW, Maisiak R, Young KR (1994). Treatment regimen and side effects of treatment measures. Am J Respir Crit Care Med 149: S44–S50.

Clark NM, Starr-Schneidkraut NJ (1994). Management of asthma by patients and families. Am J Respir Crit Care Med 149: S54–S66.

Cockroft DW, Swystun VA (1996). Asthma control versus asthma severity. J Allergy Clin Immunol 98: 1016–8.

D'Souza W, Crane J, Burgess C, et al (1994). Community-based asthma care: trial of a "credit card" self-management plan in a New Zealand Maori community. Eur Respir J 7: 1260–5.

D'Souza W, Burgess C, Ayson M, et al (1996). Trial of a "credit card" asthma self-management plan in a "high risk" group of patients with asthma. J Allergy Clin Immunol 97: 1085–92.

Dyer CAE, Sinclair AJ (1997). A hospital-based case-control study of quality of life in older asthmatics. Eur Respir J 10: 337–41.

Ehnert B, Lau-Schadendorf S, Weber A, et al (1992). Reducing domestic exposure to dust mite allergen reduces bronchial hyperreactivity in sensitive children with asthma. J Allergy Clin Immunol 90: 135–8.

Enright PL, Lebowitz MD, Cockroft DW (1994). Physiologic measures: pulmonary function tests. Am J Respir Crit Care Med 149: S9–S18.

Gergen PJ, Weiss KB (1990). Changing patterns of asthma hospitalization among children: 1979 to 1987. JAMA 264: 1688–92.

Geubelle F, Borlee-Hermans G, Leclerq-Foucart J (1971). Hyperreactivity of the bronchial tree to histamine in asthmatic children and its variations. Bull Eur Physiopathol Respir 7: 839–40.

Gottlieb DJ, Beiser AS, O'Connor GT (1995). Poverty, race, and medication use are correlates of asthma hospitalization rates: a small area analysis in Boston. Chest 108: 28–35.

Graham H (1989). Women and smoking in the United Kingdom: the implications for health promotion. Health Promotion 3: 371–82.

Haahtela T, Järvinen M, Kava T, et al (1991). Comparison of a β_2-agonist, terbutaline, with an inhaled corticosteroid, budesonide, in newly detected asthma. N Engl J Med 325: 388–92.

Hilton S, Sibbald B, Anderson HR, Freeling P (1986). Controlled evaluation of the effects of patient education on asthma morbidity in general practice. Lancet 1: 26–9.

Horn CR, Cochrane GM (1989). An audit of morbidity associated with chronic asthma in general practice. Resp Med 83: 71–5.

Hyland ME (1991a). The living with asthma questionnaire. Resp Med 85 (suppl B): 13–6.

Hyland ME, Finnis S, Irvine SH (1991b). A scale for assessing quality of life in adult asthma sufferers. J Psychosom Res 35: 99–110.

Ignacio-Garcia JM, Gonzalez-Santos P (1995). Asthma self-management education program by home monitoring of peak flow. Am J Respir Crit Care Med 151: 353–9.

Jones PW, Quirk FH, Baveystock CM (1991). The St George's Respiratory Questionnaire. Respir Med 85: 25–31.

Jones PW, Quirk FH, Baveystock CM, Littlejohns P (1992). A self-complete measure of health status for chronic airflow limitation: The St George's Respiratory Questionnaire. Am Rev Respir Dis 145: 1321–7.

Jones PW (1995). Quality of life measurement in asthma. Eur Respir J 8: 885–7.

Jones PW, and the Nedocromil Sodium Quality of Life Study Group (1994). Quality of life, symptoms and pulmonary function in asthma: long-term treatment with nedocromil sodium examined in a controlled multicentre trial. Eur Respir J 7: 55–62.

Josephs LK, Gregg I, Holgate ST (1990). Does non-specific bronchial responsiveness indicate the severity of asthma? Eur Respir J 3: 220–7.

Juniper EF, Guyatt GH, Epstein RS, et al (1992). Evaluation of impairment of health-related quality of life in asthma: development of a questionnaire for use in clinical trials. Thorax 47: 76–83.

Juniper EF, Guyatt GH, Ferrie PJ, Griffith LE (1993). Measuring quality of life in asthma. Am Rev Respir Dis 147: 832–8.

Juniper EF, Guyatt GH, Willan A, Griffith LE (1994). Determining a minimal important change in a disease-specific quality of life questionnaire. J Clin Epidemiol 47: 81–7.

Juniper EF, Johnson PR, Borkhoff CM, et al (1995). Quality of life in asthma clinical trials: comparison of salmeterol and salbutamol. Am J Respir Crit Care Med 151: 66–70.

Kaplan RM, Atkins CJ, Timms R (1984). Validity of a well-being scale as an outcome measure in chronic obstructive pulmonary disease. J Chron Dis 37: 85–95.

Kaplan RM, Atkins CJ (1989). The well-year of life as a basis for patient decision making. Patient Educ Couns 13: 281–95.

Katz PP, Yelin EH, Smith S, Blanc PD (1997). Perceived control of asthma: development and validation of a questionnaire. Am J Respir Crit Care Med 155: 577–82.

Kerstjens HAM, Brand PLP, Hughes MD, et al (1992). A comparison of bronchodilator therapy with or without inhaled corticosteroid therapy for obstructive airways disease. N Engl J Med 327: 1413–8.

Kirshner B, Guyatt GH (1985). A methodologic framework for assessing health indices. J Chron Dis 38: 27–36.

Lahdensuo A, Haahtela T, Herrala J, et al (1996). Randomised comparison of guided self-management and traditional treatment of asthma over one year. BMJ 312: 748–52.

Lebowitz MD (1996). Age, period, and cohort effects: Influences on differences between cross-sectional and longitudinal pulmonary function results. Am J Respir Crit Care Med 154: S273–S277.

Marks GB, Dunn SM, Woolcock AJ (1992). A scale for measurement of quality of life in adults with asthma. J Clin Epidemiol 45: 461–72.

Marks GB, Dunn SM, Woolcock AJ (1993). An evaluation of an asthma quality of life questionnaire as a measure of change in adults with asthma. J Clin Epidemiol 46: 1103–11.

Mayo PH, Richman J, Harris HW (1990). Results of a program to reduce admissions for adult asthma. Ann Intern Med 112: 864–71.

Nelson HS, Szefler SJ, Martin RJ (1991). Regular inhaled beta-adrenergic agonists in the treatment of bronchial asthma: beneficial or detrimental. Am Rev Respir Dis 144: 249–50.

Neukirch F, Liard R, Segala C, et al (1992). Peak expiratory flow variability and bronchial responsiveness to methacholine. Am Rev Respir Dis 146: 71–5.

O'Connor GT, Weiss ST (1994). Clinical and symptom measures. Am J Respir Crit Care Med 149: S21–S28.

Paggiaro PL, Moscato G, Giannini D, et al (1997). Relationship between peak expiratory flow (PEF) and FEV_1. Eur Respir J 10(Suppl 24): 39s–41s.

Partridge MR (1995). Delivering optimal care to the person with asthma: what are the key components and what do we mean by patient education? Eur Respir J 8: 298–305.

Picado C (1996). Classification of severe asthma exacerbations: a proposal. Eur Respir J 9: 1775–8.

Pomare E, Tutengaehe H, Ramsden I, et al (1992). Asthma in Maori people. N Z Med J 105: 469–70.

Power C, Manor O, Fox J (1991). Health and Class: the Early Years. London: Chapman Hall.

Richards JM, Hemstreet MP (1994). Measures of life quality, role performance, and functional status in asthma research. Am J Respir Crit Care Med 149: S31–S39.

Romieu I, Meneses F, Ruiz S, et al (1996). Effects of air pollution on the respiratory health of asthmatic children living in Mexico City. Am J Respir Crit Care Med 154: 300–7.

Rubinfeld AR, Pain MCF (1976). Perception of asthma. Lancet 1: 882–4.

Rutten-Van Mölken M, Custers F, Van Doorslaer EKA, et al (1995). Comparison of performance of four instruments in evaluating the effects of salmeterol on asthma quality of life. Eur Respir J 8: 888–98.

Ryan G, Latimer KM, Dolovich J, Hargreave FE (1982). Bronchial responsiveness to histamine: relationship to diurnal variation of peak flow rate, improvement after bronchodilator, and airway calibre. Thorax 37: 423–9.

Sears MR, Taylor DR, Print CG, et al (1990). Regular inhaled beta-agonist treatment in bronchial asthma. Lancet 336: 1391–6.

Shields MC, Griffin KW, McNabb WL (1990). The effect of a patient education program on emergency room use for inner-city children with asthma. Am J Public Health 80: 36–8.

Sibbald B (1989). Patient self care in acute asthma. Thorax 44: 97–101.

Tinkelman D, Reed C, Nelson H, Offord K (1993). Aerosol beclomethasone dipropionate compared with theophylline as primary treatment of chronic mild to moderately severe asthma in children. Paediatrics 92: 64–76.

Van Ganse E, Van der Linden PD, Leufkens HGM, et al (1995). Asthma medications and disease exacerbations: an epidemiological study as a method for asthma surveillance. Eur Respir J 8: 1856–60.

Vollmer WM, Osborne ML, Buist AS (1993). Temporal trends in hospital-based episodes of asthma care in a health maintenance organization. Am Rev Respir Dis 147: 347–53.

Vollmer WM, Osborne ML, Buist AS (1994). Uses and limitations of mortality and health care utilization statistics in asthma research. Am J Respir Crit Care Med 149: S79–S87.

Ware JE (1993). SF-36 Health Survey, Manual and Interpretation Guide. Boston: The Health Institute.

Williams SJ, Bury MR (1989). Impairment, disability and handicap in chronic respiratory illness. Soc Sci Med 29: 609–16.

Windom HH, Burgess CD, Crane J, et al (1990). The self-administration of inhaled beta agonist drugs during severe asthma. N Z Med J 103: 205–7.

Yoon R, McKenzie DK, Bauman A, Miles DA (1991). Characteristics of attenders and non-attenders at at an asthma education programme. Thorax 46: 886–90.

Yoon R, McKenzie DK, Bauman A, Miles DA (1993). Controlled trial evaluation of an asthma education programme for adults. Thorax 48: 1110–6.

6

Measuring Asthma Risk Factors

This chapter reviews methods of measuring exposure to some of the major risk factors for asthma. We do not present a systematic review of epidemiological findings or a detailed technical exposition of exposure measurement techniques. Rather, the intention is to review the general approaches used for exposure assessment in studies of the major asthma risk factors. We commence by considering the general issues of defining and measuring exposure and dose. Strictly speaking, *exposure* refers to the presence of a substance in the environment, whereas *dose* refers to the amount of substance that reaches susceptible targets within the body, but we use the term exposure to refer to both concepts, as well as other attributes or agents that may be risk factors for asthma (e.g., demographic factors, genetic factors). We stress that the prime consideration in asthma epidemiology studies is usually to obtain exposure information of similar accuracy for the groups being compared. We then review approaches to exposure assessment that have been used in studies of the major asthma risk factors including demographic factors, genetic factors and early life events, atopy, indoor environment, outdoor environment, occupational exposures, and other risk factors.

General Considerations

Exposure and dose

Asthma epidemiology studies typically involve measuring the effect of an exposure (e.g., air pollution) on a particular outcome (e.g., asthma, severe asthma, asthma hospital admission, asthma death) in a population. Strictly speaking, the term *exposure* refers to the presence of a substance (e.g., house dust mite allergen) in the external environment, whereas the term *dose* refers to the amount of substance that reaches susceptible targets within the body, such as the airways. In some situations (e.g., in a coal mine) measurements of external exposures may be strongly correlated with internal dose, whereas in other situations (e.g., indoor exposure to house dust mite allergen) the dose may depend on individual lifestyle and activities and may therefore be only weakly correlated with the environmental exposure levels. However, in this chapter we use the term exposure in the very general sense to denote any attribute or agent that may increase the risk of experiencing the outcome under study. It includes demographic factors (age, gender, ethnicity, social class), and genetic factors, as well as environmental risk factors (measured externally and/or internally).

Exposure levels can be assessed with regard to the *intensity* of the substance in the environment (e.g., allergen concentration in the air) and the *duration* of time for which exposure occurs. The risk of developing sensitization to allergen may be much greater if the duration of exposure is long and/or the exposure is intense, and the total *cumulative exposure* may therefore be important. On the other hand, once a person has become sensitized, the intensity of exposure may be crucial in provoking an acute attack, and such attacks may occur after exposure of a relatively short duration. For protracted etiologic processes, the time pattern of exposure may be important and it is possible to assess this by examining the separate effects of exposures in various time windows prior to the occurrence and recognition of clinical disease (Pearce, 1992a). For example, several studies have found that exposure to environmental tobacco smoke in the first years of life may be as relevant as current exposures with regard to current asthma symptoms (e.g., Shaw et al, 1994). Similarly, recent work suggests that occupational asthma is most likely to occur after about 1 to 3 years of exposure to a sensitizing agent (Antó et al, 1996).

Comparability of exposure information

Epidemiological studies rarely have optimal exposure data and often rely on relatively crude measures of exposure. The key issue is that the exposure data need not be perfect, but it should be of similar quality for the various groups being compared. Provided that this principle is followed, then misclassification of exposure will be nondifferential (see Chapter 3). Nondifferential information bias generally biases the relative risk estimate toward the null value of 1.0 (Copeland et al, 1977; Dosemeci, 1990). Hence, nondifferential information bias tends to produce "false negative" findings and is of particular concern in studies that find a negligible association between exposure and disease. However, as noted in Chapter 3, one important condition is needed to ensure that exposure misclassification produces bias toward the null: the exposure classification errors must be independent of other errors. Without this condition, nondifferential exposure misclassification can produce bias in any direction (Chavance et al, 1992; Kristensen, 1992).

Thus, it is important to ensure that (1) the exposure data are of similar quality in the groups being compared (i.e., that misclassification is non-differential) and (2) the data are of the best possible quality (i.e., that misclassification is kept to a minimum). There is often no benefit (and there may be substantial problems of bias) in collecting more detailed exposure information if this is only available for one of the groups being compared (e.g., for cases but not for controls).

General approaches to exposure assessment

Methods of exposure measurement include personal interviews or self-administered questionnaires (completed either by the study participant or by a proxy respondent), diaries, observation, routine records, physical or chemical measurements on the environment, or physical or chemical measurements on the person (Armstrong et al, 1992). Measurements on the person can relate either to exogenous exposure (e.g., airborne dust) or internal dose (e.g., plasma cotinine); the other measurement options (e.g., questionnaires) all relate to exogenous exposures.

Questionnaires and environmental measurements. Traditionally, exposure to most nonbiological risk factors (e.g., cigarette smoking) has been measured with questionnaires, and this approach has a long history of successful use in epidemiology. Questionnaires may be self-administered (e.g., postal questionnaires) or interviewer-administered (e.g., in telephone or face-to-face interviews) and may be completed by the study subject or by a proxy (e.g., parental completion of questionnaires in a childhood asthma study). The validity of questionnaire data also depends on the structure, format, content, and wording of questionnaires, as well as methods of administration and selection and training of interviewers (Armstrong et al, 1992). Questionnaires may be combined with environmental exposure measurements (e.g., pollen counts, industrial hygiene surveys) to obtain a quantitative estimate of individual exposures. Questionnaires and environmental measurements have good validity and reproducibility with regard to current exposures and are likely to be superior to biological markers with respect to historical exposures (see below).

Biomarkers. More recently, there has been increasing emphasis on the use of molecular markers of internal dose (Schulte, 1993). In fact, there are a number of major limitations of currently available biomarkers of exposure (Armstrong et al, 1992), particularly with regard to historical exposures (Pearce et al, 1995). For example, serum levels of micronutrients reflect recent rather than historical dietary intake (Willett, 1990). Some biomarkers are better than others in this respect (particularly markers of exposure to biological agents), but even the best markers of chemical exposures usually reflect only the last few weeks or months of exposure. On the other hand, with some biomarkers it may be possible to estimate historical levels provided that certain assumptions are met. For example, it may be possible to estimate historical levels of exposure to pesticides (or contaminants) from current serum levels provided that the exposure period is known and the half-life is known. Similarly, information on recent exposures can be used if it is reasonable to assume that exposure levels (or at least relative exposure levels) have remained stable over time (this may be particularly relevant in occupational studies), and have not been affected by lifestyle changes, or by the occurrence of the disease. However, if the aim is to measure historical exposures, then historical information on exposure surrogates may be more valid than direct measurements of current exposure or dose levels. This situation has long been recognized in occupational epidemiology, where the use of work history records in combination with a job-exposure matrix (based on historical exposure measurements of work areas rather than individuals) is usually considered to be more valid than current exposure measurements (whether based on environmental measurements or biomarkers) if the aim is to estimate historical exposure levels (Checkoway et al, 1989). On the other hand, some biomarkers have potential value in validation of questionnaires that can then be used to estimate historical exposures. Furthermore, biomarkers of internal dose may have relatively good validity in studies involving an acute effect of exposure such as the triggering of specific asthma attacks.

A more fundamental problem of measuring internal dose with a biomarker is that it is not always clear whether one is measuring the exposure, the biological effect, or some stage of the disease process itself (Saracci, 1984). Thus the findings may be uninterpretable in terms of the causal association between exposure and disease. When it is known that the "biologically effective dose" is the most appropriate measure, then the use of appropriate biomarkers clearly has some scientific advantages. However, choosing the appropriate biomarker is a major dilemma, and biomarkers are frequently chosen on the basis of an incomplete or erroneous understanding of the etiologic process (or simply because a particular marker can be measured). An environmental exposure (e.g., tobacco smoke) may involve hundreds of different chemicals, each of which may produce hundreds of measurable biological responses (there are exceptions to this, of course, such as environmental lead exposure, but most environmental exposure involves complex mixtures). A biomarker typically measures one of the biological responses to one of the chemicals. If the chosen biomarker measures the key etiological factor, then it may yield relatively good exposure data; however, if a biomarker is chosen that has little relationship to the etiological component of the complex exposure mixture, then the biomarker will yield relatively poor exposure data.

A further major problem with the use of biomarkers is that the resulting expense and complexity may drastically reduce the study size, even in a case-control study, and therefore greatly reduce the statistical power for detecting an association between exposure and disease.

Thus, questionnaires and environmental measurements will continue to play a major role in exposure assessment in asthma epidemiology, but biomarkers may be expected to become increasingly useful over time, as new techniques are developed. The emphasis should be on using "appropriate technology" to obtain the most practical and valid estimate of the etiologically relevant exposure. The appropriate approach (questionnaires, environmental measurements, or biological measurements) will vary from study to study, and from exposure to exposure within the same study (or within the same complex chemical mixture—for example, in tobacco smoke).

Demographic Factors

There are a variety of demographic factors that are associated with asthma, including age (Anderson et al, 1992), gender (Anderson et al, 1992), birth order (Shaw et al, 1994), season of birth (Aberg, 1989), ethnicity (Cunningham et al, 1996a), region (Aberg et al, 1989), and country (ECRHS, 1996). Age is the demographic factor that is most strongly related to asthma symptom prevalence: symptoms usually decline at or before the onset of puberty (Balfour-Lynn (1985), and puberty may be delayed in atopic children (and hence in asthmatic children), but the reasons for these patterns are unclear (Silverman, 1995).

In most instances, information on demographic factors can be obtained in a straightforward manner from routine health care records or with questionnaires. Armstrong et al (1992) argue that although in interviews it is common practice to place demographic questions at the beginning, this may not be advisable, because they are often of low interest to the respondents and certain demographic questions (e.g., ethnicity, socioeconomic status) may be considered threatening by some respondents.

In studies focusing on ethnicity, the etiologically relevant definition will depend on the extent to which an ethnic difference is considered to be due to genetic and/or cultural and environmental factors, but the available information will vary from country to country depending on historical and cultural considerations. For example, in New Zealand, Maori ethnicity is defined as "a person who has Maori ethnicity and chooses to identify as

Maori" (Pomare et al, 1992), whereas some countries use solely biologically based definitions (Polednak, 1989).

Socioeconomic status poses more significant measurement problems. It can be measured in a variety of ways, including occupation, income, and education (Liberatos et al, 1988; Berkman and MacIntyre, 1997). These measures may pose problems in some demographic groups; for example, occupation and income may be poor measures of socioeconomic status in women, for whom the total family situation may reflect their socioeconomic status better than their individual situation, and measures of socioeconomic status in children must be based on the situation of the parents or the total family situation. Nevertheless, the various measures of socioeconomic status are strongly correlated with each other, and asthma epidemiology studies are usually based on whichever measures are available, unless socioeconomic status is the main focus of the research and it is necessary to obtain more detailed information.

Studies in the 1960s and 1970s (e.g., Mitchell et al, 1973) suggested that asthma is more common in children in the higher social classes. However, there has been less evidence of social class differences as the diagnosis of asthma has become more widespread (Littlejohns and MacDonald, 1993), even though diagnostic labeling of wheezing in adults differs by social class (Littlejohns et al, 1989). In contrast, severe asthma appears to be more common in children in disadvantaged socioeconomic (Mielck et al, 1996) and ethnic groups (Pomare et al, 1992), and low socioeconomic status is associated with hospital admissions for asthma (Watson et al, 1996) and with reduced lung function in adults (Steinberg and Becklake, 1986). This could represent either a greater prevalence of asthma in disadvantaged groups, or increased severity due to environmental factors (e.g., environmental tobacco smoke, nutrition), or inadequate disease management and inadequate access to health care (Pomare et al, 1992; Littlejohns and MacDonald, 1993).

Genetic Factors and Early Life Events

Genetic factors

Asthma appears to be multifactorial in origin and influenced by multiple genes and environmental factors (Panhuysen et al, 1995; Collaborative Study on the Genetics of Asthma, 1997). Asthma genetic studies are further complicated by the difficulties in defining the asthma "phenotype" (Sandford et al, 1996) and the fact that this phenotypic expression may vary with age (Panhuysen et al, 1995). Thus, asthma is a complex genetic disorder that is not inherited in the simple mendelian fashion that is characteristic of single-gene disorders. A particular genetic factor may increase susceptibility to the effects of an environmental exposure and may thereby affect one or more aspects of the complex etiological process involved in asthma, but whether this genetic potential is expressed will depend on whether sufficient exposure to the environmental factor occurs. Furthermore, it has been proposed that some nonallergic forms of asthma may have no genetic basis (Sandford et al, 1996). Investigating possible genes for atopy or bronchial hyperresponsiveness (BHR), the underlying immunological and physiological components that often characterize clinical asthma, is also fraught with difficulties, as control of both IgE production and BHR is also multifactorial (Zamel et al, 1996), and neither is synonymous with asthma. Moreover, the increasing prevalence of asthma indicates that genetic factors alone are unlikely to account for a substantial proportion of asthma cases (Cullinan and Newman Taylor, 1994). Nevertheless, genetic susceptibility to changing environmental exposures may play an important role in changes in asthma prevalence, and a genetic predisposition may be responsible for determining specific disease manifestation in atopic individuals (Edfors-Lubs, 1971). Furthermore, knowing the gene products that are important in asthma could be important in providing new potential targets for therapeutic interventions, and identifying high-risk populations for early intervention (Hall, 1997).

Familial concordance. It is well established that people with a family history of asthma are more likely to develop asthma themselves (Horwood et al, 1985), and parental asthma is a stronger predictor of asthma in the offspring than parental atopy (Von Mutius and Nicolai, 1996). However, this association is not necessarily due to genetic factors, and could merely reflect similar lifestyles and exposures in family members (Sandford et al, 1996). For example, one study found that a person whose spouse developed asthma was also more likely to develop asthma (Smith et al, 1967), presumably due to common environmental exposures. Nevertheless, parental asthma is an important risk factor (and potential confounder) that is usually measured in asthma risk factor studies (using the methods discussed in Chapter 4).

Twin concordance. Some indication of the possible contribution of genetic factors in asthma is given by studies of twins. For example, Edfors-Lubs (1971) analyzed data on 7000 twin pairs from the Swedish Twin Register and found that concordance of asthma in monozygotic twins was greater than in dizygotic twins. However, the concordance was still only 19%, and even this may in part be due to similar environmental exposures in monozygotic twins, including a common intrauterine environment (Godfrey et al, 1994). Other large population studies have yielded similar findings, but this may be because these studies have determined asthma on the basis of questionnaires or hospital and pharmacy records, whereas smaller studies with more intensive diagnostic methods have generally yielded higher concordance (Sandford et al, 1996).

Example 6.1

Sibbald et al (1980) conducted an asthma prevalence study in relatives of 77 asthmatic and 87 control children attending a London general practice. The history of asthma in the parents and siblings of probands (i.e., the asthmatic and non-asthmatic children) was obtained through interview with one or more family members and through medical records. Table 6.1 shows that 13% of first-degree relatives of asthmatics were found to have asthma, compared with 4% of relatives of the controls (OR=3.9, 95% CI 1.9–8.3). The association was stronger in relatives of children with atopy (OR=5.1) than in relatives of children without atopy (OR=2.7); it was also stronger for parents (OR=5.1) than for siblings (OR=2.7). Among the relatives of asthmatics, atopic asthma (10%) was more common than nonatopic asthma (3%), irrespective of the atopic status of the proband (not shown in table), whereas atopic asthma (3%) and nonatopic asthma (3%) were equally common in relatives of the non-asthmatics. The authors concluded that these findings support the hypothesis that asthma and atopy are inherited independently, and that although atopy may not predispose to asthma, it may enhance a genetic susceptibility to the condition, thus increasing the likelihood that it will be expressed (Sibbald et al, 1980).

Segregation and linkage analysis. Segregation analysis tests explicit models of inheritance in families—for example, by observing the frequency of the

Table 6.1. Prevalence of asthma in first-degree relatives of children with asthma and non-asthmatic controls

	Relatives of cases	Relatives of controls	Odds ratio	95% CI
ATOPIC CASES AND CONTROLS				
Parents	18% (23/128)	3% (2/76)	8.1	1.8–51.4
Siblings	9% (11/124)	4% (2/53)	2.5	0.5–16.9
All relatives	13% (34/252)	3% (4/129)	4.9	1.6–16.6
NONATOPIC CASES AND CONTROLS				
Parents	15% (4/26)	5% (5/98)	3.4	0.7–16.3
Siblings	4% (1/26)	3% (2/75)	1.5	0.0–22.0
All relatives	10% (5/52)	4% (7/173)	2.5	0.7–9.4
ALL CASES AND CONTROLS				
Parents	17% (27/154)	4% (7/174)	5.1	2.0–13.3
Siblings	8% (12/150)	3% (4/128)	2.7	0.8–10.2
All relatives	13% (39/304)	4% (11/302)	3.9	1.9–8.3

Source: Adapted from Sibbald et al (1980).

condition in offspring and siblings and comparing it to the distribution expected on the basis of various modes of inheritance. Linkage analysis uses DNA marker data to follow the transmission of genetic information between generations in order to determine if a genetic marker is linked to a gene involved in a particular disease (Panhuysen et al, 1995; Sandford et al, 1996). In combined segregation and linkage analysis, the model of inheritance is determined simultaneously with the linkage test, using linkage, if present, to define the model.

For a trait as common as atopy, large families selected randomly, without reference to atopy, need to be studied to enable population frequencies to be determined and to provide material for genetic analysis. The ideal marker is highly polymorphic, can be typed to polymerase chain reaction (PCR), and is located within a candidate locus that is far from other marker loci. Attention has particularly focused on chromosomes 5 and 11, both of which may contain genes relevant to asthma and atopy (Meyers and Bleecker, 1995; Doull et al, 1996). However, studies investigating linkage to candidate loci may be affected by bias introduced through the methods of acquiring the probands, the broad and variable definitions of atopy, the assumption of a simple mendelian pattern of inheritance, and the lack of appreciation of antigen-specific factors such as HLA-D encoded immune responses. As a result, as with many genetic studies of other major disorders, there have been problems of failing to replicate reported genetic linkage in atopy—for example, in the major "atopy gene" located on 11q13 (Cookson et al, 1989, 1993; Morton, 1992; Van Herwerden et al, 1995).

Example 6.2

In an attempt to address the disputed findings of a single major autosomal dominant "atopy gene" linked to D11 S97 on chromosome 11q13, Lawrence et al (1994) collected data on 131 nuclear families with at least three children, randomly selected from general practice registers, without regard to atopy or asthma. Seven indices were formed by stepwise principal components analysis, from which atopy and asthma were defined. As the correlation matrix showed that atopy could be well described in terms of total serum IgE, this measurement was used in subsequent analysis. Application of the randomly collected family data strongly rejected any single locus model, including those proposed previously (Cookson et al, 1989, 1993). Comingling analysis was consistent with a small number of loci determining atopy. To probe the region around 11q13, three highly informative polymorphic markers (D11 S534, D11 S527, and D11 S480) were chosen with multiplex PCR and fluorescent gene scanning employed to identify the amplified products (Watson et al, 1995). Path analysis also did not support paternal imprinting, which had previously been proposed (Cookson et al, 1993). The authors concluded that these findings cast doubt on the validity of previously reported findings of linkage with the β-chain of the high affinity IgE receptor on 11q13.

Sib-pair analysis. Sib-pair analysis enables the assessment of the evidence for linkage without having to define the mode of inheritance (Shah and Green, 1994; Sandford et al, 1996). the analysis is done on pairs of affected siblings within a family. If a particular marker is unlinked to the disease gene, then there is a 50:50 chance that the pair will share the specific marker allele, whereas levels of allele sharing of greater than 50% indicate possible linkage of the marker to the disease gene. This deviation can be observed irrespective of the mode of inheritance.

Association studies. Association studies can be used to assess the importance of a candidate gene for asthma in the general population, rather than in familial studies (Sandford et al, 1996). These are essentially population-based asthma prevalence case-control studies in which asthmatic cases and non-asthmatic controls are compared with regard to the presence of known polymorphisms within specific genes. Because asthma is a multifactorial disease, an etiologically relevant gene will usually not be absent in a control sample and will usually not be universally present in the cases; that is, a particular gene will usually be neither necessary nor sufficient for asthma to occur but will increase the risk of developing the disease, and this will be reflected in an odds ratio that is elevated but that is not infinity. It should be stressed that such studies involve the same methodological issues as other asthma epidemiology studies; in particular, they should ideally be based on random general population samples, and it is necessary to collect information on potential confounders and to control for them in the analysis.

Example 6.3

Reihsaus et al (1993) studied 51 patients with moderate to severe asthma and 56 normal subjects. The "cases" were enrolled from the Allergy and Pulmonary Clinics at Duke University Medical Center, whereas the source of the controls was not specific. Blood was drawn from both groups and the authors examined the gene encoding the β_2-adrenergic receptor (β_2AR). They discovered nine different point mutations, four of which caused amino acid substitutions. None of these mis-sense mutations were more common in cases than in controls, but, one (substitution of glycine for arginine at position 16) was associated with more severe asthma. For example, of patients who required continuous oral corticosteroids, 75% were homozygous for Arg161 Gly16 compared with 53% of all cases and 59% of controls. The authors concluded that an alteration in the gene encoding for β_2AR plays an accessory role in the pathogenesis of asthma in certain patients. However, it is notable that this alteration was also common in non-asthmatics and would be causally involved only in a minority of severe asthma cases (the attributable risk for severe asthma is about 35% to 40%).

Intrauterine environment and early life events

There is now a large body of epidemiological evidence that the intrauterine environment may have effects that increase the risk of chronic disease in adult life (Barker, 1993). This may be either due to direct effects, for example nutritional deficiency in utero may adversely affect airways growth, or alternatively it may be due to maternal nutrition during pregnancy leading to programming of the developing immune system.

Birthweight and head circumference. Birthweight and head circumference are markers of the intrauterine environment that are routinely measured and recorded in birth records. Thus they are particularly useful for epidemiological studies. Barker et al (1991) found that low birthweight was associated with lower average values of FEV_1 in adulthood, independently of smoking, age, social class, and recorded lower respiratory tract infection in infancy. Rona et al (1993), in a study of 5573 children aged 5 to 11 years, found that respiratory symptoms such as wheeze were associated with length of gestation but not birthweight, whereas lung function was related to birthweight but not gestational age.

Example 6.4

Seidman et al (1991) studied male recruits to the Israeli army who were born between 1964 and 1971. A diagnosis of asthma was made on the basis of medical history and lung function measurements. Table 6.2 shows the association between birthweight and asthma at age 17 years. The group with low birthweights (<2500 g) had a significantly increased risk of developing asthma by age 17 years compared with the reference group, who had birthweights in the range of 3000 to 3499 g. The authors concluded that low birthweight may be a risk factor for developing asthma during childhood and adolescence.

Table 6.2. Birth weight and asthma at age 17 years in Israeli army recruits born between 1964 and 1971

Birthweight (g)	n	Percent with asthma	Odds ratio*	95% CI
<2000	223	5.8%	1.4	0.8–2.6
2000–2499	781	5.3%	1.5	1.1–2.1
2500–2999	3311	4.1%	1.1	0.9–1.4
3000–3499	8369	3.6%	1.0[†]	—
3500–3999	5160	3.4%	1.0	0.8–1.2
4000–4499	1584	3.5%	1.1	0.8–1.5
4500+	244	3.9%	1.3	0.7–2.7

*adjusted for birth order, paternal education, maternal age, and ethnicity.
[†]Reference category.
Source: Adapted from Seidman et al (1991).

More recently, Godfrey et al (1994) have found that a raised total serum IgE concentration in adult life (which is associated with an increased asthma risk) was associated with an increased head circumference at birth, independently of gestational age at birth, birthweight, and the mother's pelvic size and parity. They suggested that these associations reflect the long-term effects of sustaining fetal brain growth at the expense of the trunk, particularly the thymus, as a result of fetal undernutrition in late gestation. On the other hand, the association of larger head circumference at birth with subsequent risk of asthma may reflect increased maternal nutrition during the relevant stages of pregnancy and especially fatty acid status, which is a major determinant of brain growth, possibly also leading to programming of the developing immune system to predispose to atopic sensitization (Fergusson et al, in press). This hypothesis is more consistent with the increases in asthma prevalence in recent decades in communities in which birthweights (Chike-Obi et al, 1996), head circumference, birth length, and other markers of maternal nutrition have increased.

Infections and immunization. Another theme of recent research into early life events is that early childhood infection may have a role in either promoting asthma or protecting against sensitization (Shaheen, 1995; Cookson and Moffatt, 1997; Holt and Sly, 1997). Bronchiolitis in infancy, for example, is a risk factor for subsequent asthma (Sigurs et al, 1995), but it is unclear whether airway hyperresponsiveness is the result of bronchiolitis or contributes to it (Bellon, 1992). On the other hand, there is some epidemiological evidence that points to protective effects of early infection with regard to atopy (Shaheen et al, 1996). In addition, several studies in children have now found negative associations of the number of siblings in the household (and particularly with the number of older siblings) with atopy (Von Mutius et al, 1994a), hay fever (Strachan, 1989), and asthma (Shaw et al, 1994; Moyes et al, 1995). The reasons for these associations are unclear, but Strachan (1989) has suggested that small family size could reduce viral disease in infancy and that this could in turn increase the risk of atopic disease at older ages. In particular, viral infections may downregulate production of IgE (Cullinan and Newman Taylor, 1994; Martinez, 1994).

It is straightforward to enquire about the number of siblings, use of childcare, and other crude surrogates for risk of infection during infancy. However, ascertaining more specific information on infections during infancy is difficult in large epidemiological studies, requiring respiratory symptom diary cards in combination with the regular collection of biological samples (e.g., Johnston et al, 1995). These methods are discussed below.

In contrast, the ascertainment of immunization history, from questionnaires, routine medical records, or serological testing, is more straightforward. Shaheen (1995) has recently suggested that immunization may promote allergic sensitization. It appears, therefore, to be at least theoretically possible that immunization may have a contributory role in the induction of allergic disease, whether through reducing the incidence of clinical infectious disease in early childhood, the direct IgE-inducing effects of some of the infectious agents themselves, the potentiating adjuvants added to vaccines, or a combination of these (Kemp et al, 1997).

Early allergen exposure. Other exposures in utero and early in life may also be important, and particular interest has been shown in the hypothesis that early exposure to allergen may increase the risk of developing atopy (Newman Taylor, 1995a) and asthma (Bjorksten et al, 1980; Taylor et al, 1973; Burney, 1992). The most consistent evidence comes from studies in the Northern hemisphere that have found associations between mite allergy and birth in autumn and winter (Morrison Smith and Springett, 1979; Warner and Price, 1978). However, less consistent results have been found for the association between month of birth and allergy to pollens, which have a much more obvious seasonality (Burney, 1992; Gregg, 1983). These exposures are considered elsewhere in this chapter.

Example 6.5

Sporik et al (1990) studied the association between dust levels of *Dermatophagoides pteronyssinus* (Der p 1) in the homes of infants and the prevalence of asthma at age 11 years. The study was based on a cohort of 95 couples with children born in 1977 or 1978 in the Poole General Hospital in Dorset (England). Of the 67 children subsequently seen at age 11, 59 had had their homes visited during infancy. There was a trend toward an increasing degree of sensitization at age 11 with greater exposure at age 1 (Table 6.3); 78% of those in the highest exposure group were atopic at age 11. The authors concluded that exposure in early childhood to house dust mite allergens was an important determinant of the subsequent development of

Table 6.3. Exposure at age 1 to house dust mites and sensitivity at age 11

Exposure to mite allergen (μg/g)	Number of children	Atopy at age 11 (%)
<2	3	0 (0%)
2–10	13	5 (38%)
11–50	34	17 (50%)
>50	9	7 (78%)

Source: Adapted from Sporik et al (1990).

asthma, but noted that the relationship was weak at age 5 and had only become apparent because the children had been followed to age 11 years.

Atopy

"Atopy" has previously been used as a poorly defined term to refer to allergic conditions that tend to cluster in families, including hay fever (allergic rhinitis), asthma, atopic eczema, and other specific and nonspecific allergic states (Burney et al, 1989).

Serum IgE

More recently, atopy has been characterized by the production of circulating IgE in response to common environmental allergens. Although atopy has sometimes been defined as "a genetic disposition" for this IgE response (NHLBI, 1992), most definitions focus on the production of IgE irrespective of the mechanism (genetic and/or environmental) by which it is produced. Nevertheless, the tendency to develop atopy may be at least partially inherited, as discussed in the previous section (Cookson and Hopkin, 1988). Prospective studies have shown that high levels of serum IgE predict the subsequent development of asthma in childhood (Foucard, 1974; Kjellman, 1976; Kjellman and Croner, 1984; Martinez et al, 1995). For example, Croner et al (1982) found that about 70% of newborn infants with elevated cord IgE levels develop definite or probable atopic disease (asthma, rhinoconjunctivitis, dermatitis, allergic urticaria, gastrointestinal allergy) before the age of 18 months compared with 4.9% of other infants. On the other hand, 56% of those who developed atopic disease had not had high cord blood IgE levels.

IgE titers are known to gradually increase with age during early childhood, before declining again during adulthood. For example, in a study of children from 160 unselected families (Gerrard et al, 1974), the geometric mean IgE titers gradually increased to maximum levels by about 12 years of age. IgE levels are also affected by tobacco smoking (Burrows et al, 1982), and men generally have higher levels than women (Barbee et al, 1981). Serum levels of total IgE have been found to be associated with asthma independently of specific IgE levels (Sunyer et al, 1996). However, specific IgE is important with regard to specific exposures, particularly in investigating epidemic outbreaks due to unusual or intermittent exposures (see Example 6.6). In the European Community Respiratory Health Survey (ECRHS), total and specific IgE was measured against *Dermatophagoides pteronyssinus*, grass, cat, Cladosporium, and a local allergen, using the Pharmacia CAP system (Burney et al, 1994).

Table 6.4. Elevated serum IgE levels against soybean antigens in cases of epidemic asthma and in controls

Soybean antigen type	Cases <0.35	Cases 0.35+	Controls <0.35	Controls 0.35+	Odds ratio	95% CI
Commercial soybean antigen	64	22	4	82	59.6	25.3–140.8
Soybean dust extract 1	73	13	5	81	90.9	38.8–213.1
Soybean dust extract 2	75	11	4	82	139.8	57.2–341.7

Source: Adapted from Sunyer et al (1989).

Example 6.6

Sunyer et al (1989) conducted a case-control study of epidemic asthma in Barcelona. The cases were 86 patients who had had emergency-room admissions for asthma during the epidemic periods, and the controls were 86 patients who had asthma but who had not had emergency room admissions during the epidemic periods. Both groups were tested for serum IgE levels against commercially prepared soybean antigens and two soybean dust extracts collected from the hold of a ship that had been unloaded during two of the epidemic outbreaks. They found very high relative risks of epidemic asthma associated with IgE for each of the three soybean preparations with odds ratios of 60 or more (Table 6.4). By contrast, there was a weaker relationship with total serum IgE: 61.6% of the cases and 38.4% of the controls had levels of 150 IU/mL or above (OR = 2.6); this illustrates the importance of measuring specific IgE in this study. The authors concluded that the findings supported a causal relationship between the release of dust during unloading of soybean at the harbor and the occurrence of asthma outbreaks, suggesting an underlying allergic mechanism.

Skin testing

A positive response to the application of a specific allergen in skin-prick testing reflects the production of specific IgE antibodies to the allergen, and is strongly related to total serum IgE (Halonen et al, 1982; Cline and Burrows, 1989; Oryszczyn et al, 1991). Skin-prick testing therefore provides a convenient test for atopy in epidemiological studies (Barbee et al, 1976; Burrows et al, 1976). It has been used to assess clinical allergic disease since the nineteenth century, and prevalences of asthma have been shown to be closely related to the frequency and severity of skin test reactions to common inhalant allergens (Burrows et al, 1976)

The prevalence of allergen skin test reactivity in general population samples varies widely according to the number of antigens used, the age of the population, the criteria used to define a positive reaction, and the choice and potency of the antigens themselves (Barbee et al, 1987), as well as between different operators. In particular, the development of skin-test reactivity to a particular antigen will depend on previous levels of allergen exposure; for example, reactivity to house dust mite allergen is strongly related to the level of exposure early in life (Sporik and Platts-Mills, 1992). Thus, a general susceptibility to the development of sensitization (either due to genetic factors, or exposures in utero or early in life) may be expressed differently depending on the major local allergen exposures.

A variety of standardized skin testing protocols have been used in epidemiological studies. The ECRHS protocol (Burney et al, 1994) specifies that skin testing be carried out using Phazets (Pharmacia Diagnostics AB, Uppsala, Sweden), which are lancets precoated with standardized lyophilized allergen extracts. A standard list of allergens was used, including *Dermatophagoides pteronyssinus*, cat, *Alternaria alternata, Cladosporium herbarum*, timothy grass, birch, *Parietaria judaica*, olive, and ragweed, with a positive control (histamine) Phazet and a negative control (uncoated) Phazet. Each area was also permitted to add up to two additional allergens of local importance.

The ISAAC skin testing protocol (Strachan, 1995) uses the ALK lancet, which has good reproducibility, precision, safety, and simplicity of application (Nelson et al, 1993). The core allergens to be tested on the left forearm are histamine (positive control), *Dermatophagoides pteronyssinus*, cat, mixed grasses, diluent (negative control), *Dermatophagoides farinae, Alternaria tenuis*, and mixed trees. Each center is also permitted to add up to eight allergens of their choice for testing on the right forearm. Skin-prick tests are to be performed in the morning hours (because of the circadian rhythm in the size of skin-prick reactions; Dreborg, 1989). A detailed protocol is specified for the sequence of allergen extracts, the placing of one drop of each skin-prick solution, and the use of a separate ALK lancet to prick vertically through each drop (Strachan, 1995). Reactions are measured 15 minutes after the pricks, with the contours of each wheal being outlined with a fine filtertip pen, then transfered to a record sheet by means of a translucent tape. The size of each wheal is calculated as the mean of the longest diameter and the diameter perpendicular to it (Strachan, 1995).

Example 6.7

Schwartz and Weiss (1995) studied the relationship between skin test reactivity and level of FEV_1 in a stratified random sample of 127 U.S. children aged 6 to 12 years with asthma or frequent wheezing. Allergen skin tests were performed for alternaria, bermuda grass, cat, dog, house dust mite, mixed long and short ragweed, oak, and rye grass allergens on an alcohol-prepped arm by applying drops of allergen to the arm and then pricking the skin under the drops by lifting the skin lightly with a 25-gauge BD needle. After 20 minutes the length and width of the flare were measured and summed. The reaction was considered to be positive if the difference in the (summed) flare for an individual allergen was 21mm or more greater than for the saline control. House dust mite allergen skin reactivity was associated with a 17% decrement in FEV_1 (95% CI −9% to −25%). In general, indoor allergens (−13%, 95% CI −6% to −20%) were associated with greater effects than outdoor allergens (−5%, 95% CI −2% to −13%).

Relationship of atopy to asthma

Although asthma and atopy are strongly associated (e.g., Zimmerman et al, 1988), they also occur independently of each other (Pearlman, 1984), and Sherman et al (1990) found that parental asthma was a stronger predictor than parental atopy for current asthma. About 80% of asthma in children and young adults is associated with evidence of atopic sensitization, but about 20% is not. Furthermore, a substantial proportion of non-asthmatics are also "atopic"; thus the proportion of asthma that is due to atopic sensitization would appear to be well below 80%. The association is also likely to vary between populations. Yemaneberhan et al (1997) found atopy to be strongly associated with asthma in urban areas, but negatively associated with asthma in rural areas of Ethiopia. On the other hand, it has been argued that some type of IgE-mediated process is involved in almost all asthma cases, even when skin-test reactivity to common allergens is not found (Burrows et al, 1989). Atopy is also strongly associated with BHR, even in children who have been asymptomatic throughout their lives (Sears et al, 1991), but they can occur independently of each other, and it has been suggested that they are independently inherited characteristics (Sibbald et al, 1980).

The degree of atopy, BHR, and allergen exposure all may form part of a variable equation that determines whether asthma occurs and how severe it is (Pearlman, 1984). For example, Clough et al (1991) found that although atopy and wheeze were both associated with greater peak expiratory flow rate (PEFR) variability in children, atopy was associated with more chronic symptoms, whereas wheeze was associated with more severe symptoms. Thus, in asthma epidemiology studies, atopy is not a surrogate measure for asthma. It is both an associated condition (which is of interest in itself), and a risk factor for developing asthma (which is why we are considering it in this chapter rather than in Chapters 4 and 5). In the latter context, atopy can often also be considered as an intermediate step in some causal pathways leading from allergen exposure to asthma—that is, it may be an intermediate factor (see Chapter 3) and a modifier of the effects of other exposures. For example, it might be inappropriate to control for atopy in a study of dust mite allergen exposure in infancy and asthma at age 5 years because the development of atopic sensitization might be considered to be an intermediate stage of the causal process leading from dust mite allergen exposure to asthma symptoms. However, atopy would also modify the effect of dust mite allergen exposure: atopic persons would be more likely to develop asthma symptoms than nonatopic persons at the same level of dust mite exposure.

Indoor Environment

Tobacco smoke

Children exposed to environmental tobacco smoke are at increased risk of asthma (e.g., Weiss et al, 1980; EPA, 1983; DHHS, 1986; NRC, 1986; Cunningham et al, 1996b; Samet and Lange, 1996), particularly when the mother is a smoker (Burr et al, 1989). The evidence is strongest for increases in severity in children who already have asthma (NRC, 1986), whereas the evidence for the initial occurrence of asthma (incidence) is less conclusive (Chen et al, 1996). Nevertheless, tobacco exposure, particularly in utero and in infancy, may enhance sensitization. This may occur through increasing allergen access to mucosal T cells through increased mucosal permeability (Venables et al, 1985), by components of tobacco smoke acting as allergens themselves (Lehrer et al, 1984), or by increased exposure to oxygen radicals that promote inflammation (Seaton et al, 1994).

Measuring tobacco smoke exposure

These findings are largely based on parental reporting or self-reporting of smoking habits (e.g., Chilmonczyk et al, 1993; Infante-Rivard, 1993), and standard questions are available for self-administered questionnaires and interviews with direct respondents and proxy respondents (Armstrong et al, 1992). However, in recent years there has been a trend for increasing use of biomarkers of tobacco smoke exposure in epidemiological studies (Schulte, 1993). In particular, the level of cotinine, the major metabolite of nicotine, can be measured in various biologic fluids (Corbo et al, 1996) and nicotine can be measured in hair samples. However, even the best currently available measures of exposure to tobacco smoke, such as plasma or urinary cotinine, appear to have similar validity to questionnaires for the measurement of current exposures (Chilmonczyk et al, 1993; Hulka, 1990; Thompson et al, 1990; Vineis, 1992), and their very short half-life makes them inferior to questionnaires in the estimation of historical exposures. Thus, except in unusual circumstances (e.g., in studies in which there may be particularly strong tendencies to underreporting of smoking by household members) measuring plasma or urinary cotinine adds little, if anything, to the information obtained from questionnaires and may impact on response rates and study costs (Pearce et al, 1995). Therefore, questionnaires continue to be the standard approach for gathering information on current levels of exposure to tobacco smoke, and remain the only option for studies of historical exposures, as there is no reliable biological marker of long-term exposure (Ashmore, 1995). However, urinary and plasma cotinine have value in the validation of smoking questionnaires (e.g., Forastiere et al, 1993), which can then be used to estimate historical exposures.

Example 6.8

Thompson et al (1990) studied 49 smokers and 184 reported nonsmokers attending a health screening center. The median urinary cotinine concentration was 1623 ng/mL in the smokers and 6 ng/mL in the nonsmokers. In smokers the cotinine levels increased with reported average cigarette consumption; in nonsmokers it increased with the reported total 7-day duration of exposure to other people's tobacco smoke. Cotinine levels were about three times higher in nonsmokers living with a partner or spouse who was a smoker than in those living with a nonsmoker. The authors concluded that the study confirmed the relation of urinary cotinine with reported tobacco smoke exposure and further validated the use of information on the smoking habits of the spouse or partner as a measure of tobacco smoke exposure in epidemiological studies of nonsmokers.

Other indoor air pollution

Little is currently known about the contribution of indoor air pollutants (other than environmental tobacco smoke) to the development of asthma. The range of potential pollutants is large, the determinants of ambient levels involve a complex interaction of lifestyle and building factors, and precise measurement of airborne or respirable concentrations is difficult. In addition, indoor air pollution may arise from both indoor and outdoor sources (Brauer et al, 1989).

Studies of indoor air pollution therefore involve many of the same exposures that are involved in studies of outdoor air pollution (see below), but routine environmental monitoring data is not available, and it is therefore necessary to collect exposure information for each specific study participant. Investigators have used a variety of exposure measurement techniques, including a variety of questions on use of gas, coal and wood for heating and cooking, as well as airborne dust sampling (e.g., Koo and Ho, 1994) and personal exposure monitors (e.g., Example 6.9). Nitrogen dioxide from burning fossil fuels has received by far the most attention (e.g., Florey et al, 1979; Dodge, 1982; Dijkstra et al, 1990; Samet and Utell, 1990; Neas et al, 1991); sulfur dioxide from burning sulfur-containing coal or gas (see *Air pollution,* below), mosquito coil smoke (Koo and Ho, 1994), and formaldehyde from wood preparation (Marbury and Kriegler, 1991) have also been considered. Particulates from open or closed wood and coal burning fires have received less attention in developed countries (Osbourne and Honicky, 1986; Dockery, 1987) but have been studied in developing countries, where very high indoor levels have been encountered (Anderson, 1974, 1979).

Example 6.9

Infante-Rivard (1993) conducted a case-control study of childhood asthma and indoor environmental risk factors in Montreal, Quebec (see also example 2.6). The cases comprised 457 children aged 3 to 4 years with a first-time diagnosis of asthma, recruited at an emergency room; controls were children with no previous diagnosis of asthma who were of the same age and the same census tract (in the urban area) or postal code (in the rural area) as the case at time of diagnosis. There was an association of asthma with maternal smoking but not with paternal smoking (Table 6.5). There was also an association with the presence of other smokers in the home. A subsample of 20% of study parents were asked to have their children wear a

Table 6.5. Case-control study of asthma prevalence and exposure to indoor airborne chemicals

Factor	Cases	Controls	Odds ratio*	95% CI
Number of cigarettes smoked per day by mother				
0	273	289	1.0[†]	—
1–20	138	135	1.1	0.8–1.5
20+	45	32	1.6	1.0–2.7
Number of cigarettes smoked per day by father				
0	297	275	1.0[†]	—
1–20	150	174	0.8	0.6–1.1
20+	10	8	1.2	0.5–3.1
Other smokers in the home				
No	392	424	1.0[†]	—
Yes	65	33	2.2	1.4–3.6
NO_2 (ppb)				
0–0.5	15	31	1.0[†]	—
0.5–10.0	11	34	0.8	0.3–1.9
10.1–15.0	8	8	2.5	0.8–8.4
15.1+	27	6	10.5	3.5–31.9

*Adjusted for various matching factors and other confounders.
[†]Reference category.
Source: Adapted from Infante-Rivard (1993).

passive nitrogen dioxide monitoring badge for 24 hours. There was a strong association of asthma prevalence with NO_2 levels, with an odds ratio of 10.5 for the highest level of NO_2 exposure (Table 6.5). The authors concluded that these findings show that indoor environmental factors, including NO_2 from gas stoves, gas heaters, and tobacco smoke, contribute to the incidence of asthma.

Indoor allergens

Most asthmatics (80%) are sensitized to at least one common allergen (Peat, 1996), and indoor allergens probably represent the most important source of stimulation of the chronic airway inflammatory process (Bjorksten, 1994). The relevant allergens may vary across countries and demographic groups; in most Western countries house dust mites, cats, other pets, cockroaches and molds are major sources of sensitization (Crane, 1995).

House dust mites   Since Voorhorst and Spieksma (1967) identified the house dust mite as a major source of allergen for asthma and allergic rhinitis in the 1960s, both the epidemiology and immunology of these allergens has received increasing interest (Platts-Mills et al, 1992). The two most important species are *Dermatophagoides pteronyssinus* and *Dermatophagoides farinae* of the family Pyroglyphidae. Twelve other members of this family have been found in domestic dust, but often in discrete geographical regions. Six species have been found exclusively in association with human habitation, whereas another 26 species live exclusively on birds or in their nests. Two other families, known as storage mites (Acaridae and Clyophagidae), have also been implicated in asthma, particularly in people handling grains and cheese (Baker, 1994).

Mites can be counted in dust samples, and by using a standard technique comparisons of the degree of infestation can be made between different environments. However, this is a slow, labor-intensive process and requires skill in recognition, although it does allow the different species to be identified and permits recognition of the life cycle stages of the mite. Live migratory mites can also be directly examined using adhesive tape; they can then be counted, using the "mobility" test developed by Bischoff et al (1992). This involves adhesive tape placed on furniture or bedding overnight; the tape can then be covered with plastic wrap for viewing on a stero microscope at 20 to 30 times normal size.

The development of ELISA techniques using monoclonal antibodies to mite allergens has led to accurate quantification of mite allergens (Chapman et al, 1983) and has opened the way for studies of environmental levels. Major and minor allergens have been identified from complex allergenic extracts of *Dermatophagoides pteronyssinus* and *Dermatophagoides farinae*. Two major allergens, Derf 1 from *D farinae* (Dandeu et al, 1982) and

Der p 1 from *D pteronyssinus* have been purified and extensively studied. Other mite allergens (groups 2, 3, and 4) have been shown to elicit IgE responses but for allergen quantification purposes have been much less widely studied. The inhalant allergen Der p 1 is a cysteine protease excreted in the feces of *D pteronyssinus*. IgE antibodies directed against this major allergen Der p 1 dominate the response of most mite-allergic patients (Chapman and Platts-Mills, 1980), making it an ideal molecule for study. A two-site monoclonal antibody (Mab) ELISA has been developed to measure group 1 allergens from *Dermatophagoides* spp: Der p 1 from *D pteronyssinus* and Der f 1 from *D farinae* (Luczynska et al, 1989).

Airborne dust mite allergen can most easily be measured using a settle technique. Small open petri dishes are left side by side, one or two meters above floor level with no overhanging shelves and where the dishes are unlikely to be disturbed by children or pets. This technique has the advantage of measuring airborne allergen and therefore most closely reflecting the allergen available for inhalation (Crane, 1995). However, most investigators have continued to use comparisons based on reservoir sampling of furniture, carpets, and bedding, as airborne methods usually only detect allergen following dust disturbance. Results can be expressed as the concentration of allergen per gram of fine dust ($\mu g/g$) as recommended by the Second International Workshop on Mite Allergens and Asthma (Platts-Mills et al, 1992), or as the amount of allergen per square meter of sampling area ($\mu g/m^2$). Exposure levels have been estimated for allergen reservoirs in the domestic environment from prevalence studies, and these have been associated with current asthma symptoms in dust mite–sensitized children (Peat et al, 1996). Exposure to >2 μg Der p 1/g of fine dust and exposure to >10 $\mu g/g$ fine dust have been associated with sensitization and exacerbations of asthma, respectively (Sporik and Platts-Mills, 1992).

Reservoir sampling requires a standardized procedure as to the area and time of dust collection. The International Study of Asthma and Allergies in Childhood (ISAAC) (Strachan, 1995) specifies that dust should be sampled from two sites within homes (e.g., the mattress or sleeping place and either the carpets, upholstery, or floor in the living room). Soft surfaces are vacuumed for two minutes per square meter, covering an area of 2 to 4 square meters, and hard surfaces are cleaned for one minute per square meter, covering an area of at least 4 square meters. Sampling is performed at a defined time, preferably three days after the last cleaning, and there is a detailed protocol for the freezing of samples for 2 days (to kill the mites), sieving of dust, and analysis of samples using radioimmunoassay (RIA) or ELISA. Results are expressed both as the concentration of allergen per gram of fine dust ($\mu g/g$) and as the amount of allergen per square meter of sampling area ($\mu g/m^2$) (Strachan, 1995).

Table 6.6. Exposure to house dust mites in 25 mite-sensitive asthmatics and 75 controls

Mite concentration (mites/0.10 g dust)	Cases	Controls	Odds ratio	95% CI
MATTRESS DUST				
0–10	7	54	1.0	—
11–100	7	11	4.9	1.5–15.9
101+	11	10	8.5	2.9–25.0
BEDROOM FLOOR DUST				
0–10	6	52	1.0	—
11–100	5	13	3.3	0.9–12.2
101+	14	10	12.1	4.2–35.3
LIVINGROOM FLOOR DUST				
0–10	14	62	1.0	—
11–100	7	11	2.8	0.9–8.4
101+	4	2	8.9	1.9–42.5

Source: Adapted from Korsgaard (1983).

Example 6.10

Korsgaard (1983) conducted a case-control study in Aarhus (Denmark) of 25 patients with newly diagnosed house dust mite asthma and 75 randomly selected controls. All 100 homes were investigated by the same researcher, and dust was collected from mattress surfaces and floors in bedrooms and living rooms by a portable vacuum cleaner. Dust sampling was standardized by time and area. Table 6.6 shows the odds ratio associated with various levels of house dust mite concentration (mites per 0.10 g dust) in mattress dust, bedroom floor dust, and living room floor dust. In each instance there was a strong dose-response relationship, with an approximately 10-fold risk of asthma prevalence associated with the highest level of dust mite concentration. The authors noted that the cases lived in older and more humid houses than the controls and concluded that this suggested possibilities for the introduction of hygienic standards for the indoor environment as a means of primary prevention of house dust mite allergy.

A wide variety of mite avoidance strategies have been considered and some have been evaluated (Harving et al, 1991; Siebers et al, 1996). For example, strict mite avoidance in the hospital (Platts-Mills et al, 1982), or at an altitude (Peroni et al, 1994) where low relative humidity prevents mite proliferation, have both been associated with improvement in asthma symptoms and a decrease in BHR. In the domestic environment, chemical control involving acaricides has produced equivocal results, possibly because of the problems of delivering acaricide in sufficient concentration (e.g., to the base of carpets) (Platts-Mills et al, 1992). Barrier protection has been the most promising approach to date (Siebers et al, 1996), with most studies having shown clinical benefits, although only three had control groups (Murray and Ferguson, 1983); this method usually involves covering mattresses with porous plastic zippered covers. More recently, some investigators have advocated alterations in humidity, including the use of mechanical ventilation systems (see Example 6.11), although this approach may not work in countries with high levels of humidity year-round (Crane, 1995). Carpets constitute the major reservoir of house dust mites (Siebers et al, 1996; Wickens et al, 1997), and removal of carpets, particularly from bedrooms, is another practical strategy for reducing exposures. Other possible approaches include freezing, steam cleaning, intensive dry vacuum cleaning, wet vacuum cleaning, and sun drying (Crane, 1995).

Example 6.11

Dorward et al (1988) conducted a randomized trial of house dust mite avoidance measures; these included an initial application of liquid nitrogen to mattresses and bedroom carpets, followed by weekly vacuuming of the bed, weekly washing of blankets, sheets and duvets, daily folding back of blankets and upper sheets or duvets, weekly damp dusting of hard surfaces, and removal of plants, soft toys, cushions and upholstered furniture from the bedroom. The 21 adult patients were randomly allocated to the intervention group, or to a control group, and 9 patients in each group completed the study. Histamine responsiveness, symptom scores, peak expiratory flow rates (PEFR) and house dust mite numbers were determined during the 2-week pretrial and 8-week trial periods. Mean mattress dust mite levels fell only slightly (from 7.0 to 4.2 mites per 0.25 m^2/min) in the control group but fell from 6.6 to 0.3 mites per 0.25 m^2/min in the avoidance group. The avoidance group showed a significant improvement in the number of hours each day spent wheezing (from 8.6 to 4.5 hours), and in PEFR in the morning (from 364 to 388 L/min) and the evening (368 to 392 L/min).

Other indoor allergens. Several common family pets such as cats, dogs, and rodents are known to produce allergens that may cause or aggravate asthma (Brunekreef et al, 1992), and clinical studies of asthmatics have found sensitization to allergens produced by these pets (e.g., Sears et al, 1989; Vanto and Koivikko, 1983). Cats may be particularly important because of their widespread occurrence and the potency of their allergens (Brunekreef et al, 1992). A number of cat allergens have been isolated, the most important being Fel d 1, the allergen protein for Felis domesticus, found predominantly in saliva and lacrimal secretions (Milligen et al, 1990). Fel d 1 is distributed by preening, in which the fur is coated in saliva and ejected into the air in the form of small (less than 2.5 μm) diameter sticky particles (Platts-Mills et al, 1986). This cat allergen is much more widely distributed in the environment than house dust mite allergen, being found in households with no history of cat ownership (Warner et al, 1991) and even in the space shuttle (Crane, 1995).

Dog allergens have been less intensively studied to date, but a monoclonal antibody to the main allergen Can f 1 has recently been developed. Can f 1 comes from hair, saliva, and dander (Blands et al, 1977). Dog allergens appear less likely to cause sensitivity, although it is unclear whether this is because of lower allergenic potential or a less ubiquitous distribution (Crane, 1995).

It is relatively straightforward to ask about pet ownership in questionnaires, but a major source of bias is the tendency for pets to be removed from the home if they are suspected of causing asthma symptoms in family members. For example, a Swedish study (Kjellman and Peterson, 1983) found that asthmatic children had a high prevalence of animal dander allergy, but asthmatic children with dander allergy had pets in the home significantly less often than asthmatic children without dander allergy or non-asthmatic children. Donnelly et al (1987) found that parents of asthmatic children were willing to give up pets but were not willing to give up tobacco smoking. This may explain why some studies (e.g., Clifford et al, 1989) have found no association, or even a negative association, between current pet ownership and current asthma symptoms. It is therefore essential to enquire about past as well as current pet ownership. For example, Brunekreef et al (1992) found a negative association of current pet ownership with current respiratory symptoms, but a positive association of past pet ownership with current respiratory symptoms.

Cockroach allergen may also be an important risk factor for asthma since cockroaches are ubiquitous in inner-city areas in many countries and are highly allergenic. Monoclonal-antibody-based assays can be used to measure allergen protein for Blattella germanica (Bla g 1 and Bla g 2) in house dust or in the air (Platts-Mills and Carter, 1997). Methods of reducing exposure to cockroach allergens are not well established, but air filtration has little role because the particles fall rapidly, and avoidance measures should focus on eliminating cockroaches (Platts-Mills and Carter, 1997).

Example 6.12

Rosenstreich et al (1997) studied 476 inner city children with asthma, aged 4 to 9 years, in 8 inner-city areas of the United States. Sensitization to cockroach, house dust mite, and cat allergens was measured by skin testing and the corresponding allergens were measured using monoclonal antibody-based enzyme-linked immuno-absorbent assays. Table 6.7 shows the findings for cockroach allergen. Children who were sensitized to cockroach allergen and exposed to high levels had 0.37 hospitalizations per year compared with 0.11 for other children (p=0.001); they had 2.56 unscheduled medical visits for asthma per year compared with 1.43 for other children (p<0.001). The authors concluded that the combination of cockroach allergy

Table 6.7. Relations between skin test sensitivity, bedroom-dust cockroach allergen levels, and morbidity due to asthma in a study of 476 inner city children

Asthma morbidity	Negative skin test		Positive skin test	
	Low allergen level (Group 1) (n=160)	High allergen level (Group 2) (n=141)	Low allergen level (Group 3) (n=77)	High allergen level (Group 4) (n=98)
Hospitalizations in past year	0.14	0.08	0.10	0.37
Unscheduled medical visits in past year	1.40	1.44	1.50	2.56
Days of wheezing in past two weeks	3.21	3.13	3.86	4.04
Nights when child lost sleep in past two weeks	1.62	1.59	1.77	1.92
Days when child's activity was reduced in past two weeks	1.89	1.90	2.04	2.13
Schooldays missed in past three months (%)	6.12	6.14	5.60	7.65
Days when care giver changed plans in past year	9.11	11.07	7.22	15.52
Nights when care giver lost sleep in past two weeks	2.08	1.98	2.11	2.33
Peak expiratory flow rate (% of predicted)	86.6	86.7	84.5	85.9

Source: Adapted from Rosenstreich et al (1997).

and exposure to high levels of this allergen may explain the high frequency of asthma-related health problems in inner city children.

Dampness and humidity

Dampness and humidity not only are features of old houses but may also occur in modern houses with tight insulation (Andrae et al, 1988) and in modern office buildings (Hoffman et al, 1993). Dampness can encourage the growth of fungal molds and house dust mites (Verhoeff et al, 1995; Pirhonen et al, 1996), as well as promoting the survival of viruses in droplet spray, and cold air can itself trigger asthma attacks (Strachan and Sanders, 1989). Several epidemiological studies have found associations between damp housing and asthma symptoms (e.g., Burr et al, 1981; Dales et al, 1991; Strachan and Sanders, 1989).

Measuring dampness and humidity

Most of these studies have relied on questionnaires about conditions in the home, particularly with regard to heating and ventilation, condensation, damp patches, and visible mold growth. For example, Dales et al (1991) investigated the association between home dampness and mold and health, in a prevalence survey of 14,799 parents (at least 21 years old) of school-aged children, and used the question "within the past year . . . have you ever had wet or damp spots on surfaces inside your present house other than in the basement (for example, on walls, wallpaper, ceilings or carpets)?" However, Dales et al (1997) found major inaccuracies and systematic reporting bias in responses to questionnaires on home dampness and mold growth. Questionnaires can be supplemented by home visits (e.g., Andrae et al, 1988; Verhoeff et al, 1995). Direct measurements of humidity levels in the home can be performed using a variety of methods, including wood blocks (Strachan and Sanders, 1989), wax-coated tongue depressors, and thermohygrometers (Wickens et al, 1997). The latter technique provides an accurate humidity measurement at a particular time, whereas wood-based methods can provide a weighted average of relative humidity over a specified time (e.g., 2 weeks) by weighing the wood and using a known equilibrium moisture content relation for the wood.

Example 6.13

Strachan and Sanders (1989) studied 778 children aged 7 years; their families received a block of hardwood with instructions to place the block in the child's bedroom for 7 days and to return it in a sealed plastic bag. The moisture content of each block was determined within 48 hours of collection and compared with that obtained by leaving the blocks in 55% humidity for 10 days. All homes in the top quintile of humidity, and a sample of the remainder, were then subjected to more detailed measurements of temperature and humidity with 7-day recordings using thermohygrographs. The investigators found no association of humidity levels with respiratory symptoms. They concluded that these findings were inconsistent with the widely held belief that indoor temperature and humidity are important determinants of respiratory health, but noted that airborne humidity may be a poor measure of the biologically relevant exposure in the microenvironments suitable for mold growth and mite survival.

Outdoor Environment

Air pollution

The role of outdoor air pollutants in asthma and other conditions has been extensively studied and debated (Barnes, 1994; Bascom et al, 1996). "Conventional" air pollution includes SO_2 and airborne particulates with a size of 10 μm or less that can be inhaled into the lung (Dockery and Pope, 1997).

More recently, attention has focused on NO_2 (see also other indoor air pollution) as the concentration of this chemical has risen in recent decades because of increasing motor vehicle use (Sunyer, 1997). An association between traffic density on residential streets and asthma symptoms has been found in studies in Germany (Duhme et al, 1996), Sweden (Pershagen et al, 1995), and the Netherlands (Oosterlee et al, 1995), but not in the United Kingdom (Livingstone et al, 1996). Ground level ozone is formed from nitrogen oxides, hydrocarbons, and sunlight. Ozone has been shown to increase the sensitivity to allergen challenge in asthmatics (Molfino et al, 1991), and exacerbations of asthma have been reported in association with fluctuations in outdoor ozone levels (Borja-Aburto and Loomis, 1997). Overall, the weight of evidence does not support a major role for outdoor air pollution as a determinant of asthma prevalence or morbidity, although the possibility of interactions between pollutants and the possibility of a very different alveloar response to ultra-fine particles (Seaton et al, 1995) suggests that further studies are required.

Types of air pollution studies. Ayres (1995) discusses six main types of epidemiological studies that have been used to examine the relationship between air pollution and asthma.

Panel studies are time series studies that follow a group of patients over a short period of time and measure day-to-day variations in air pollution levels and asthma symptoms. These are particularly relevant for air pollution because, unlike many other risk factors for asthma, air pollution levels can vary markedly from day to day; and, provided that an exposure on a particular day does not have very extended effects (e.g., more than a few days), it is possible to study the day-to-day variation in asthma symptoms and to relate it to the day-to-day variation in air pollution levels.

Example 6.14

Pope et al (1991) studied changes in respiratory health associated with daily changes in fine particulate pollution (PM_{10}) in Utah Valley, Utah. Participants included two samples: (1) 34 relatively healthy school students aged 9 to 11 years who had reported asthma symptoms and/or diagnosed asthma in a school-based prevalence survey and (2) 21 patients aged 8 to 72 years who were receiving medical treatment for asthma. Participants completed daily symptom diaries and performed peak expiratory flow rate (PEFR) measurements three times just before bedtime, with the highest reading being recorded. PM_{10} monitoring was conducted by the Utah State Department of Health, with monitoring stations at three sites in the valley. PM_{10} levels from the most centrally located site were used, except for 8 days during which data were not available from that site and data from a second site was

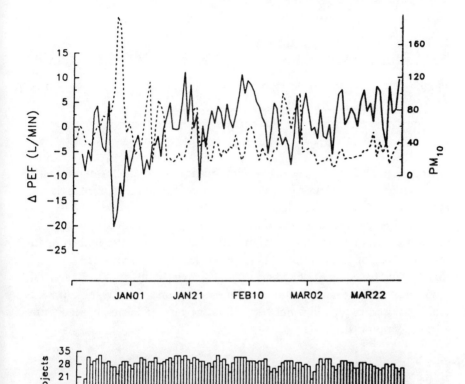

Figure 6.1. Daily PM_{10} levels (broken line), mean peak expiratory flow deviations (solid line), and daily number of participants in a school-based sample, December 13, 1989, through March 31, 1990. (Source: Pope et al, 1991.)

used. Figure 6.1 shows the daily PM_{10} levels, mean peak expiratory flow deviations, and daily number of participants in the school-based sample. In this sample, elevated PM_{10} levels of 150 $\mu g/m^3$ over 3 consecutive days were associated with a decrease in mean PEFR of 15.5 L/min (i.e., about 6%).

Opportunistic studies include summer camp studies. These have involved studying children in summer camps spending more time than usual out-of-doors in recreational activities in a non-urban location in which they may be exposed to higher or lower than usual levels of outdoor air pollutants (e.g., particulates).

Event studies examine a particular unusual pollution episode. Studies of major air pollution episodes have reported increased symptoms and an increase in hospital admissions for asthma (Wardlaw, 1993), and the well-

Table 6.8. Asthma emergency visits by quartile of PM_{10}

Range ($\mu g/m^3$)	PM_{10} Concentration ($\mu g/m^3$)	Emergency visits per day	95% CI
6–17	13.0	6.24	5.34–7.80
17–24	20.3	6.59	5.71–7.46
24–36	29.6	7.61	6.71–8.50
36–103	55.3	8.00	—

Source: Adapted from Schwartz et al (1993).

known United Kingdom smogs (from burning fossil fuels) of the early 1950s were associated with increased respiratory mortality, but these deaths rarely involved asthmatics (Scott, 1953).

Routinely collected data such as mortality and hospital admission data can be used to examine changes in mortality or admission rates and to relate them to levels of air pollution. These are analogous to panel studies, except that they are based on a defined geographical area (or the catchment area for a hospital) rather than a group of diagnosed asthmatics, and the outcome under study is asthma hospital admission or death, rather than changes in asthma symptoms.

Example 6.15

Schwartz et al (1993) studied emergency room visits for asthma from eight hospitals in the Seattle metropolitan area during the Septemeber 1988 to September 1990. Air quality data were obtained from the Washington State Department of Ecology and the Puget Sound Air Pollution Control Agency. Sulfur dioxide (SO_2) values were obtainable only from an industrial site. Daily light-scattering (b_{sp}) and PM_{10} values were available from a residential site in a wood-burning neighborhood. Table 6.8 shows that there was a strong association of the mean daily number of asthma hospital emergency visits by quartile of PM_{10}. This association was confirmed in Poisson regression analyses, controlling for weather, season, time trends, age, hospital, and day of the week; the strongest association was obtained when using the mean of the previous 4 days PM_{10}. The authors noted that an association was observed even though the mean PM_{10} levels were quite low, and they commented that increased attention should be given to the control of particulate matter air pollution.

Cross-sectional studies (e.g., urban/rural studies) compare the prevalence of symptoms in polluted and less-polluted areas (e.g. Von Mutius et al, 1992, 1994b). Such studies suffer from the usual problems of geographically based ecologic studies, in that the areas compared may differ markedly with regard to other risk factors for asthma, in addition to their differing air pollution levels. Thus, there may be substantial confounding. For example, Devereux et al (1996) report a study of asthma prevalence in rural West

Cumbria and urban Newcastle upon Tyne. They found very similar prevalences of symptoms and BHR in the two areas, despite markedly different
levels of air pollution from vehicle exhausts; however, they commented that
it was possible that an air pollution effect in Newcastle had been balanced
by asthmagenic effects of other asthmagenic agents in West Cumbria.

Finally, *longitudinal studies* of asthma incidence (or repeated prevalence
surveys—see Example 6.16) are particularly useful for examining whether
air pollution causes or limits the disease, whereas the other study designs
often focus on the exacerbation of the disease. Longitudinal studies can also
be used to relate long-term changes in lung function to air pollution levels,
although difficulties may arise because other determinants of pulmonary
function also change over time (Dockery and Brunekreef, 1996).

Example 6.16

Hsieh and Shen (1988) conducted asthma prevalence surveys, using the same methodology, in schoolchildren aged 7 to 15 years in Taipei, Taiwan, in 1974 and 1985.
They found that the prevalence of childhood asthma (defined as at least three
recurrent, paroxysmal attacks of wheezing and dyspnea in the previous 12 months)
increased from 1.3% in 1974 to 5.1% in 1985. Air pollution from SO_2, NO_2 and
particulates decreased during the same period (Fig. 6.2). The authors concluded
that childhood asthma was becoming a major problem in Asian Pacific countries, as
it was already in Western countries, and that the increase in asthma prevalence could
not be explained by air pollution.

Measuring air pollution. Levels of pollution have traditionally been measured by the "black smoke method" in which air is drawn through a filter
paper and the density of the stain in measured. However, most urban pollu-

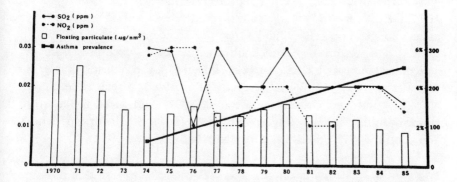

Figure 6.2. Changes in air pollution and prevalence of bronchial asthma in Taipei from
1970 to 1985. (Source: Hsieh and Shen, 1988.)

tion is now from vehicle exhausts and is less black, and pollution levels are now usually measured by the mass of particles that pass through a size-selective orifice with a 50% collection efficiency at $10\mu m$ diameter (PM_{10}) (Seaton et al, 1995). In epidemiological studies, measurements can be made by the direct approach, in which personal monitors are worn or carried by study subjects (Ashmore, 1995). Alternatively, indirect estimates of individual exposure can be obtained by combining environmental pollutant concentration measures with information on the time-activity patterns of individuals (Ashmore, 1995). However, in many epidemiological studies, exposure estimates are based entirely on environmental measures and it is assumed that all individuals living in the relevant area receive the same daily exposure levels. Thus there is considerable potential for non-differential misclassification of exposure, particularly because routine monitoring networks are often located in heavily polluted areas (Maynard, 1995) and may not reflect average population levels of exposure (Coggon, 1995).

Airborne allergens

Airborne allergens include various pollens and spores, their derivatives, and material from other sources including plant sap, anther linings, and leaf leachate (Emberlin, 1995), as well as material of insect origin (Kino et al, 1987). Although some studies have focused on routine climatic changes (e.g., Suzuki et al, 1988) or seasonal patterns (e.g., Reid et al, 1986), most studies of airborne allergens have involved investigating epidemic asthma outbreaks—for example, brief epidemic increases in hospital admissions or emergency room visits for asthma. Studies of such epidemic outbreaks fall into two main groups: effects of thunderstorms and exposures from the agricultural history. Several asthma epidemic outbreaks have been linked to thunderstorms, including studies in Birmingham (Packe and Ayres, 1985), Melbourne (Morrison, 1960; Egan, 1985), and London (Murray et al, 1994; Celenza et al, 1996). The airborne allergens involved are believed to include fungal spores (Packe and Ayres, 1986) and pollen grains (Suphioglu et al, 1992). Asthma epidemic outbreaks linked to exposures from the agricultural industry include outbreaks linked to soybean dust in Barcelona (Antó et al, 1989), Cartagena (Navarro et al, 1993), Naples (D'Amato et al, 1994), and New Orleans (White et al, 1997), and outbreaks linked to castor bean dust in Ohio (Figley and Elrod, 1928), South Africa (Mendes and Cintra, 1954), and Brazil (Ordman, 1955).

Strategies for studying airborne allergens

Antó (1995) outlines five steps that may be followed in investigating such epidemic outbreaks: (1) descriptive studies within well-defined time/space coordinates to estimate the magnitude of the outbreak and to search for a potential time/space pattern, (2) a process of hypothesis generation, (3) complete etiological studies when a firm hypothesis is available, (4) prevention or prediction if a suitable factor has been implicated, followed by intervention studies if an intervention has been implemented, and (5) clinical epidemiological and mechanistic studies on epidemic asthma for specific issues of scientific relevance.

This approach was followed in the investigation of the Barcelona soybean asthma epidemic outbreak (Antó and Sunyer, 1990). After an initial report on six outbreaks (Ussetti et al, 1983), a monitoring system was established and a detailed report was published on the eighth epidemic outbreak (Antó et al, 1986), which showed that the epidemic was unlikely to be due to air pollution or unusual levels of pollen or fungal spores. It was subsequently observed that at least three epidemics had occurred on days on which soybeans were unloaded in the harbor, and this hypothesis was tested in a study of 13 asthma epidemic days (Antó et al, 1989), and a case-control study in which epidemic cases and nonepidemic asthma controls were tested for specific IgE levels to soybean (Sunyer et al, 1989). Finally, further outbreaks were prevented by installing filters on the soybean silos (Antó et al, 1993).

Once a hypothesis has been developed as to the likely cause(s) of the outbreaks (step 2) then the study design options are the same as for studies of outdoor air pollution (see above). The methodological issues involved are also similar, and individual exposures can, once again, be estimated by direct methods (personal monitoring), or indirect methods (environmental monitoring combined with information on individual activities), provided that further epidemic outbreaks can be anticipated and the relevant exposures measured. However, one important advantage in studies of airborne allergens is the potential to test for sensitization in patients involved in epidemic outbreaks (see Example 6.6 and Example 6.17).

Example 6.17

O'Hollaren et al (1991) conducted skin tests for reactivity to *Alternaria alternata* in 11 patients with episodes of respiratory arrest and 99 asthmatic controls without a history of respiratory arrest; cases and controls were all identified through Mayo Clinic records, all patients came from the American Midwest, and all episodes of respiratory arrest occurred in summer or early fall. Of the 11 patients with respiratory arrest, 10 had positive skin-puncture tests for sensitivity to alternaria, compared to 31 of the 99 controls; this yielded an age-adjusted odds ratio of 189.5 (95% CI 6.5–5535.8). The authors concluded that exposure to *alternaria alternata* is a risk factor for respiratory arrest in children and young adults with asthma.

Occupational Exposures

Occupational causes of asthma

Occupational asthma is "asthma that is caused, in whole or part, by agents encountered at work" (Burge, 1995). It was documented as long ago as 1713 by Ramazzini, who described grain dust asthma (Chan-Yeung and Lam, 1986). Nowadays, there are more than 200 known occupational causes of asthma, and asthma is the most common occupational respiratory disease in developed countries (Chan-Yeung, 1995). For example, asthma was the most common disease category and accounted for 28% of cases reported to the United Kingdom Surveillance of Work-related and Occupational Respiratory Diseases (SWORD) project (Meredith et al, 1991). Estimates of the proportion of adult asthma that is thought to be occupational in origin range from 2% to 15% in the United States, 15% in Japan (Chan-Yeung and Malo, 1994), 5% in Spain (Kogevinas et al, 1996), 2% to 3% in New Zealand (Fishwick et al, 1997), and 2% to 6% in the United Kingdom (Meredith and Nordman, 1996).

Occupational asthma has important similarities with other forms of asthma in which a given population is exposed to a specific allergen from a particular point in time (e.g., soybean epidemic asthma; Antó et al, 1996). Thus occupational asthma, in which the exposure is often relatively well defined in place and time, and in which removal of the exposure is often possible, may serve as a useful model for some forms of asthma in the general population. In particular, several studies have shown the importance of avoidance of exposure, and other standard occupational hygiene techniques, in occupational asthma (rather than improving asthma management while permitting exposure to continue), and that occupational asthma can lead to permanent asthma even after removal from exposure (e.g., Burge, 1982).

Occupational asthma with a "latency period" involves a variable time, depending on the agent involved (Malo et al, 1992), in which sensitization takes place, whereas occupational asthma without a latency period may be termed irritant-induced asthma (Malo and Cartier, 1996). Typically, the onset of occupational asthma may occur 1 to 3 years after initial exposure, although some exposures may induce occupational asthma in some workers in less than one month (Antó et al, 1996). One study has reported that intermittent exposure to high levels involves a greater risk than steady exposure to lower levels (Luo et al, 1988). In many instances the mechanisms involved in occupational asthma are unknown. Some workplace agents can directly induce asthma by effects similar to those of pharmacologic agonists (Chan-Yeung and Lam, 1986), but most (perhaps more than 80%) occupational exposures probably cause asthma through sensitization and IgE-mediated mechanisms, and almost all patients with occupational asthma have evidence of BHR (Burney et al, 1989). Tobacco smokers may be particularly sensitive to some occupational allergens (Zetterstrom et al, 1981). However, the positive predictive value of atopy in occupational asthma is low (e.g., Malo et al, 1990a,b; Slovak and Hill, 1981) and it has been argued screening for atopy in high-risk workplaces is not justified (Chan-Yeung and Malo, 1995).

The diagnosis of occupational asthma normally relies on a combination of sources of information. The presence of work-related respiratory symptoms is usually suggestive of occupational asthma. These are symptoms that are reported to be worse at work and better on rest days and holidays. However, the latter may not be present in established cases of occupational asthma, as 1 to 2 rest days may not be sufficient to ease symptoms. In addition, it is important to consider less common symptoms of occupational asthma, including cough and sputum production. Unfortunately, the most widely used questionnaires (including those of the UK Medical Research Council and the American Thoracic Society) were not originally designed to identify cases of asthma, although validated questionnaires are now available (Newman Taylor, 1995b). The subsequent confirmation of a diagnosis of occupational asthma rests on aspects of a full occupational and medical history, documented changes (or work effect) in lung function and the assessment of nonspecific (e.g., to methacholine or histamine) and specific bronchial challenge. However, the most appropriate initial confirmatory test is serial peak expiratory flow rate (PEFR) measurement (Gannon and Burge, 1997).

Epidemiological studies are usually based on respiratory symptom questionnaires, particularly with regard to work-related chest tightness, wheeze, and shortness of breath. However, only about half of workers considered to have occupational asthma from questionnaire responses will have this diagnosis confirmed by other means (Malo et al, 1991). Thus, in epidemiological studies it may be important to investigate some workers further with serial measures of lung function across the working day and throughout the working week.

The most common method of recording serial measures of lung function is for the worker to record peak expiratory flow (PEF). There are many strategies used to diagnose occupational asthma using this technique (Moscato et al, 1995), but most include measurement (best of three recorded, with a minimum of four daily readings) at work and at least one period away from work. Various patterns of abnormality are found in occupational asthma, ranging from progressive deterioration through a working week to a more prolonged "week to week" deterioration (Moscato et al,

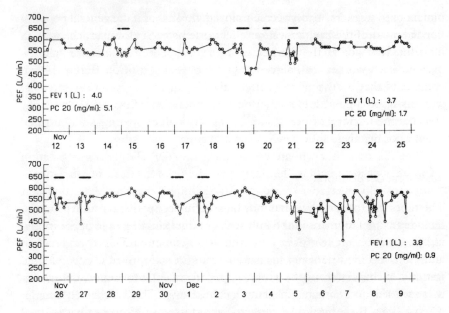

Figure 6.3. Daily variations in individual peak expiratory flow rates (PEFR) with periods at work shown by the dark horizontal lines. Values of FEV$_1$ and PC$_{20}$ assessed in the laboratory are also shown. (Source: Desjardins et al, 1994.)

1995). The key is to establish a work effect on the PEF that can clearly be distinguished from rest periods.

For example, Figure 6.3 shows recordings made of PEFR and FEV$_1$ in a 35 year old male aluminum-plant worker who was a lifelong non-smoker with no history of asthma or atopy at time of hire (Desjardins et al, 1994). The figure shows greater variability of PEFR and lower mean values during periods at work in the potrooms.

Specific bronchial challenge remains the standard for confirming a diagnosis of occupational asthma (Pepys and Hutchcroft, 1975), but this is usually impractical for epidemiological studies, and in clinical practice the diagnosis can usually be made without this investigation. There are also small risks involved with antigen challenge, but it does provide definitive evidence that a specific agent is the cause of a worker's asthma. Skin-prick testing to various occupationally encountered antigens can also be used to identify specific causes of occupational asthma.

Occupational asthma studies rely on the availability of an "available" working population, and have therefore most often involved cross-sectional studies, or a series of cross-sectional studies, in active workers. These may be invalid for comparing symptom prevalence or mean lung function, determining long-term trends in lung function over time, between exposed and nonexposed workers, or between employed workers and the general population, because of the healthy worker effect (see below). However, changes in lung function across the working day can be studied with more validity because each worker then serves as his or her own control. Burge (1995) comments that a drop in peak flow or FEV_1 of more than 15% across a working shift is good evidence of occupational asthma provided that suitable control exposures are made. However, failure to find such a drop should not be taken as evidence against occupational asthma.

Measuring occupational exposures

The types of exposure data that may be used in occupational asthma studies include (1) employment in the industry, (2) duration of employment in the industry, (3) ordinally ranked jobs or tasks, (4) quantified job-specific data, and (5) quantified personal measurements (Checkoway et al, 1989). The first step in characterizing the workplace environment is to identify the agents that are likely to be toxic (Checkoway et al, 1989). This is relatively simple when a study is motivated by concerns about agents of known toxicity, but reports of symptoms or illness (e.g., chest tightness, phlegm production) can suggest problems with agents that are not known to cause respiratory disease. The second step in characterizing the environment is to establish the most relevant exposure routes for the agents of concern. Measures of current exposure levels will usually then be based on direct exposure (or dose) measurements. The various measurement techniques are reviewed in industrial hygiene texts (e.g., Cralley and Cralley, 1982) and will not be discussed here.

Information on past exposures is usually based on routine employment records in combination with industrial hygiene surveys of typical levels of exposure in various jobs or tasks (Gamble and Spirtas, 1976), supplemented by records of production methods and materials purchased, and information on historical work practices. The sources of data for a job-exposure matrix (JEM) include industrial hygiene sampling data, process descriptions and flow charts, plant production records, inspection and accident reports, engineering documentation, and biological monitoring data (Checkoway et al, 1989). The major concerns with such information are the completeness of the data and the ability to combine information from different time periods when different exposure measurement methods may have been used (Checkoway et al, 1989). The epidemiologist must be particularly concerned with the reasons that sampling was performed (Gardiner, 1995). In particular, industrial hygienists usually concentrate on the most heavily exposed workers and the areas where concentrations are believed to be highest. Thus, assignment of exposures to unmonitored workers, jobs, or worker areas may be difficult. The physical location of measurement devices

Table 6.9. Prevalence of asthma symptoms by history of exposure in 703 hard metal workers in Japan

	Exposure	n	Symptom prevalence (%)
MEN			
	Non-exposed	263	6.1%
	Formerly exposed	75	10.7%
	Currently exposed	242	13.6%
	Currently or formerly exposed	317	12.9%
WOMEN			
	Non-exposed	91	8.8%
	Formerly exposed	1	0%
	Currently exposed	27	11.1%
	Currently or formerly exposed	28	10.7%

can also severely affect the measurements. Although personal monitoring devices should yield more precise exposure measurements, workers may change their work practices (e.g., wearing protective equipment or taking greater precautions) as a result of wearing a device (or as a result of illness in cases in a case-control study), and the measurements may not be generalizable to other workers in the same jobs and work areas. Furthermore, there may be serious problems with the generalizability of measurements from personal biological monitoring (see above). The key issue is that the exposure information should be of comparable quality for the various groups being compared (see above), and this is often more readily achieved by workplace area measurements rather than personal monitoring.

Example 6.18

Kusaka et al (1996) studied the entire workforce (n=703) of a Japanese corporation producing hard metal tools. Table 6.9 shows that the prevalence of asthma symptoms was higher in currently exposed workers than in formerly exposed and non-exposed workers. Positive IgE reaction against cobalt was found in seven men (2.0%) all of whom reported asthma symptoms.

The healthy worker effect

A major issue in occupational studies is the healthy worker effect (Mc-Michael, 1976). The typically lower relative risk of death or chronic disease in an occupational cohort occurs because relatively healthy individuals are likely to gain employment and to remain employed. These effects were first described by William Ogle in 1885 (Fox and Collier, 1976) when he outlined the two major difficulties in studying occupational mortality. One was that "some occupations may repel, while others attract, the unfit at the age of starting work" while the other was the "considerable standard of muscular strength and vigour to be maintained." The healthy worker effect is particularly strong for deaths from respiratory disease, and it is also of major concern in studies of nonfatal respiratory disease, including asthma. The healthy worker effect may be particularly strong at older ages (Fox and Collier, 1976; Musk et al, 1978).

Selection occurs at two time points (Pearce et al, 1986, 1992a): selection into the workforce at time of hire (which is influenced by good health) and selection out of the workforce at time of termination of employment (which is influenced by poor health). The initial selection occurs at time of hire in that relatively healthy persons are more likely to seek and to be offered employment; the most direct way to partially control for this phenomenon is to stratify on initial employment status—that is, to compare the asthma morbidity of a particular workforce with that of other employed persons rather than with a general population sample (which includes invalids and the unemployed). The second key aspect of the health worker effect is the selection of unhealthy persons out of the workforce; this problem can be partially addressed by considering each worker's employment status (i.e., active or nonactive worker) at a particular time and controlling for it as a confounder (Pearce, 1992b; Steenland and Stayner, 1991). Furthermore, the strength of the healthy worker effect tends to diminish with increasing time since first employment; this problem can be addressed by controlling for length of follow-up.

Thus, there are at least three aspects of the healthy worker effect (Fox and Collier, 1976): (1) the selection of healthy persons into employment, (2) the selection of unhealthy persons out of the workforce, and (3) the length of time the population has been followed. These three aspects of the healthy worker effect can in part be delimited, and controlled for, by several time-related factors. These time-related factors thus have important implications for the design and analysis of occupational asthma studies. Although the use of an internal reference group will control for initial employment status and therefore for the initial selection into employment (aspect 1 of the healthy worker effect), it will not necessarily eliminate other forms of bias, particularly in cross-sectional prevalance studies. This is of particular concern in occupational asthma epidemiology studies because most of them are cross-sectional (Malo and Cartier, 1996). Furthermore, Krzyanowski and Kauffmann (1988) have noted that most studies have focused on industrial groups with high levels of exposure, and that these groups may be particularly affected by selection effects (Graham and Graham-Tomasi, 1985). For example, Petsonk et al (1995) found that miners with the longest duration of work at the coal face had a low prevalence of BHR compared with miners who had never worked at the coal face (12% compared with 39%) and that miners with BHR were consistently less likely, throughout their careers, to have worked in dusty jobs. Studies in these groups may therefore underestimate the effects of exposure because the most affected workers may have changed jobs. By contrast, Krzyanowski and Kauffmann (1988) studied a community-based sample and found significant associations of wheezing with relatively low levels of nonindustrial occupational exposures to dusts, gases, and chemical fumes.

Example 6.19

Eisen et al (1995) studied the effects of low-level granite dust exposure in 618 Vermont granite workers followed for 5 years with annual lung function tests. The group included 353 "survivors" and 265 "dropouts" without data in the final survey because of retirement, termination, nonparticipation, or test failure. The two groups were similar at baseline with respect to age, height, and previous exposure, but the dropouts had worked for fewer years, smoked more "pack-years," and had a slightly lower FEV_1 at baseline. In the survivor population, the pattern of decline in FEV_1 in relation to smoking status was consistent with other reports in healthy working populations, with an average rate of decline of 44 mL/year that was unrelated to past and current dust exposure. However, the dropout population lost FEV_1 at an average of 69 mL/year and the rate of decline was associated with both past and current dust exposure. The authors commented that these results provide an illustration of bias due to the healthy worker effect and an example of the failure to detect a true work-related health effect in a study based only on a survivor population.

Other Exposures

A variety of other "lifestyle" factors are known to influence disease risk. Apart from tobacco smoke (see above), the lifestyle factors that have received the most attention in asthma epidemiology studies are diet and viral exposures.

Diet

Several dietary factors, including dietary sodium (Burney, 1987), selenium (Malmgren et al, 1986; Beasley et al, 1991), and antioxidant intake (Soutar et al, 1997), have been found to influence the development of asthma symptoms (Burney, 1995). It has been hypothesized that changes in the diet in Western countries in the past few decades, involving reductions in antioxidant intake, may be responsible for a reduction in host resistance to allergens and a rise in atopic disease (Seaton et al, 1994). However, a recent prospective study found that antioxidant supplementation during adult-hood was not an important determinant of adult-onset asthma (Troisi et al, 1995). Diet during pregnancy may also be relevant to the findings on birthweight and head circumference (see *Intrauterine environment and early life events,* above). Duration of breast feeding may also be of interest, al-though this has not generally been found to be strongly related to asthma risk (Cogswell et al, 1987).

Methods of measuring dietary intake in epidemiological studies have been reviewed in detail by Willett (1990) and by Armstrong et al (1992). The standard questionnaire methods are retrospective food frequency ques-tionnaire and dietary diaries (food records). The latter approach facilitates the collection of information on food items that are quickly forgotten, and does not require the study participants to attempt to summarize their usual eating patterns. The main limitation is that only current intake is measured, and diaries will only be good measures of past exposures if current and past dietary intake are highly correlated (Armstrong et al, 1992). In addition, food records require some skill, time, and commitment on the part of study participants. Willett et al (1985) found that the validity of micronutrient intake from a 1-week dietary diary was greater than that of a retrospective food frequency questionnaire, using as the standard three other 1-week diaries completed over a 1-year period; however, the expense of diet diaries was an important consideration in choosing between the two methods (Arm-strong et al, 1992).

The alternative approach is biological measurements of dietary intake, but even the best available methods do not represent purely the effect of diet, because other factors influence the biological measurements. For exam-ple, serum levels of vitamin E are affected by cholesterol levels, and it is necessary to adjust for this in studies of serum vitamin E levels (Armstrong et al, 1992). Furthermore, biomarkers of dietary intake suffer from the same limitations as other biomarkers of exposure (see *General approaches to expo-sure assessment*), particularly with regard to historical exposures and the possibility of decreased response rates. Nevertheless, biomarkers of dietary intake may be of value in some asthma epidemiology studies, particularly in longitudinal studies involving repeated sampling.

Example 6.20

Schwartz and Weiss (1990) studied dietary factors and their relation to respiratory symptoms, in an analysis of data from the Second National Health and Nutrition Examination Survey (NHANES II), which included 9074 persons aged 30 to 74 years throughout the United States. Estimates of nutrient intake were based on 24-hour

Table 6.10. Association of dietary factors with wheezing in the Second
National Health and Nutrition Examination Survey, 1976–1980

	Odds ratio	95% CI
Smoking (10 pack-years)	1.2	1.1–1.4
Family income (tertile change)	0.6	0.5–0.7
Northeast US	0.7	0.5–0.8
Southern US	0.8	0.5–0.9
Calories (2 SD change)	1.3	1.0–1.7
Niacin (2 SD change)	0.7	0.6–0.9
Zinc:copper (2 SD change)	0.7	0.6–0.8
Serum vitamin C (2 SD change)	0.7	0.6–0.9

Source: Adapted from Schwartz and Weiss (1990).

dietary recall, which was analyzed using a current nutrient data bank. Information on asthma symptoms was obtained with an interviewer-administered medical history questionnaire. Several dietary factors were found to be negatively associated with wheezing (Table 6.10), including niacin, serum vitamin C, and the serum zinc to copper ratio. The authors concluded that these dietary constituents may influence the occurrence of respiratory symptoms in adults, independently of cigarette smoking.

Viruses

As noted in *Intrauterine environment and early life events* (above), infections during infancy may protect against the development of sensitization and asthma. On the other hand, some viral infections during the first year of life may increase the risk of developing asthma (e.g., Pullan and Hey, 1992), and infections during childhood may cause exacerbations of asthma and provoke episodes of wheezing in children who already have the condition (Welliver et al, 1981; Stenius-Aarniala, 1987). In children under 5 years of age, respiratory syncytial virus (RSV) and parainfluenza (PI) are the most common pathogens, whereas in older children rhinovirus and influenza A are more important. Viral respiratory tract infections are less commonly associated with exacerbations of asthma in adults (Burney et al, 1989), although they may account for up to 40% of severe exacerbations (Beasley et al, 1988). Viral infections may provoke an IgE response and respiratory syncytial virus (RSV) produces such a response in 70% of children (Burney, 1992), although the persistence of the response appears to be determined by the host, and virsuses do not appear to play a major part in the sensitization process (Cogswell et al, 1982).

Unfortunately, measuring viral infections is not straightforward in epidemiological studies. Respiratory symptom diary cards can be used to record upper respiratory symptoms (e.g., Johnston et al 1995); these include runny nose; sneezing; blocked or stuffy nose; itchy, sore, or watery eyes; sore throat; hoarse voice; fever or shivering; and headaches or face aches. However, it is not straightforward to relate these symptom reports to viral infections. Until recently, studies employing the standard identification techniques of immunofluorescence, serology, and cell culture have identified viral infections in 10% to 50% of exacerbations of asthma in childhood. More recently, with the development of polymerase chain reaction (PCR) technology for identifying rhinovirus and coronavirus infections (which are responsible for the majority of common colds and are difficult to detect), viruses have been identified in up to 85% of asthmatic episodes (Johnston et al, 1995). However, these techniques require intensive monitoring and the collection of nasal and/or serum samples, and they may be impractical and/or too expensive for large-scale epidemiological studies (see Example 6.28).

Example 6.21

Johnston et al (1995) conducted a prospective community-based study of the role of virus infections as a cause of asthma exacerbations in 108 children aged 9 to 11 years. The study participants kept a daily diary card of upper and lower respiratory tract symptom scores and peak flow rates for a total period of 13 months. On reporting an exacerbation, children were visited at home, with nasal and serum samples taken for virus identification. Using standard techniques, respiratory viruses were identified in 43% of exacerbations of asthma. With the addition of PCR technology to identify rhinoviruses, viruses were detected in 80% to 85% of asthmatic episodes. The authors concluded that upper respiratory viral infections are associated with 80% to 85% of asthma exacerbations in school-age children. However, the authors also noted that the study did not include a control group, because they thought that it would be difficult to recruit asymptomatic children "to an intensive and invasive study of this type," indicating that these methods may not be suitable for routine epidemiological use.

Summary

Methods of exposure measurement include personal interviews or self-administered questionnaires (completed either by the study participant or by a proxy respondent), diaries, observation, routine records, physical or chemical measurements of the environment, or physical or chemical measurements of the person. Measurements of the person can relate either to exogenous exposure (e.g., airborne dust) or to internal dose (e.g., plasma cotinine); the other measurement options (e.g., questionnaires) all relate to exogenous exposures. Traditionally, exposure to most nonbiological risk factors (e.g., cigarette smoking) has been measured with questionnaires (either self-administered or interviewer-administered), and this approach has a long history of successful use in epidemiology. Questionnaires may be combined with environmental exposure measurements (e.g., pollen counts, industrial hygiene surveys) to obtain a quantitative estimate of individual exposures. More recently, there has been increasing emphasis on the use of molecular markers of internal dose (Schulte, 1993). However, questionnaires and environmental measurements have good validity and reproducibility with regard to current exposures and are likely to be superior to biological markers with respect to historical exposures. The emphasis should be on using "appropriate technology" to obtain the most practical and valid estimate of the etiologically relevant exposure. The appropriate approach (questionnaires, environmental measurements or biological measurements) will vary from study to study, and from exposure to exposure within the same study (or within the same complex chemical mixture—e.g., in tobacco smoke). The prime consideration is to obtain exposure information of similar accuracy and high validity for the groups being compared in a manner that is practical and acceptable to study participants and that thereby yields high response rates.

References

Aberg N (1989). Birth season variation in asthma and allergic rhinitis. Clin Exp Allergy 19: 643–8.

Aberg N, Enstrom I, Lindberg U (1989). Allergic diseases in Swedish school children. Acta Paediatr Scand 78: 246–52.

Anderson HR (1974). The epidemiological and allergic features of asthma in the New Guinea Highlands. Clin Allergy 4: 171–83.

Anderson HR (1979). Respiratory abnormalities, smoking habits and ventilatory capacity in a highland community in Papua New Guinea: prevalence and effect on mortality. Int J Epidemiol 8: 127–35.

Anderson HR, Pottier AC, Strachan DP (1992). Asthma from birth to age 23: incidence and relation to prior and concurrent disease. Thorax 47: 537–42.

Andrae S, Axelson O, Bjorksten B, et al (1988). Symptoms of bronchial hyperreactivity and asthma in relation to environmental factors. Arch Dis Child 63: 473–8.

Antó JM (1995). Asthma outbreaks: an opportunity for research? Thorax 50: 220–2.

Antó JM, Sunyer J (1990). Epidemiological studies of asthma epidemics in Barcelona. Chest 98: 185S–190S.

Antó JM, Sunyer J, and the Barcelona Asthma Collaborative Group (1986). A point source asthma outbreak. Lancet 1: 900–3.

Antó JM, Sunyer J, Rodriguez-Roisin R, et al (1989). Community outbreaks of asthma associated with inhalation of soybean dust. N Engl J Med 320: 1097–1102.

Antó JM, Sunyer J, Reed CE, et al (1993). Preventing asthma epidemics due to soybeans by dust-control measures. N Engl J Med 329: 1760–3.

Antó JM, Sunyer J, Newman-Taylor AJ (1996). Comparison of soybean epidemic asthma and occupational asthma. Thorax 51: 743–9.

Armstrong BK, White E, Saracci R (1992). Principles of Exposure Measurement in Epidemiology. New York: Oxford University Press.

Ashmore M (1995). Human exposure to air pollutants. Clin Exp Allergy 25 (suppl 3): 12–22.

Ayres JG (1995). Epidemiology of the effects of air pollutants on allergic disease in adults. Clin Exp Allergy 25 (suppl 3): 47–51.

Baker A (1994). Domestic mites and allergens. Allergy News 6: 3–4.

Balfour-Lynn L (1985). Childhood asthma and puberty. Arch Dis Child 60: 231.

Barbee RA, Lebowitz MD, Thompson HC, Burrows B (1976). Immediate skin test reactivity in a general population sample. Ann Intern Med 84: 129–33.

Barbee RA, Halonen M, Lebowitz M, Burrows B (1981). Distribution of IgE in a community population sample: correlations with age, sex and allergen skin test reactivity. J Allergy Clin Immunol 68: 106–11.

Barbee RA, Kaltenborn W, Lebowitz MD, Burrows B (1987). Longitudinal changes in allergen skin test reactivity in a community population sample. J Allergy Clin Immunol 79: 16–24.

Barker DJP (ed) (1993). Fetal and infant origins of adult disease. London: British Medical Journal.

Barker DJP, Godfrey KM, Fall C, et al (1991). Relation of birthweight and child-hood respiratory infection to adult lung function and death from chronic obstructive airways disease. BMJ 303: 671–5.

Barnes PJ (1994). Air pollution and asthma. Postgraduate Medical Journal 70: 319–25.

Bascom R, Bromberg PA, Costa DA, et al (1996). Health effects of outdoor air pollution. Am J Respir Crit Care Med 153: 3–50.

Beasley R, Coleman ED, Hermon Y, et al (1988). Viral respiratory tract infection and exacerbations of asthma in adult patients. Thorax 43: 679–83.

Beasley R, Thomson C, Pearce NE (1991). Selenium, glutathione peroxidase and asthma. Clin Exp Allergy 21: 157–9.

Bellon G (1992). From acute viral bronchiolitis in infancy to asthma in childhood. Pediatrics 47: 263–8.

Berkman LF, MacIntyre S (1997). The measurement of social class in health studies: old measures and new formulations. In: Kogevinas M, Pearce N, Susser M, Boffetta P (eds). Socioeconomic Factors and Cancer. Lyon: IARC, pp 51–64.

Bischoff E, Fischer A, Liebenberg B (1992). Assessment of mite numbers: new methods and results. Exp Appl Acarol 16: 1–14.

Bjorksten B (1994). Risk factor in early childhood for the development of atopic diseases. Allergy 49: 400–7.

Bjorksten F, Suoniemi I, Koski V (1980). Neonatal birch pollen contact and subsequent allergy to birch pollen. Clin Allergy 10: 585–91.

Blands J, Loewenstein H, Weeke B (1977). Characterisation of extract of dog hair and dandruff from six different dog breeds by quantitative immunoelectrophoresis (CRIE). Acta Allergo 32: 147–50.

Borja-Aburto VH, Loomis D (1997). Outdoor Air III: Ozone. In: Steenland K, Savitz DA (eds). Topics in environmental epidemiology. New York: Oxford University Press, pp 184–199.

Brauer M, Koutrakis P, Spengler J (1989). Personal exposures to acidic aerosols and gases. Environ Sci Tech 23: 1408–12.

Brunekreef B, Groot B, Hoek G (1992). Pets, allergy and respiratory symptoms in children. Int J Epidemiol 21: 338–42.

Burge PGS (1982). Occupational asthma in electronic workers caused by colophony fumes: follow-up of affected workers. Thorax 37: 348–53.

Burge PGS (1995). Occupational asthma. In: Brewis RAL, Corrin B, Geddes GM, Gibson GJ (eds). Respiratory Medicine. 2nd ed. London: WB Saunders, pp 1262–80.

Burney PGJ (1987). A diet rich in sodium may potentiate asthma. Chest 91: 143S–148S.

Burney PGJ (1992). Epidemiology. Br Med Bull 48: 10–22.

Burney PGJ (1995). Asthma: epidemiology. In: Brewis RAL, Corrin B, Geddes DM, Gibson GJ. Respiratory Medicine. 2nd ed. London: WB Saunders, pp. 1098–1107.

Burney PGJ, Anderson HR, Burrows B, et al (1989). Epidemiology. In: Holgate ST, Howell JBL, Burney PGJ, et al (eds). The Role of Inflammatory Processes in Airway Hyperresponsiveness. Oxford: Blackwell Scientific.

Burney PGJ, Luczynska C, Chinn S, et al (1994). The European Community Respiratory Health Survey. Eur Respir J 7: 954–60.

Burr ML, St Leger AS, Yarness JWG (1981). Wheezing, dampness and coal fires. Community Med 3: 205–9.

Burr ML, Miskelly FG, Butland BK, et al (1989). Environmental factors and symptoms in infants at high risk of allergy. J Epidemiol Community Health 43: 125–32.

Burrows B, Lebowitz MD, Barbee RA (1976). Respiratory disorders and allergy skin-test reactions. Ann Intern Med 84: 134–9.

Burrows B, Halonen M, Lebowitz MD, et al (1982). The relationship of serum immunoglobulin E, allergy skin tests, and smoking to respiratory disorders. J Allergy Clin Immunol 70: 199–204.

Burrows B, Martinez FD, Halonen M, et al (1989). Association of asthma with serum IgE levels and skin-test reactivity to allergens. N Engl J Med 320: 271–7.

Celenza A, Fothergill J, Kupek E, Shaw RJ (1996). Thunderstorm associated asthma: a detailed analysis of environmental factors. BMJ 312: 604–7.

Chan-Yeung M (1995). Assessment of asthma in the workplace. Chest 108: 1084–1117.

Chan-Yeung M, Lam S (1986). Occupational asthma. Am Rev Respir Dis 133: 686–703.

Chan-Yeung M, Malo J-L (1995). Epidemiology of occupational asthma. In: Busse W, Holgate S (eds). Asthma and Rhinitis. Oxford: Blackwell Scientific, pp. 44–57.

Chapman M, Platts-Mills T (1980). Purification and characterisation of the major allergen from Dermatophagoides pteronyssinus—antigen PI. J Immunol 125: 592–7.

Chapman M, Rowntree S, Mitchell E, et al (1983). Quantitative assessment of IgG and IgE antibodies to inhalant allergens in patients with atopic dermatitis. J Allergy Clin Immunol 72: 27–33.

Chavance M, Dellatolas G, Lellouch J (1992). Correlated nondifferential misclassifications of disease and exposure: application to a cross-sectional study of the relationship between handedness and immune disorders. Int J Epidemiol 21: 537–46.

Checkoway HA, Pearce NE, Crawford-Brown DJ (1989). Research Methods in Occupational Epidemiology. New York: Oxford University Press.

Chen Y, Rennie DC, Dosman JA (1996). Influence of environmental tobacco smoke on asthma in nonallergic and allergic children. Epidemiology 7: 536–9.

Chike-Obi U, David RJ, Coutinho R, Wu S-Y (1996). Birth weight has increased over a generation. Am J Epidemiol 144: 563–9.

Chilmonczyk BA, Salmun LM, Megathlin KN, et al (1993). Association between exposure to environmental tobacco smoke and exacerbations of asthma in children. N Engl J Med 328: 1665–9.

Clifford RD, Radford M, Howell JB, Holgate ST (1989). Prevalence of respiratory symptoms among 7 and 11 year-old school children and association with asthma. Arch Dis Child 64: 419–24.

Cline MG, Burrows B (1989). Distribution of allergy in a population sample residing in Tucson, Arizona (1989). Thorax 44: 425–31.

Clough JB, Williams JD, Holgate ST (1991). Effect of atopy on the natural history of symptoms, peak expiratory flow, and bronchial responsiveness in 7 and 8 year old children with cough and wheeze. Am Rev Respir Dis 143: 755–60.

Cogswell JJ, Halliday DF, Alexander JR (1982). Respiratory infections in the first year of life in children at risk of developing atopy. BMJ 284: 1011–3.

Cogswell JJ, Mitchell EB, Alexander J (1987). Parental smoking, breast feeding, and respiratory infection in development of allergic diseases. Arch Dis Child. 62: 338–44.

Coggon D (1995). Assessment of exposure to environmental pollutants. Occup Environ Med 52: 562–4.

Collaborative Study on the Genetics of Asthma (CSGA) (1997). A genome-wide search for asthma susceptibility loci in ethnically diverse populations. Nature Genetics 15: 389–92.

Cookson WOCM, Hopkin JM (1988). Dominant inheritance of atopic IgE responsiveness. Lancet 1: 86–7.

Cookson WOCM, Moffatt MF (1997). Asthma: an epidemic in the absence of infection? Science 275: 41–2.

Cookson WOCM, Sharp PA, Faux JA, Hopkin JM (1989). Linkage between IgE responses underlying asthma and rhinitis and chromosome iiq. Lancet 1: 1292–4.

Cookson WOCM, et al (1993). Maternal inheritance of atopic IgE responsiveness on chromosome 11q. Lancet 340: 381–4.

Copeland KT, Checkoway H, McMichael AJ, et al (1977). Bias due to misclassification in the estimation of relative risk. Am J Epidemiol 105: 488–95.

Corbo GM, Agabiti N, Forastiere F, et al (1996). Lung function in children and adolescents with occasional exposure to environmental tobacco smoke. Am J Respir Crit Care Med 154: 695–700.

Cralley, LV, Cralley LJ (1982). Patty's Industrial Hygiene and Toxicology, 3rd rev ed, vol 3. New York: Wiley.

Crane J (1995). Asthma and the indoor environment. Wellington, New Zealand: Public Health Commission.

Croner S, Kjellman NIM, Eriksson B, Roth A (1982). IgE screening in 1701 newborn infants and the development of atopic disease during infancy. Arch Dis Child 57: 364–368.

Cullinan P, Newman Taylor AJ (1994). Asthma in children: environmental factors. BMJ 308: 1585–6.

Cunningham J, Dockery DW, Speizer FE (1996a). Race, asthma and persistent wheeze in Philadelphia schoolchildren. Am J Public Health 86: 1406–9.

Cunningham J, O'Connor GT, Dockery DW, Speizer FE (1996b). Environmental tobacco smoke, wheezing, and asthma in children in 24 communities. Am J Respir Crit Care Med 153: 218–24.

Dales RE, Burnett R, Zwanenburg (1991). Adverse health effects among adults exposed to home dampness and molds. Am Rev Respir Dis 143: 505–9.

Dales RE, Miller D, McMullen E (1997). Indoor air quality and health: validity and determinants of reported home dampness and molds. Int J Epidemiol 26: 120–5.

D'Amato G, Liccardi G, Cazzola M (1994). Environment and development of respiratory allergy. I. Outdoors. Monaldi Arch Chest Dis 5: 406–11.

Dandeu J, Le Mao J, Rabillon J, et al (1982). Antigens and allergens of Dermatophagoides farinae mites II. Purification of Ag 11, a major allergen in Dermatophagoides farinae. Immunology 46: 679–87.

DHHS (Department of Health and Human Services) (1986). The health consequences of involuntary smoking: a report of the Surgeon General. Washington, DC: DHHS.

Desjardins A, Bergeron J-P, Ghezzo H, et al (1994). Aluminium potroom asthma confirmed by monitoring of forced expiratory volume in one second. Am J Respir Crit Care Med 150: 1714–7.

Devereux G, Ayatollahi T, Ward R, et al (1996). Asthma, airways responsiveness and air pollution in two contrasting districts of Northern England. Thorax 51: 169–74.

Dijkstra L, Houthuijs D, Brunekreef B (1990). Respiratory health effects of the indoor environment in a population of Dutch children. Am Rev Respir Dis 123: 479–85.

Dockery D (1987). Associations of health status with indicators of indoor air pollution from an epidemiologic study in six US cities. In: Indoor Air 1987. Seifert. Berlin: Institute for Water, Soil and Air Hygiene, pp 203–7.

Dockery DW, Brunekreef B (1996). Longitudinal studies of air pollution effects on lung function. Am J Respir Crit Care Med 154: S250–S256.

Dockery DW, Pope CA (1997). Outdoor air I: Particulates. In: Steenland K, Savitz DA (eds). Topics in environmental epidemiology. New York: Oxford University Press, pp. 119–166.

Dodge R. (1982). The effects of indoor pollution on Arizona children. Arch Environ Health 37: 151–5.

Donnelly JE, Donnelly WJ, Thong YHTI (1987). Parental perceptions and attitudes towards asthma and its treatment: a controlled study. Soc Sci Med 24: 431–7.

Dorward AJ, Colloff MJ, MacKay NS, et al (1988). Effect of house dust mite avoidance measures on adult atopic asthma. Thorax 43: 98–102.

Dosemeci M, Wacholder S, Lubin JH (1990). Does nondifferential misclassification of exposure always bias a true effect toward the null value? Am J Epidemiol 132: 746–8.

Doull IJM, Lawrence S, Watson M, et al (1996). Allelic association of gene markers on chromosomes 5q and 11q with atopy and bronchial hyperresponsiveness. Am Rev Respir Crit Care Med 153: 1280–4.

Dreborg S (ed) (1989). Skin tests used in type I allergy testing. Position paper prepared by the subcommittee on skin tests of the European Academy of Allergology and Clinical Immunology. Allergy 44 (suppl): 22–30, 52–9.

Duhme H, Weiland SK, Keil U, et al (1996). The association between self-reported symptoms of asthma and allergic rhinitis and self-reported traffic density on street of residence in adolescents. Epidemiology 7: 578–82.

Edfors-Lubs ML (1971). Allergy in 7000 twin pairs. Acta Allergologica 26: 249–85.

Egan P (1985). Weather or not. Med J Aust 142: 330.

Eisen EA, Wegman DH, Louis TA, et al (1995). Healthy worker effect in a longitudinal study of one-second forced expiratory volume (FEV1) and chronic exposure to granite dust. Int J Epidemiol 24: 1154–62.

Emberlin J (1995). Interaction between air pollutants and aeroallergens. Clin Exp Allergy 25 (suppl 3): 33–9.

EPA (Environmental Protection Agency) (1983). Repiratory health effects of passive smoking: lung cancer and other disorders. Washington, DC: EPA.

European Community Respiratory Health Survey (ECRHS) (1996). Variations in the prevalence of respiratory symptoms, self-reported asthma attacks, and use of asthma medication in the European Community Respiratory Health Survey (ECRHS). Eur Respir J 9: 687–95.

Fergusson D, Crane J, Beasley R, Horwood LJ (in press). Perinatal factors and atopic disease in childhood. Clin Exper Allergy.

Figley KD, Elrod RH (1928). Endemic asthma due to castor bean dust. JAMA 90: 79–82.

Fishwick D, Pearce N, D'Souza W, et al (1997). Occupational asthma in New Zealanders: a population-based study. Occup Environ Med 54: 301–6.

Florey C, Melia R, Chinn S (1979). The relation between respiratory illness in primary school-children and the use of gas for cooking III. Nitrogen dioxide, respiratory illness and lung function. Int J Epidemiol 8: 347–53.

Forastiere F, Agabiti N, Dell'orco V, et al (1993). Questionnaire data as predictors of urinary cotinine levels among non-smoking adolescents. Arch Environ Health 48: 230–4.

Foucard T (1974). A follow-up study of children with asthmatic bronchitis. II. Serum IgE and eosinophil counts in relation to clinical course. Acta Paediatr Scand 63: 129.

Fox AJ, Collier PF (1976). Low mortality rates in industrial cohort studies due to selection for work and survival in the industry. Br J Prev Soc Med 30: 225–30.

Gamble JF, Spirtas R (1976). Job classification and utilization of complete work histories in occupational epidemiology. J Occup Med 18: 399–404.

Gannon PFG, Burge PS (1997). Serial peak expiratory flow measurement in the diagnosis of occupational asthma. Eur Respir J 10 (suppl 24): 57s–63s.

Gardiner K (1995). Needs of occupational exposure sampling strategies for compliance and epidemiology. Occup Environ Med 52: 705–8.

Gerrard JW, Horne S, Vickers P, et al (1974). Serum IgE levels in parents and children. J Pediatr 85: 660–663.

Godfrey KM, Barker DJP, Osmond C (1994). Disproportionate fetal growth and raised IgE concentration in adult life. Clin Exp Allergy 24: 641–8.

Graham S, Graham-Tomasi R (1985). Achieved status as a risk factor in epidemiology. Am J Epidemiol 122: 553–8.

Gregg I (1983). Epidemiological aspects. In: Clark TJK, Godfrey S (eds). Asthma. London: Chapman Hall.

Hall IP (1997). The future of asthma. BMJ 314: 45–9.

Halonen M, Barbee RA, Lebowitz MD, Burrows B (1982). An epidemiologic study of the interrelationships of total serum immunoglobulin E, skin-test reactivity, and eosinophilia. J Allergy Clin Immunol 69: 221–8.

Harving H, Hansen L, Korsgaard J, et al (1991). House dust mite allergy and antimite measures in the indoor environment. Allergy 46 (suppl 11): 33–8.

Hoffman RE, Wood RC, Kreiss K (1993). Building-related asthma in Denver office workers. Am J Public Health 83: 89–93.

Holt PG, Sly PD (1997). Allergic respiratory disease: strategic targets for primary prevention during childhood. Thorax 52: 1–4.

Horwood LJ, Fergusson DM, Shannon FT (1985). Social and familial factors in the development of early childhood asthma. Pediatrics 75: 859–68.

Hsieh K-H, Shen J-J (1988). Prevalence of childhood asthma in Taipei, Taiwan and other Asian Pacific countries. J Asthma 25: 73–82.

Hulka BS (1990). Methodologic issues in molecular epidemiology. In: Hulka BS, Wilcosky TC, Griffith JD (eds). Biological Markers in Epidemiology. New York: Oxford University Press, pp 214–26.

Infante-Rivard C (1993). Childhood asthma and indoor environmental risk factors. Am J Epidemiol 137: 834–4.

Johnston SL, Pattemore PK, Sanderson G, et al (1995). Community study of role of virus infections in exacerbations of asthma in 9–11 year old children. BMJ 310: 1225–9.

Kemp T, Pearce N, Fitzharris P, Crane J, Fergusson D, St George I, Wickens K, Beasley R (1997). Is infant immunization a risk factor for childhood asthma and allergy? Epidemiol 8:678–80.

Kino T, Chihara J, Fukuda K, et al (1987). Allergy to insects in Japan. III: High frequency of IgE antibody responses to insects (Moth, butterfly, caddis fly, and chironomid) in patients with bronchial asthma and immunochemical quantitation of the insect-related airborne particles smaller than 10 μm in diameter. J Allergy Clin Immunol 79: 857–66.

Kjellman NIM (1976). Predictive value of high IgE levels in children. Acta Paediatr Scand 65: 465–471.

Kjellman B, Petterson R (1983). The problem of furred pets in childhood atopic disease. Allergy 38: 65–73.

Kjellman NIM, Croner S (1984). Cord blood IgE determination for allergy prediction—A follow-up to seven years of age in 1,651 children. Ann Allergy 53: 167–171.

Kogevinas M, Antó JM, Soriano JB, et al (1996). The risk of asthma attributable to occupational exposures: a population-based study in Spain. Am J Respir Crit Care Med 154: 137–43.

Koo LC, Ho JH-C (1994). Mosquito coil smoke and respiratory health among Hong Kong Chinese: results of three epidemiological studies. Indoor Environ 3: 304–10.

Korsgard J (1983). Mite asthma and residency: a case-control study on the impact of exposure to house-dust mites in dwellings. Am Rev Respir Dis 128: 231–5.

Kristensen P (1992). Bias from nondifferential but dependent misclassification of exposure and outcome. Epidemiology 3: 210–5.

Krzyzanowski M, Kauffmann F (1988). The relation of respiratory symptoms and ventilatory function to moderate occupational exposure in a general population. Int J Epidemiol 17: 397–406.

Kusaka Y, Iki M, Kumagai S, Goto S (1996). Epidemiological study of hard metal asthma. Occup Environ Med 53: 188–93.

Lawrence S, Beasley R, Doull I, et al (1994). Genetic analysis of atopy and asthma as quantitative traits and ordered polychotomies. Ann Human Genet 58: 359–68.

Lehrer S, Barbandi F, Taylor J, et al (1984). Tobacco smoke sensitivity—is there an immunologic basis? J Allergy Clin Immunol 73: 240–5.

Liberatos P, Link BG, Kelsey JL (1988). The measurement of social class in epidemiology. Epidemiol Rev 10: 87–121.

Littlejohns P, Ebrahim S, Anderson HR (1989). The prevalence and diagnosis of chronic respiratory symptoms in adults. BMJ 298: 1556–60.

Littlejohns P, MacDonald LD (1993). The relationship between severe asthma and social class. Respir Med 87: 139–43.

Livingstone AE, Shaddick G, Grundy C, Elliott P (1996). Do people living near inner city main roads have more asthma needing treatment? BMJ 312: 676–7.

Luczynska C, Arruda L, Platts-Mills T, et al (1989). A two-site monoclonal antibody ELISA for the quantification of the major Dermatophagoides spp allergens Der p 1 and Der f 1. J Immunol Methods 118: 227–35.

Luo JCJ, Nelson K, Eischbein A (1988). Persistent reactive airways dysfunction after exposure to toluene diisocyanate. Br J Ind Med 47: 239–41.

McMichael AJ (1976). Standardised mortality ratios and the "healthy worker effect": scratching below the surface. J Occup Med 18: 165–8.

Malmgren R, Unge G, Zetterstrom O, et al (1986). Lowered glutathione peroxidase activity in asthmatic patients with food and aspirin intolerance. Allergy 41: 43–45.

Malo J-L, Cartier A (1996). Occupational asthma. In: Harber P, Schenker M, Balmes J (eds). Occupational and Environmental Respiratory Disease. St Louis, MI: Mosby, pp 420–32.

Malo J-L, Cartier A, L'Archevêque J, et al (1990a). Prevalence of occupational asthma and immunological sensitization to pollution among health personnel in chronic care hospitals. Am Rev Respir Dis 142: 1359–66.

Malo J-L, Cartier A, L'Archevêque J, et al (1990b). Prevalence of occupational asthma and immunological sensitization to guar gum among employees at a carpet-manufacturing plant. J Allergy Clin Immunol 86: 562–9.

Malo J-L, Ghezzo H, L'Archevêque J, et al (1991). Is the clinical history a satisfactory means of diagnosing occupational asthma? Am Rev Respir Dis 143: 528–32.

Malo J-L, Ghezzo H, D'Aquino C, et al (1992). Natural history of occupational asthma: relevance of type of agent and other factors on the rate of development of symptoms in subjects with disease. J Allergy Clin Immunol 90: 937–44.

Marbury M, Kriegler R (1991). Formaldehyde. In: Samet J, Spengler JD (eds). Indoor Air Pollution: A Health Perspective. London: Johns Hopkins University Press, pp 223–251.

Martinez F (1994). Role of viral infections in the inception of asthma and allergies during childhood: could they be protective? Thorax 49: 1189–91.

Martinez FD, Wright AL, Taussig LM, et al (1995). Asthma and wheezing in the first six years of life. N Engl J Med 332: 133–8.

Maynard RL (1995). Concentrations of air pollutants in the UK. Clin Exp Allergy 25 (suppl 3): 22–32.

Mendes E, Cintra U (1954). Collective asthma, simulating an epidemic, provoked by castor-bean dust. J Allergy 25: 253–9.

Meredith S, Nordman H (1996). Occupational asthma: measures of frequency from four countries. Thorax 51: 435–40.

Meredith SK, Taylor VM, McDonald JC (1991). Occupational respiratory disease in the United Kingdom 1989: a report to the British Thoracic Society and the Society of Occupational Medicine by the SWORD project group. Br J Ind Med 48: 292–8.

Meyers DA, Bleecker ER (1995). Approaches to mapping genes for allergy and asthma. Am J Respir Crit Care Med 152: 411–3.

Mielke A, Reitmeir P, Wjst M (1996). Severity of childhood asthma by socioeconomic status. Int J Epidemiol 25: 388–93.

Milligen F, Vroom T, Aalberse R (1990). Presence of Felis Domesticus allergen I in the cat's salivary and lacrimal glands. Int Arch Allergy Appl Immunol 92: 375–8.

Mitchell RG, Dawson B (1973). Educational and social characteristics of children with asthma. Arch Dis Child 48: 467–71.

Molfino N, Wright S, Katz I, et al (1991). Effects of low concentrations of ozone on inhaled allergen responses in asthmatic subjects. Lancet 338: 199–203.

Morrison I (1960). It happened one night. Med J Aust 1: 850–1.

Morrisson Smith J, Springett VH (1979). Atopic disease and month of birth. Clin Allergy 9: 153–7.

Morton NE (1992). Major loci for atopy? Clin Exp Allergy 22: 1041–3.

Moscato G, Godnic-Cvar J, Maestrelli P, for the Subcommittee on Occupational Allergy of European Academy of Allergy and Clinical Immunology (1995). Statement on self-monitoring of peak expiratory flows in the investigation of occupational asthma. J Allergy Clin Immunol 96: 295–301.

Moyes CD, Waldon J, Dharmalingam R, et al (1995). Respiratory symptoms and environmental factors in schoolchildren in the Bay of Plenty. N Z Med J 108: 358–61.

Murray A, Fergusson A (1983). Dust free bedrooms in the treatment of asthmatic children with house dust or house dust mite allergy: a controlled trial. Pediatrics 71: 418–22.

Murray V, Venables K, Laing-Morton T, et al (1994). Epidemic of asthma possibly related to thunderstorms. BMJ 309: 131–2.

Musk AW, Monson RR, Peters JM, et al (1978). Mortality among Boston fire-fighters, 1915–1975. Br J Ind Med 35: 104–8.

NRC (National Research Council) (1986). Environmental tobacco smoke: measuring exposures and assessing health effects. Washington, DC: National Academy Press.

Navarro C, Márquez M, Hernando L, et al (1993). Epidemic asthma in Cartagena, Spain and its association with soybean sensitivity. Epidemiology 4: 76–9.

Neas L, Dockery D, Ware J, Spengler J, Speizer F, Ferris B (1991). Association of indoor nitrogen dioxide with respiratory symptoms and pulmonary function in children. Am J Epidemiol 134: 204–19.

Nelson HS, Rosloniec DM, McCall LI, Ilké D (1993). Comparative performance of five commerical prick skin test devices. J Allergy Clin Immunol 92: 750–6.

Newman Taylor A (1995a). Environmental determinants of asthma. Lancet 345: 296–9.

Newman Taylor A (1995b). Asthma. In: McDonald C (ed). Epidemiology of Work Related Diseases. London: BMJ Publishing, pp 117–42.

NHLBI (1992). International consensus report on diagnosis and treatment of asthma. National Heart, Lung and Blood Institute. Washington, DC: DHHS.

O'Hollaren MT, Yunginger JW, Offord KP, et al (1991). Exposure to an aeroallergen as a possible precipitating factor in respiratory arrest in young patients with asthma. N Engl J Med 324: 359–63.

Oosterlee A, Drijver M, Lebret E, Brunekreef (1995). Chronic respiratory symptoms in children and adults living along streets with high traffic density. Occup Environ Med 53: 241–7.

Ordman D (1995). An outbreak of bronchial asthma in South Africa, affecting more than 200 persons, caused by castor bean dust from an oil-processing factory. Int Arch Allergy 7: 10–24.

Oryszczyn M-P, Annesi I, Neukirch F, et al (1991). Relationships of total IgE level, skin prick test response, and smoking habits. Ann Allergy 67: 355–9.

Osbourne J, Honicky R (1986). Chronic respiratory symptoms in young children and indoor heating with a wood burning stove. Am Rev Respir Dis 133: 300 (abstract).

Packe GE, Ayres JG (1985). Asthma outbreak during a thunderstorm. Lancet 2: 199–204.

Packe GE, Ayres JG (1986). Aeroallergen skin sensitivity in patients with severe asthma during a thunderstorm. Lancet 1: 850–1.

Pannett B, Coggon D, Acheson RED (1985). A job exposure matrix for use in population based studies in England and Wales. Br J Ind Med 42: 777–83.

Panhuysen CIM, Meyers DA, Postma DS, Bleecker ER (1995). The genetics of asthma and atopy. Allergy 50: 863–9.

Pearce N, Checkoway H, Shy CM (1986). Time-related factors as potential confounders and effect modifiers in studies based on an occupational cohort. Scand J Work Environ Health 12: 97–107.

Pearce N (1992a). Methodological problems of time-related variables in occupational cohort studies. Rev Epidemiol Santé Publique 40: S43–S54.

Pearce NE (1992b). Time-related confounders and intermediate variables in epidemiologic studies. Epidemiology 3: 279–81.

Pearce N, Sanjose S, Boffetta P, et al (1995). Limitations of biomarkers of exposure in cancer epidemiology. Epidemiology 6: 190–4.

Pearlman DS (1984). Bronchial asthma: a perspective from childhood to adulthood. Am J Dis Chest 138: 459–66.

Peat JK (1996). Prevention of asthma. Eur Respir J 9: 1545–55.

Peat JK, Tovey E, Toelle BG, et al (1996). House dust mite allergens: a major risk factor for childhood asthma in Australia. Am J Respir Crit Care Med 153: 141–6.

Pepys J, Hutchroft B (1975). Bronchial provocation tests in etiologic diagnosis and analysis of asthma. Am Rev Respir Dis 112: 829–59.

Peroni DG, Boner AL, Vallone G, et al (1994). Effective allergen avoidance at high altitude reduces allergen-induced bronchial hyperresponsiveness. Am J Respir Crit Care Med 149: 1442–6.

Pershagen G, Rylander E, Norberg S, et al (1995). Air pollution involving nitrogen dioxin exposure and wheezing bronchitis in children. Int J Epidemiol 24: 1147–53.

Petsonk EL, Daniloff EM, Mannino DM, et al (1995). Airway responsiveness and job selection: a study in coal miners and non-mining controls. Occup Environ Med 52: 745–9.

Pirhonen I, Nevalainen A, Husman T, Pekkanen J (1996). Home dampness, moulds and their influence on respiratory infections and symptoms in adults in Finland. Eur Respir J 9: 2618–22.

Platts-Mills T, Tovey E, Mitchell E, et al (1982). Reduction of bronchial hyper-reactivity during prolonged allergen avoidance. Lancet 2: 675–8.

Platts-Mills TAE, Carter MC (1997). Asthma and indoor exposure to allergens. N Engl J Med 336: 1382–4 (editorial).

Platts-Mills T, Heyman P, Longbottom J, et al (1986). Airborne allergens associated with asthma: particle size measurements with a cascade impactor. J Allergy Clin Immunol 77: 850–7.

Platts-Mills T, Thomas W, Aalberse R, et al (1992). Dust mite allergens and asthma: report of a second international workshop. J Allergy Clin Immunol 89: 1046–60.

Polednak AP (1989). Racial and Ethnic Differences in Disease. New York: Oxford University Press.

Pomare E, Tutengaehe H, Ramsden I, et al (1992). Asthma in Maori people. N Z Med J 105: 469–70.

Pope CA, Dockery DW, Spengler JD, Raizenne ME (1991). Respiratory health and PM_{10} pollution: a daily time series analysis. Am Rev Respir Dis 144: 668–74.

Pullan CR, Hey EN (1982). Wheezing, asthma, and pulmonary dysfunction 10 years after infection with respiratory syncytial virus in infancy. BMJ 284: 1665–9.

Reihsaus E, Innis M, MacIntyre N, Liggett SB (1993). Mutations in the gene encoding for the β_2-adrenergic receptor in normal and asthmatic subjects. Am J Respir Cell Mol Biol 8: 334–9.

Reid MJ, Moss RB, Hsu Y-P, et al (1986). Seasonal asthma in northern California: allergic causes and efficacy of immunotherapy. J Allergy Clin Immunol 78: 590–600.

Rona RJ, Gulliford MC, Chinn S (1993). Effects of prematurity and intrauterine growth on respiratory health and lung function in children. BMJ 306: 817–20.

Rosenstreich DL, Eggleston P, Kattan M, et al (1997). The role of cockroach allergy and exposure to cockroach allergen in causing morbidity among inner-city children with asthma. N Engl J Med 336: 1356–63.

Samet JM, Utell MJ (1990). The risk of nitrogen dioxide: what have we learned from epidemiological and clinical studies? Toxicol Ind Health 6: 247–62.

Samet JM, Lange P (1996). Longitudinal studies of active and passive smoking. Am J Respir Crit Care Med 154: S257–S265.

Sanford A, Weir T, Paré P (1996). The genetics of asthma. Am Rev Respir Crit Care Med 153: 1749–65.

Saracci R (1984). Assessing exposure of individuals in the identification of disease determinants. In: Berlin A, Draper M, Hemminki K, Vainio H (eds). Monitoring Human Exposure to Carcinogenic and Mutagenic Agents. Lyon: IARC.

Schulte PA (1993). A conceptual and historical framework for molecular epidemiology. In: Schulte P, Perera FP. Molecular Epidemiology: Principles and Practices. New York: Academic Press, pp 3–44.

Schwartz J, Weiss ST (1990). Dietary factors and their relation to respiratory symptoms. Am J Epidemiol 132: 67–76.

Schwartz J, Weiss ST (1995). Relationship of skin test reactivity to decrements in pulmonary function in children with asthma or frequent wheezing. Am J Respir Crit Care Med 152: 2176–80.

Schwartz J, Slater D, Larson TV, et al (1993). Particulate air pollution and hospital emergency room visits for asthma in Seattle. Am Rev Respir Dis 147: 826–31.

Scott J (1953). Fog and deaths in London, December 1952. Public Health Reports 68: 474–9.

Sears MR, Herbison GP, Holdaway MD, et al (1989). The relative risks of sensitivity to grass pollen, house dust mite and cat dander in the development of childhood asthma. Clin Exp Allergy 19: 419–24.

Sears MR, Burrows B, Flannery EM, et al (1991). Relation between airway responsiveness and serum IgE in children with asthma and in apparently normal children. N Engl J Med 325: 1067–71.

Seaton A, Godden DJ, Brown K (1994). Increase in asthma: a more toxic environment or a more susceptible population? Thorax 49: 171–4.

Seaton A, MacNee W, Donaldson K, Godden D (1995). Particulate air pollution and acute health effects. Lancet 345: 176–8.

Seidman DS, Laor A, Gale R, et al (1991). Is low birth weight a risk factor for asthma during adolescence? Arch Dis Childhood 66: 584–7.

Shah S, Green JR (1994). Disease susceptibility genes and the sib-pair method: a review of recent methodology. Ann Hum Genet 58: 381–95.

Shaheen SO (1995). Changing patterns of childhood infection and the rise in allergic disease. Clin Exp Allergy 25: 1034–1037.

Shaheen SO, Aaby P, Hall AJ, et al (1996). Measles and atopy in Guinea-Bissau. Lancet 347: 1792–6.

Shaw R, Woodman K, Crane J, et al (1994). Risk factors for asthma in Kawerau children. N Z Med J 107: 387–91.

Sherman CB, Tosteson TD, Tager IB, et al (1990). Early childhood predictors of asthma. Am J Epidemiol 132: 83–95.

Sibbald B (1980). Genetic basis of sex differences in the prevalence of asthma. Br J Dis Chest 74: 93–4.

Siebers RW, Fitzharris P, Crane J (1996). Beds, bedrooms, bedding, and bugs: anything new between the sheets? Clin Exp Allergy 26: 1225–7.

Sigurs N, Bjarnason R, Sigurbergsson F, et al (1995). Asthma and immunoglobulin E antibodies after respiratory syncytial virus bronchiolitis: a prospective cohort study with matched controls. Pediatrics 95: 500–5.

Silverman M (1995). Childhood asthma and other wheezing disorders. In: Brewis RAL, Corrin B, Geddes GM, Gibson GJ (eds). Respiratory Medicine. 2nd ed. London: WB Saunders, pp 1239–61.

Slovak AJ, Hill RN (1981). Laboratory animal allergy: a clinical survey of an exposed population. Br J Ind Med 38: 38–41.

Smith JM, Knowles LA (1967). Epidemiology of asthma and allergic rhinitis. II. In a university-centered community. Am Rev Respir Dis 92: 31–8.

Soutar A, Seaton A, Brown K (1997). Bronchial reactivity and dietary antioxidants. Thorax 52: 166–70.

Sporik R, Holgate T, Platts-Mills T, Cogswell JJ (1990). Exposure to house-dust mite allergen (Der p I) and the development of asthma in childhood. N Engl J Med 323: 502–7.

Sporik R, Platts-Mills T (1992). Epidemiology of dust-mite-related disease. Exp Appl Acarol 16: 141–51.

Steenland K, Stayner L (1991). The importance of employment status in occupational cohort mortality studies. Epidemiology 2: 418–23.

Steinberg M, Becklake MR (1986). Socio-environmental factors and lung function: a review of the literature. S Af Med J 70: 2704.

Stenius-Aarniala B (1987). The role of infection in asthma. Chest 91: 157S–160S.

Strachan DP (1989). Hay fever, hygiene, and household size. BMJ 299: 1259–60.

Strachan DP (1995). International Study of Asthma and Allergies in Childhood (ISAAC). Phase II modules. London: St George's Hospital Medical School.

Strachan DP, Sanders CH (1989). Damp housing and childhood asthma: respiratory effects of indoor air temperature and relative humidity. J Epidemiol Community Health 43: 7–14.

Sunyer J (1997). Outdoor Air II: Nitrogen dioxide. In: Steenland K, Savitz DA (eds). Topics in environmental epidemiology. New York: Oxford University Press, pp 167–183.

Sunyer J, Antó JM, Rodrigo M-J, et al (1989). Case-control study of serum immunoglobulin-E antibodies reactive with soybean in epidemic asthma. Lancet 1: 179–82.

Sunyer J, Antó JM, Castellsagué J, et al (1996). Total serum IgE is associated with asthma independently of specific IgE levels. Eur Respir J 9: 1880–4.

Suphioglu C, Singh MB, Taylor P, et al (1992). Mechanism of grass-pollen-induced asthma. Lancet 339: 569–72.

Suzuki S, Kamakura T, Tadokoro K, et al (1988). Correlation between the atmospheric conditions and the asthmatic symptom. Int J Biometeorol 32: 129–33.

Taylor B, Normal A, Orgel H, et al (1973). Transient IgA deficiency and pathogenesis of infantile atopy. Lancet 2: 111–3.

Thompson SG, Stone R, Nanchahal K, Wald NJ (1990). Relation of urinary cotinine concentrations to cigarette smoking and to exposure to other people's smoke. Thorax 45: 356–61.

Troisi RJ, Willett WC, Weiss ST, et al (1995). A prospective study of diet and adult-onset asthma. Am J Respir Crit Care Med 151: 1401–8.

Ussetti P, Roca J, Agusti AGN, et al (1983). Asthma outbreaks in Barcelona. Lancet 2: 280–1.

Van Herwerden L, Harrap SB, Wong ZYH, et al (1995). Linkage of high-affinity IgE receptor gene with bronchial hyperreactivity, even in absence of atopy. Lancet 346: 1262–5.

Vanto T, Koivikko A (1983). Dog hypersensitivity in asthmatic children. Acta Paediatr Scand 72: 571–5.

Venables K, Topping M, Howe W, et al (1985). Interaction of smoking, and atopy in producing IgE antibody against hapten protein conjugate. Br Med J 290: 201–4.

Verhoeff AP, Van Strien RT, Van Wijnen JH, Brunekreef B (1995). Damp housing and childhood respiratory symptoms: the role of sensitisation to dust mites and molds. Am J Epidemiol 141: 103–10.

Vineis P (1992). Uses of biochemical and biological markers in occupational epidemiology. Rev Epidemiol Sante Publique 40: S63–S69.

Verhoeff AP, Van Strien RT, Van Wijnen JH, Brunekreef B (1995). Damp housing and childhood respiratory symptoms: the role of sensitization to dust mites and molds. Am J Epidemiol 141: 103–10.

Von Mutius E, Fritzsch C, Weiland SK, et al (1992). Prevalence of asthma and allergic disorders among children in united Germany: a descriptive comparison. BMJ 305: 1395–9.

Von Mutius E, Martinez FD, Fritzsch C, et al (1994a). Skin test reactivity and number of siblings. BMJ 308: 692–5.

Von Mutius E, Martinez FD, Fritzsch C, et al (1994b). Prevalence of asthma and atopy in two areas of West and East Germany. Am J Respir Crit Care Med 149: 358–64.

Von Mutius E, Nicolai T (1996). Familial aggregation of asthma in a South Bavarian population. Am J Respir Crit Care Med 153: 1266–72.

Voorhorst T, Spieksma FM, Varekamp H, et al (1967). The house dust mite (Dermatophagoides pteronyssinus) and the allergens it produces: identity with the house dust mite allergen. J Allergy 39: 325–39.

Wardlaw A (1993). The role of air pollution in asthma. Clin Exp Allergy 23: 81–96.

Warner JO, Price JF (1978). House dust mite sensitivity in childhood asthma. Arch Dis Child 53: 710–3.

Warner J, Little S, Polloch I, et al (1991). The influence of exposure to house dust mite, cat, pollen and fungal allergens in the home in primary sensitisation in asthma. Pediatr Allergy Immunol 1: 79–86.

Watson JP, Cowen P, Lewis PA (1996). The relationships between asthma admission rates, routes of admission, and socieconomic deprivation. Eur Respir J 9: 2087–93.

Watson M, Lawrence S, Collins A, et al (1995). Exclusion from proximal 11q of a common gene with a megaphenic effect on atopy. Ann Hum Genet 59: 403–11.

Weiss ST, Tager IB, Speizer FE, Rosner B (1980). Persistent wheeze: its relation to respiratory illness, cigarette smoking, and level of pulmonary function in a population sample of children. Am Rev Respir Dis 122: 697–707.

Welliver RC, Wong DT, Sun M, et al (1981). The development of respiratory syncytial virus–specific IgE and the release of histamine in nasopharyngeal secretions after infection. N Engl J Med 305: 841–6.

White MC, Etzel RA, Olson DR, Goldstein IF (1997). Reexamination of epidemic asthma in New Orleans, Louisiana, in relation to the presence of soy at the harbor. Am J Epidemiol 145: 432–8.

Wickens K, Martin I, Pearce N, et al (1997). House dust mite allergen levels in public places in New Zealand. J Allergy Clin Immunol 99: 587–93.

Willett W (1990). Nutritional Epidemiology. New York: Oxford University Press.

Willett WC, Sampson L, Stampfer MJ, et al (1985). Reproducibility and validity of a semiquantitative food frequency questionnaire. Am J Epidemiol 122: 51–65.

Yemaneberhan H, Bekele Z, Venn A, et al (1997). Prevalence of wheeze and asthma in relation to atopy in urban and rural Ethiopia. Lancet 350: 85–90.

Zamel N, McClean PA, Sandell PR, et al (1996). Asthma on Tristan de Cunha: looking for the genetic link. Am Rev Respir Crit Care Med 153: 1902–6.

Zetterstrom O, Osterman K, Machado L, Johansson SGO (1981). Another smoking hazard: raised serum IgE concentration and increased risk of occupational allergy. BMJ 283: 1215–7.

Zimmerman B, Feanny S, Reisman J, et al (1988). Allergy in asthma. I. The dose relationship of allergy to severity of childhood asthma. J Allergy Clin Immunol 81: 63–70.

Part III
ASTHMA MORTALITY

7

Studying Time Trends
in Asthma Deaths

The epidemics of asthma deaths in the 1960s and 1970s have provided the main motivation for studies of time trends in asthma deaths. We begin by briefly reviewing the background to these studies, before proceeding to discuss the methodological issues and approaches involved. These include (1) assessing possible artifactual explanations for an increase in mortality and (2) assessing possible explanations for a real increase in mortality, including considering whether an increase is due to a change in prevalence or incidence (or whether there has been an increase in the case fatality rate), considering whether some demographic groups are particularly affected by an increase in mortality; and using this information to consider possible causal explanations for an increase in mortality. These approaches lead on to the formal analytical epidemiological studies of asthma deaths that are discussed in the next chapter.

Introduction

It was once held that "the asthmatic pants into old age" and that asthmatics rarely died of their disease (Osler, 1901). This is now known to be incorrect, but asthma deaths were certainly very rare in the first half of this century (Speizer and Doll, 1968; Beasley et al, 1990; Baumann and Lee, 1990). Since that time, the patterns of asthma mortality have become considerably more complex (Pearce et al, 1991, 1994). In contrast to the relatively stable asthma death rates during the first half of this century (Fig. 7.1), asthma mortality increased dramatically in at least six developed countries in the 1960s: England and Wales, Scotland, Ireland, New Zealand, Australia, and Norway. The time trends are shown in Figure 7.2 for three of the epidemic countries (England and Wales, Australia, and New Zealand), and for two countries that did not experience epidemics (the United States and Germany). In the 1970s and 1980s a second asthma mortality epidemic oc-

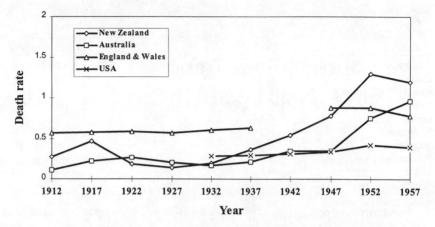

Figure 7.1. Asthma mortality in persons aged 5 to 34 years in New Zealand, Australia, England and Wales, and the USA 1910–1960.

curred in New Zealand, but not in other countries. In recent years attention has also focused on the possible causes of the gradual increase in mortality (Fig. 7.2) that appears to have occurred in a number of countries during the 1970s and 1980s (Burney, 1986; Buist, 1988; Sly, 1988; Jackson et al, 1988; La Vecchia et al, 1992; Weiss and Wagener, 1990; Foucard and Graff-Lonnevig, 1994). Table 7.1 shows increases in asthma mortality in

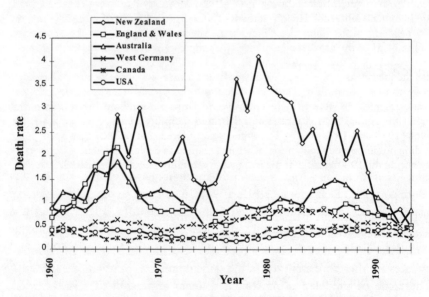

Figure 7.2. International patterns of asthma mortality in persons aged 5 to 34 years, 1960–1990.

Table 7.1. Asthma mortality per 100,000 per year in persons aged 5 to 34 years in 10 countries in 1975–1977 and 1985–1987

Country	1975–1977	1985–1987	Percent increase
Australia	0.86	1.42	65%
Canada	0.33	0.47	42%
England and Wales	0.57	0.90	58%
France	0.24	0.51	113%
Japan	0.44	0.59	34%
Singapore	0.75	0.88	17%
Sweden	0.37	0.54	46%
Switzerland	0.31	0.45	45%
USA	0.19	0.40	111%
West Germany	0.59	0.78	32%

Source: Beasley et al (1997).

persons aged 5 to 34 years in 10 countries between 1975 and 1977 and 1985 and 1987. All of the countries considered experienced increases in mortality, ranging from 17% in Singapore to 113% in France, although recent data suggest that mortality may now be declining again in some countries (Beasley et al, 1997).

Example 7.1

Weiss and Wagener (1990) examined asthma mortality among persons aged 5 to 34 years in the United States during 1968–1987. Mortality data were obtained from the National Center for Health Statistics (NCHS) using a file of mortality data on US residents in 48 states (i.e., excluding Hawaii and Alaska) and the District of Columbia. For the time trend analyses two simple models were considered: a linear model and a log-linear model. Both fit the data well, but the investigators decided to use the log-linear model because this provided a measure of the percentage change in death rates per annum. They found that asthma mortality decreased by 7.8% per year during the 1970s, but increased by 6.2% per year during the 1980s. Figure 7.3 shows the annual mortality rates and the fitted mortality trends, on a log scale, for 1968–1978 and 1979–1986. The authors considered that neither changes in ICD coding nor improved recognition of asthma seemed to explain the increasing mortality during the 1980s, and that the increase in mortality therefore appeared to be real.

In this chapter we will not consider detailed statistical methods for analyzing time trends in asthma deaths; mathematical modeling methods and issues are reviewed in depth in a number of standard texts (e.g., Kleinbaum et al, 1988). Mortality data are a special type of incidence data, and mortality rates are therefore analyzed in the same manner as other incidence rates. These can be modeled using weighted linear regression (if a linear trend with time is hypothesized) or log-linear regression (if an exponential trend with time is hypothesized). However, it should be stressed that studies of

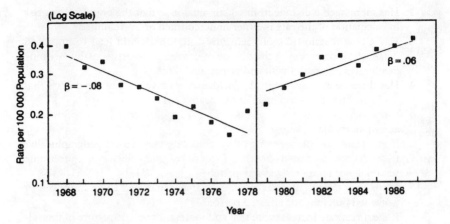

Figure 7.3 Trends in US asthma mortality among persons aged 5 to 34 years in the United States during 1968–1986. (Source: Weiss and Wagener, 1990.)

time trends, and particularly nonepidemic time trends, suffer from the same limitations as other ecologic analyses and provide relatively weak evidence as to causal associations (Greenland and Robins, 1994). In particular, many factors may change over time (asthma prevalence, sales of asthma drugs, sales of television sets), and there are therefore considerable difficulties in establishing causality on the basis of time trends alone, particularly if only a gradual increase in mortality has occurred. However, analyses of such trends may still provide important descriptive information (see Example 7.1). Our emphasis here will be on considering epidemic increases in asthma mortality (particularly the 1960s epidemics), and we will stress that in this context analyses of time trends should primarily be used as part of a process of generating hypotheses as to the possible causes of the epidemic increases; these hypotheses should then be tested in more formal epidemiological studies (Chapter 8).

As Stolley and Lasky (1993a) note, any explanation for the 1960s epidemics must account for several key features including (1) that the epidemic of deaths among asthmatics began abruptly, (2) that the epidemic affected only some countries and spared others, and (3) that asthma mortality had been remarkably constant in most countries until the epidemic began. Stolley and Lasky (1993a) list nine questions that should be considered by an epidemiologist attempting to ascertain the causes of such an increase in mortality:

1. Is the increase in death rates real or an artifact of reporting practices or nosologic changes? Has there been a change in nosology, nomenclature, or coding practices over the course of the presumed epidemic and what is the possible effect of such changes?

2. Has there been a change in the denominator so that the population at risk in calculation of the rate is either undercounted or overcounted?
3. Has a new diagnostic tool been introduced that could lead to improved diagnosis or detection of the disease of interest, thus artifactually elevating death rates compared with earlier periods?
4. Has there been a change in the incidence or prevalence of the disease that could account for the change in the death rates?
5. Is the increase in death rates uniform in all groups at risk or concentrated among particular groups?
6. If the deaths are plotted on a "spot map," do they cluster geographically?
7. If deaths are examined month by month, do they cluster or concentrate seasonally or temporally in any pattern?
8. Has a new treatment been introduced that could lead to an improved or worsened outcome for affected persons?
9. If the death rate increases are real and represent the true picture of mortality, what working hypotheses can explain this unusual phenomenon?

These questions naturally fall into two groups. Questions 1 through 3 involve assessing the validity of the reported increase in mortality. The subsequent questions involve assessing possible explanations for a real increase in mortality, including considering whether the increase is due to a change in prevalence or incidence (prevalence is the most relevant measure in this instance because it provides the "denominator" population at risk for asthma death) or whether an increase in the case fatality rate has occurred (question 4), considering whether some demographic groups are particularly affected by the increase in mortality (questions 5 through 7, and using this information to consider possible causal explanations for the increase in mortality (questions 8 and 9). These two groups of questions are considered in the next two sections. We focus on studies of epidemics of asthma deaths, but where relevant we also consider issues of studying more gradual increases in asthma mortality.

Assessing the Validity of Time Trends

Of the types of possible bias listed by Stolley and Lasky (1993a), an undetected change in the denominator is not a plausible explanation for the asthma mortality epidemics, because the time trends are based on national census data and national death data. However, the other possible biases are relevant to time trends in asthma mortality. In particular, the key methodological issues in assessing the validity of such time trends are (1) the accuracy of death certificates, (2) changes in disease classification, and (3) changes in diagnostic fashion (Jackson, 1993). In each instance we conclude that these factors could account for gradual changes in death rates over time, but could not account for epidemic increases. In particular, Speizer et al (1968a) conducted a detailed examination of the mortality trends in the 5 to 34 age group in England and Wales, and concluded that the epidemic was real and was not due to changes in death certification, disease classification, or diagnostic practice, and similar conclusions were reached by Jackson et al (1982) with regard to the second epidemic in New Zealand.

Accuracy of death certificates

The first consideration in assessing time trends in asthma mortality is the accuracy of the death certificate information on asthma deaths. Almost all comparative studies of asthma mortality have been confined to the 5 to 34 age group because the diagnosis of asthma mortality is more firmly established in this group (British Thoracic Association, 1984; Jackson et al, 1982; Sirken et al, 1987). For example, Sears et al (1986) studied asthma deaths in New Zealand during 1981–1983 and found that in patients aged less than 35 years, the recorded information was considered accurate in 98% of all certified deaths, and in 100% of deaths coded as asthma in national mortality data; the corresponding estimates for those aged 65 years or more were 44% and 55%, respectively (Fig. 7.4).

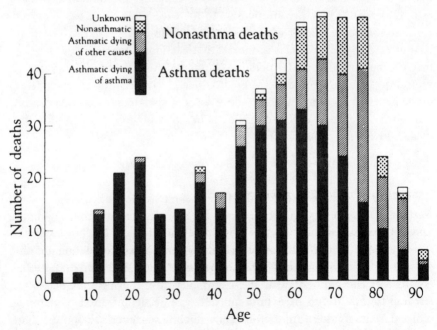

Figure 7.4. Accuracy of certification of asthma deaths, as judged by a review panel of physicians, of 492 cases with 'asthma' in part I of the death certificate or on the coroner's report of cause of death. (Source: Sears, 1990.)

Table 7.2. Comparability of International Classification of Diseases coding by the Office of Population Censuses and Surveys (OPCS), and panel classification of asthma deaths

	Panel's assessment		
OPCS coding	Asthma was cause of death	Other cause of death	Total
Asthma death	77	24	101
Other cause of death	12	34	46
Total	89	58	147

Source: British Thoracic Association (1984).

Example 7.2

The Research Committee of the British Thoracic Association studied asthma deaths in adults aged 15 to 64 years in the West Midland and Mersey regions during 1979 (British Thoracic Association, 1984). Death certificates recording the word asthma were received for 153 persons. Information was obtained from relatives, family doctors, hospital doctors, case notes and pathologists reports. All of the information was then reviewed by three physicians without knowledge of the certified cause of death. The panel was unable to agree about the role of asthma in five deaths, and for one other death insufficient information was available. For the other 147 deaths, Table 7.2 compares the panel's assessment of cause of death with that coded by the national Office of Population Censuses and Surveys (OPCS). Overall, 89 patients were considered by the panel to have died of asthma; and in 77 (87%) of these cases the death certificates were considered to have been correctly coded. As with other similar studies, the agreement was much greater in the younger age groups (90% in the 15 to 44 years age group, 76% in the 45 to 54 years group, and 61% in the 55 to 64 years group). On the other hand, 24 of the 58 deaths that were not considered by the panel to have been due to asthma were coded as asthma by the OPCS. Thus, the total number of 101 deaths coded as being due to asthma represented a net overestimate of 13% when compared to the panel's coding of 89 deaths as being due to asthma.

Most studies of this type have examined only the possibility of false-positive reporting (i.e., deaths from other causes being falsely attributed to asthma). A New Zealand study (Jackson et al, 1982) found that false-negative reporting (i.e., asthma deaths being falsely assigned to other categories) appeared to be very rare; in 66 cases in which death was attributed to disorders that could have been confused with asthma, only one person was considered to have died with asthma, but even in this case death could not be confidently attributed to asthma. However, a more recent study in the United Kingdom (Guite and Burney, 1996) found that four of 22 asthma deaths had been incorrectly certified as non-asthma deaths: two as deaths from chronic obstructive pulmonary disease (COPD) and two as deaths from cardiovascular disease. A recent study in Minnesota (Hunt et al,

1993) also found significant false-negative reporting in older asthmatics (see Example 7.3). Nevertheless, given the accuracy of death rates in the 5 to 34 age group, it is clear that inaccuracies in death certificates could not explain epidemic increases occurring over a period of just a few years.

Example 7.3

Hunt et al (1993) reviewed the complete medical records of 339 deaths from a cohort of 5241 Rochester residents who received medical treatment for asthma between 1964 and 1983. For each death, they used a physician-reviewer to identify whether asthma was an immediate or underlying cause (part I of the death certificate) or a contributing cause (part II of the death certificate). Where there was disagreement between the death certificate and the reviewer, the case was reviewed by a panel consisting of the physician-reviewer and four other physicians certified in allergy and critical care medicine. Of the 339 deaths, the panel considered that asthma was the underlying cause of death in 53 instances; of these, only 22 deaths were listed as asthma on the death certificate, a sensitivity of 42% (22/53). Of the other 286 deaths that the panel considered were not due to asthma, the death certificate listed asthma as a cause of death in four instances, a specificity of 99% (282/286). The authors concluded that in this population, death certificate diagnosis of asthma had a low sensitivity but a high specificity, and that death certificate data may have underestimated asthma-related mortality. However, in this population the median age at death was 74 years, with an interquartile range of 63 to 82 years. Considerably lower rates of misclassification have been found in studies of younger asthmatics (e.g. Sears et al, 1986).

Changes in disease classification

Changes in disease classification are also of concern when examining time trends in asthma mortality. The International Classification of Diseases (ICD) has gone through several major changes in coding practices for asthma deaths since the early 1900s. These largely involved changes in the coding of deaths due to "asthma and bronchitis," which were assigned to bronchitis during some periods and to asthma during others (Table 7.3). However, these changes have primarily affected the data for the older age groups, and they appear to have had little effect on the key trends in the 5 to 34 years age group (Jackson, 1993). For example, the most important revision occurred with the change from ICD-4 to ICD-5, when the method of coding the underlying cause of death was changed, but no major changes in mortality rates occurred. A further significant change occurred with the change from ICD-8 to ICD-9. However, an analysis of death registrations in New Zealand (Jackson et al, 1988) found that the maximum possible increase that could be attributed to the change was approximately 5%,

Table 7.3. Changes to coding of asthma deaths during this century and years of use of each code in New Zealand

Classification	Years	Comments
Bertillon	1908–1922	"Asthma and bronchitis" coded according to which was judged to be underlying cause of death
ICD 3	1923–1929	"Asthma and bronchitis" coded according to which was judged to be underlying cause of death
ICD 4	1930–1939	"Asthma and bronchitis" coded according to which was judged to be underlying cause of death
ICD 5	1940–1949	"Asthma and bronchitis" coded as bronchitis "Asthmatic bronchitis" coded as asthma
ICD 6	1950–1958	"Asthma and bronchitis" coded as asthma
ICD 7	1959–1967	"Asthma and bronchitis" coded as bronchitis, unless the asthma was specified as allergic
ICD 8	1968–1978	"Asthma and bronchitis" coded as bronchitis.
ICD 9	1979–1988	"Asthma due to bronchitis" coded as bronchitis "Bronchitis due to asthma" coded as asthma

Source: Beasley et al (1990).

and a similar estimate was obtained in the United Kingdom (Lambert, 1981). Thus, changes in disease classification could account for modest changes in death rates but could not account for epidemic increases.

Example 7.4

In the eighth revision of the International Classification of Diseases (ICD), asthma with mention of bronchitis was coded as bronchitis, whereas under the ninth revision, it was coded as asthma unspecified. Jackson et al (1988) discuss a bridge coding exercise conducted in New Zealand, in which all deaths in the 5 to 34 years age group that were identified in an asthma mortality survey (Sears et al, 1986) were independently coded under both the eighth and ninth revisions of the ICD codes. It was found that the difference in the number of deaths coded as due to asthma was only 2.4%. It was therefore concluded that the change in ICD coding in 1979 could not have accounted for the dramatic rise in asthma deaths in New Zealand which commenced in 1976 and peaked during 1977–1982.

Changes in diagnostic fashion

The effects of changes in diagnostic fashion over time are more difficult to quantify, although several attempts have been made by simultaneously examining time trends in other respiratory diseases that could be confused with asthma (Jackson, 1993). In general, investigators have found that changes in diagnostic fashion could not account for the asthma mortality epidemics (see Example 7.5). However, it is not possible to exclude changes in diagnostic fashion as an explanation for more gradual changes in asthma

Table 7.4. Death rates from respiratory diseases in the 5 to 34 years age group in England and Wales, 1959–1965

Diagnostic category	Year						
	1959	1960	1961	1962	1963	1964	1965
Bronchitis	0.65	0.57	0.66	0.67	0.65	0.62	0.66
Chronic respiratory disease	0.45	0.49	0.39	0.40	0.38	0.39	0.40
Pneumonias	2.61	2.15	2.24	2.47	2.15	2.04	1.93
Asthma	0.66	0.68	0.89	1.00	1.40	1.76	2.05

Source: Speizer et al (1968a).

mortality. Diagnostic fashion may be a more important source of bias in international comparisons than in comparisons of time trends within a single country. For example, asthma deaths may be underestimated in some populations in the United States (see Example 7.3), and Burney (1989) found major differences in the certification of two ambivalent case histories by physicians from eight European countries.

Example 7.5

Speizer et al (1968a) considered the possibility that a change in diagnostic criteria could account for the sudden epidemic of asthma mortality in England and Wales in the early 1960s. The compared the trends in asthma deaths with those for a variety of other respiratory diseases during 1959–1965 (Table 7.4). No appreciable change took place in the death rates from bronchitis and other chronic respiratory diseases; some decrease occurred for pneumonias, but this was less than half of the increase in asthma deaths over the same period. The number of deaths attributed to bronchitis for which asthma was mentioned on the death certificate did not decrease, as would have been expected if doctors had tended to attribute the underlying cause to asthma alone rather than to asthma and bronchitis. Furthermore, the number of asthma deaths that were certified by coroners increased more rapidly than asthma deaths in general. Thus, if the increase were an artifact then one would have to postulate that there had been a greater diagnostic change among pathologists than among clinicians, or that there had been a change in the type of case referred to coroners. Both these possibilities appeared most unlikely. Speizer et al (1968a) therefore concluded that the increase in mortality from asthma in the 5 to 34 years age group was largely real and was not due to changes in diagnostic fashion.

Assessing Possible Explanations for Time Trends

If it is assumed that an increase in asthma deaths is real, then attention shifts to assessing the possible explanations for the increase.

Has there been a change in asthma prevalence or incidence?

The first issue to consider is whether the increase in mortality is due to an increase in asthma prevalence (or in the prevalence of severe asthma) or whether there has been a change in the case fatality rate. Changes in asthma prevalence over time can be assessed using the methods described in Chapter 4. In fact, in both epidemics (Speizer et al, 1968a; Jackson et al, 1982) there was little evidence available on whether or not asthma prevalence had changed (and virtually no information on asthma incidence). However, in both instances it was considered highly unlikely that the epidemics could be due to changes in asthma prevalence because the evidence that was available did not indicate any dramatic increase in prevalence; the epidemics had commenced so abruptly after a long period of stable asthma death rates; and the epidemic countries were scattered around the world, while neighboring countries had not experienced epidemics. Thus, although increasing asthma prevalence could certainly account for gradual changes in mortality over time, it could not account for such epidemic increases. Therefore although direct information on changes in asthma prevalence was not available, this was considered to be a highly unlikely explanation for the epidemics, and attention therefore shifted to considering possible explanations for a change in the case fatality rate.

Does the increase in mortality affect particular groups?

The first step in considering possible explanations for an increase in case fatality is to examine whether the increase in mortality is concentrated in particular demographic groups. This is the standard "descriptive epidemiology" approach of considering variations in mortality by person, place, or time (Stolley and Lasky's questions 5 through 7). For example, as noted above, the epidemic occurred in some countries and not others, and occurred after a long period of relatively stable asthma death rates. There was less information available on characteristics of the patients who died, but Speizer et al (1968a) noted that the increase in mortality was greatest in the 10 to 19 years age group and that "at these ages children have begun to act independently and may be particularly prone to misuse a self-administered form of treatment."

What hypotheses might explain these changes in the case fatality rate?

Thus in both the 1960s and 1970s epidemics, it appeared that the increases in mortality were real and were due to an increase in the case fatality rate;

Table 7.5. Case series of asthma deaths

Location	Years	Age group	Source of cases	n	Reference
UNITED KINGDOM					
Cardiff	1963–74	All	Outside hospital	90	MacDonald et al (1976a)
Cardiff	1963–74	All	Hospital	53	MacDonald et al (1976b)
England/Wales	1968	5–34	All deaths	184	Speizer et al (1968b)
Greater London/ SE Lancashire	1968–69	5–34	All deaths	52	Fraser et al (1971)
London	1971	35–64	Hospital	38	Cochrane and Clark (1975)
Birmingham	1975–77	All	All deaths	53	Ormerod et al (1980)
West Midlands/ Mersey	1979	15–64	All deaths	90	British Thoracic Association (1982)
UNITED STATES					
Oregon	1982	34–90	Hospital	41	Barger et al (1988)
AUSTRALIA					
South Australia	1988–91	All	All deaths	80	Campbell et al (1994)
Victoria	1986–87	All	All deaths	168	Robertson et al (1990)
NEW ZEALAND					
Auckland	1980–81	All	All deaths	22	Wilson et al (1981)
New Zealand	1981–83	0–69	All deaths	271	Sears et al (1985)

the most likely explanation was that there had been some change in medical management that had occurred relatively suddenly in some countries, but not in others.

The 1960s epidemics. With regard to the 1960s epidemics, it was noted that the sudden increase in deaths had followed the introduction of pressurized beta agonist aerosols in the early 1960s, and that the increase in mortality paralleled the increase in sales (Inman and Adelstein, 1969). These initial observations were complemented by a number of case series reports. Table 7.5 summarizes a number of such case series of asthma deaths (we have included only reports listing at least ten deaths).

Example 7.6

Fraser et al (1971) examined the circumstances preceding death in asthma deaths in the 5 to 34 years age group in Greater London and the South-East Lancashire conurbation in the period February 1, 1968, to January 31, 1969. Copies of death certificates for 52 asthma deaths were provided by local registrars of births and deaths, and the General Register Office in London. Interviews were conducted with general practitioners for 51 of the deaths, and with next-of-kin for 42 of the deaths, and necropsy reports were obtained in 45 cases. The authors found that death was sudden and "unexpected" in 84% of patients. They concluded that excessive inhalation of bronchodilators might have been a factor in approximately one third of the deaths. The duration of the terminal episode in the patients who used drugs excessively was longer than in other patients, and it was possible that the excessive users found an effective dose for a time, but then reached and failed to recognize a state in which they were unable to respond to bronchodilators.

Case reports cannot in themselves establish the cause of an increase in mortality, but they can suggest possible hypotheses or identify phenomena that need to be explained. In the 1960s mortality epidemics, it was known that the deaths were often sudden and unexplained, most occurred outside the hospital (Anonymous 1972), direct information on drug usage was scanty, and the likely mechanism of death was unknown. However, it was noted that the relief of symptoms could enable a patient to tolerate worsening hypoxia and to unduly delay seeking medical help (Speizer et al, 1968b). It was also argued that both chronic and acute side effects of inhaled beta agonists could occur, and that direct toxicity could occur in certain circumstances because isoprenaline (one of the most commonly used beta agonists at the time) is a nonselective beta agonist (Beasley et al, 1991). Thus, the case reports, and other available information, were consistent with a possible role of beta agonist aerosols in the epidemics, and Inman and Adelstein (1969) concluded that:

> the excess deaths . . . were likely to have been the result of overuse of pressurized aerosols and that the subsequent decline in mortality has resulted from a greater awareness by doctors and patients of the dangers of overuse.

However, although the time trends seemed to be consistent with the hypothesis that the epidemics were due to the introduction of beta agonist aerosols, the geographic patterns were inconsistent with this hypothesis because the epidemics did not occur in some countries, including the United States, in which beta agonist aerosol sales were also available. These anomalies were eventually clarified by Stolley (1972), who noted that a high dose formulation of isoprenaline (isoprenaline forte), which contained five times the dose per administration of other isoprenaline aerosols, had been licensed in only eight countries (Table 7.6). Six of these (England and Wales, Ireland, Scotland, Australia, New Zealand, and Norway) had mortality epidemics that coincided with the introduction of the drug, and in the other two countries (the Netherlands and Belgium) the preparation was introduced relatively late and sales volumes were low. Overall, there was a strong posi-

Table 7.6. Cross-classification of countries by presence or absence of an epidemic of asthma mortality and presence or absence of sales of isoprenaline forte aerosols

Epidemic of asthma mortality in the 1960s	Isoprenaline forte aerosols		
	Available	Not available	Total
Present	6	0	6
Absent	2	6	6
Total	8	6	14

Source: Stolley and Schinnar (1978).

tive correlation internationally between the asthma mortality rate and isoprenaline forte sales in these eight countries, whereas no mortality epidemics occurred in countries in which isoprenaline forte was not licensed, such as Sweden, Canada, West Germany, and the United States (Stolley, 1972). Thus, the time trend evidence was inconsistent with a general effect of beta agonist aerosols but was highly consistent with the hypothesis that the epidemic was due to the high-dose beta agonist aerosol isoprenaline forte.

Some anomalies still remained in the time trend data, but these were generally minor. For example, Gandevia (1973) found no correlation between beta agonist aerosol sales and asthma mortality in Australia when sales were examined on a state-by-state basis. However, Campbell (1976) subsequently reanalyzed the same data and found that there was a remarkably high correlation in each of the four most populated states until 1966. After that time, widespread publicity about the mortality epidemic, and the elimination of nonprescription availability of beta agonist aerosols, was followed by a decrease in the death rate independently of isoprenaline forte sales. Similar phenomena had been noted in other epidemic countries (Pearce et al, 1991). Formal analytical epidemiological studies (see Chapter 8) were never mounted because the epidemic declined before there was time to conduct them. Nevertheless, the weight of evidence was highly consistent with the isoprenaline forte hypothesis. Thus, death from bronchodilator aerosols was designated one of the most important adverse drug reactions since thalidomide (Venning, 1983).

However, the potential hazards of beta agonist aerosols are now disputed in many texts and reviews (Anonymous, 1979; Buist, 1988; Paterson and Musk, 1987). For example, Benatar (1986) argues that:

> For many years the hypothesis that sudden death from asthma resulted from the use of aerosol bronchodilators was widely believed within the medical profession and the lay public . . . subsequent studies refuted these reports.

In fact, very little new evidence has appeared since 1972, with the exception of further analyses conducted by Stolley and Schinnar (1978), which strengthened Stolley's original conclusions (see Example 7.7). The process of "reinterpretation" of the 1960s epidemic was based on the minor anomalies in the time trend data, which were emphasized, and to some extent exaggerated, in subsequent reviews (Benatar, 1986; Esdaile et al, 1987; Lanes and Walker, 1987); these did not provide any significant new data but merely referenced other reviews for support (Stolley and Lasky, 1993b). In addition, other factors such as delays in seeking medical help began to receive greater emphasis, and it was argued that "errors of omission are a much more frequent cause of death than errors of commission" (Read, 1968). However, delays in starting appropriate treatment can themselves be caused by overtreatment with beta agonists (Jackson, 1985), and acute toxicity is most likely to occur in the presence of such delays. Furthermore, it is very difficult to envisage how (non-drug-induced) delays could have spontaneously occurred and then regressed in some countries but not in others. Thus, the "errors of omission" theory is inconsistent with the key features of the epidemics (Stolley and Lasky, 1993a).

Example 7.7

Stolley and Schinnar (1978) carried out a multiple regression analysis of time trends in drug sales and asthma mortality, using data from six countries during 1962–1974. These showed a strong correlation between sales of isoprenaline forte and asthma deaths in the countries in which the high-dose preparation had been marketed; there was no significant correlation between asthma deaths and sales of regular isoprenaline, orciprenaline, or other beta agonist aerosols. Figure 7.5 shows the time trends in drug sales and asthma mortality in England and Wales (which experienced a mortality epidemic) and Figure 7.6 shows the corresponding data for the United States (which did not experience an epidemic). In England and Wales there was a strong parallel in sales of regular isoprenaline and those of isoprenaline forte, and its was therefore not possible to separate their relative contributions to the mortality epidemic; the death rate strongly paralleled the rise and fall in sales of both formulations. In the United States, isoprenaline forte was not available, and the death rate remained stable and then fell slightly during the period that other six countries were experiencing mortality epidemics.

The second New Zealand epidemic. Similar issues and controversies accompanied the analyses of the second New Zealand asthma mortality epidemic. The initial case report (Wilson et al, 1981) involved 22 asthma deaths in Auckland, including 16 patients in whom death was seen to be sudden and unexpected. Keating et al (1984) then analyzed trends in sales of asthma drugs in Australia, New Zealand, and the United Kingdom during 1975–1981, and found that there had been a striking increase in per capita sales of beta agonist aerosols and oral theophyllines in all three countries, with the greatest increase occurring in New Zealand. However, the striking increase in beta agonist sales in New Zealand (Fig. 7.7) commenced in 1979, whereas the epidemic of deaths commenced in 1976. Furthermore, appreciable in-

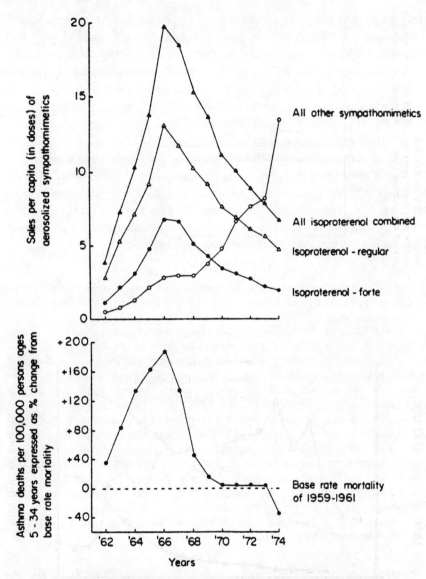

Figure 7.5. Asthma mortality per 100,000 persons aged 5 to 34 years in relation to per capita sales of beta agonist aerosols in England and Wales during 1962–1974. (Source: Stolley and Schinnar, 1978.)

creases in sales had also occurred in Australia and the United Kingdom, and no epidemics of deaths had occurred. Thus, it seemed most unlikely that the general increase in beta agonist sales (as a class) was the cause of the New Zealand epidemic. However, it was subsequently noted (Crane et al, 1989) that the New Zealand time trends were more consistent with an effect of the high-dose beta agonist fenoterol (see Example 7.8).

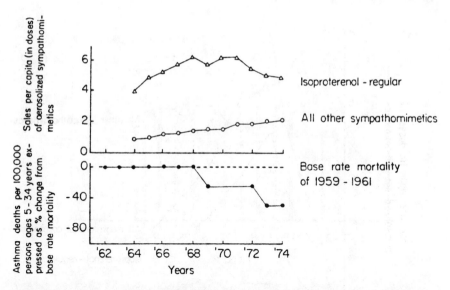

Figure 7.6 Asthma mortality per 100,000 persons aged 5 to 34 years in relation to per capita sales of beta agonist aerosols in the United States during 1962–1974. (Source: Stolley and Schinnar, 1978.)

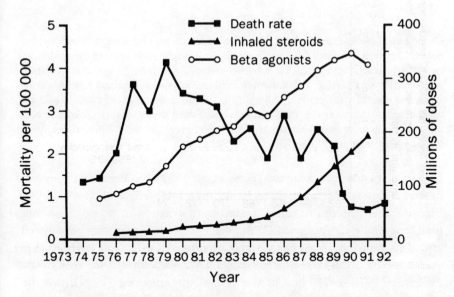

Figure 7.7. Time trends in asthma mortality among persons aged 5 to 34 years in New Zealand during 1974–1990 and total sales of inhaled beta agonists (doses) and inhaled corticosteroids (100 μg equivalents). (Source: Pearce et al, 1995.)

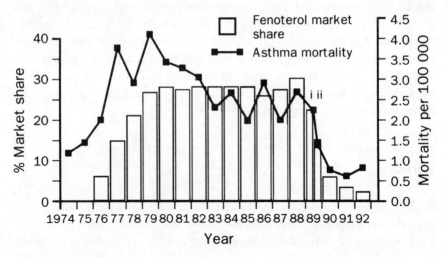

Figure 7.8. Time trends in asthma mortality among persons aged 5 to 34 years in New Zealand during 1974–1992 and fenoterol market share. (Source: Pearce et al, 1995.)

Example 7.8

Crane et al (1989) examined the New Zealand time trend data and found a close parallel between fenoterol sales and asthma deaths in the early years of the epidemic; by 1979 fenoterol accounted for a market share of nearly 30%, and mortality had increased threefold. After 1979, the fenoterol market share remained relatively constant, but mortality fell gradually (Fig. 7.8), possibly due to other changes in asthma management. Pearce et al (1995) subsequently found that mortality fell by one half after warnings were issued about the safety of fenoterol in mid-1989 and remained low in subsequent years (Fig. 7.8).

One criticism of such analyses (Haas et al, 1992) has been that they are based on fenoterol market share rather than total fenoterol doses sold. If Figure 7.8 were redrawn using the latter information, it would show that total fenoterol sales increased during the 1980s while mortality initially fell and then remained reasonably stable during 1983–1988. Therefore, the evidence would still be consistent with a role of fenoterol at the start of the epidemic (1976–1979) and at the end of the epidemic (1989), but the evidence for the intermediate period (1980–1988) would be less consistent. A major problem with such an analysis, however, is that total beta agonist sales increased markedly after 1979 following a switch to regular use of inhaled beta agonists for most asthmatics (Fig. 7.7). There is little information available on patterns of prescribing, but it is very likely that this increase in sales was almost entirely to mild asthmatics who were switched from use "as required" to regular use of beta agonists, whereas severe asthmatics, who were at much greater risk of death and also at much greater risk from fenoterol, were already using beta agonists regularly (use "as required" equates to regular use in this group) and were less affected by this change in prescribing practice. Thus, when comparing the effects of a particular beta agonist (e.g., fenoterol) with others in the same class, it is more reliable to examine trends in market share (within the class of inhaled beta agonists) rather than trends in total sales.

Summary

Studies of time trends, and particularly nonepidemic time trends, suffer from the same limitations as other ecological analyses and provide relatively weak evidence of causal associations. Thus analyses of time trends should primarily be used as part of a process of generating hypotheses as to the possible causes of the epidemic increases. The stages in this process include (1) assessing possible artifactual explanations for an increase in mortality and (2) assessing possible explanations for a real increase in mortality, including considering whether an increase is due to a change in prevalence or incidence (or whether there has been an increase in the case fatality rate), considering whether some demographic groups are particularly affected by an increase in mortality, and using this information to consider possible causal explanations for an increase in mortality. These approaches lead to the formal analytical epidemiological studies of asthma deaths that are discussed in the next chapter.

References

Anonymous (1982). Asthma deaths: a questions answered. BMJ 2: 443–4 (editorial).

Anonymous (1979). Fatal asthma. Lancet 2: 337–8 (editorial).

Barger LW, Vollmer WM, Felt RW, Buist AS (1988). Further investigation into the recent increase in asthma death rates: a review of 41 asthma deaths in Oregon in 1982. Ann Allergy 60: 31–9.

Baumann A, Lee S (1990). Trends in asthma mortality in Australia, 1911–1986. Med J Aust 153: 366 (letter).

Beasley R, Smith K, Pearce NE, et al (1990). Trends in asthma mortality in New Zealand, 1908–1986. Med J Aust 152: 570–3.

Beasley R, Pearce NE, Crane J, et al (1991). Asthma mortality and inhaled beta agonist therapy. Aust N Z J Med 21: 753–63.

Beasley R, Pearce N, Crane J (1997). International trends in asthma mortality. In: The Rising Trends in Asthma. Ciba Foundation Symposium 206. Chichester: Wiley, pp 140–56.

Benatar SR (1986). Fatal asthma. N Engl J Med 314: 423–9.

British Thoracic Association (BTA) (1982). Deaths from asthma in two regions of England. BMJ 285: 1251—5.

British Thoracic Association (BTA) (1984). Accuracy of death certificates in bronchial asthma. Thorax 39: 505–9.

Buist AS (1988). Is asthma mortality increasing? Chest 93: 449–50 (editorial).

Burney PGJ (1986). Asthma mortality in England and Wales: evidence for a further increase, 1974–84. Lancet 2: 323–6.

Burney PGJ (1989). The effect of death certification practice on recorded national asthma mortality rates. Rev Epidemiol Santé Publique 37: 385–9.

Campbell AH (1976) Mortality from asthma and bronchodilator aerosols. Med J Aust 1: 386–91.

Campbell DA, MacLennan G, Coates JR, et al (1994). A comparison of asthma deaths and near-fatal asthma attacks in South Australia. Eur Respir J 7: 490–7.

Cochrane GM, Clark TJH (1975). A survey of asthma mortality in patients between ages 35 and 64 in the Greater London hospitals in 1971. Thorax 30: 300–5.

Crane J, Pearce N, Flatt A, et al (1989). Prescribed fenoterol and death from asthma in New Zealand, 1981–1983: a case-control study. Lancet 1: 917–22.

Esdaile JM, Feinstein AR, Horwitz RI (1987). A reappraisal of the United Kingdom epidemic of fatal asthma. Arch Intern Med 147: 543–9.

Foucard T, Graff-Lonnevig V (1994). Asthma mortality rate in Swedish children and young adults 1973–88. Allergy 49: 616–9.

Fraser PM, Speizer FE, Waters DM, et al (1971). The circumstances preceding death from asthma in young people in 1968 to 1969. Brit J Dis Chest 65: 761–84.

Gandevia B (1973). Pressurized sympathomimetic aerosols and their lack of relationship to asthma mortality in Australia. Med J Aust 1: 273–7.

Greenland S, Robins J (1994). Ecologic studies—biases, misconceptions, and counterexamples. Am J Epidemiol 139: 747–60.

Guite HF, Burney PGJ (1996). Accuracy of recording of deaths from asthma in the UK: the false negative rate. Thorax 51: 924–8.

Haas JF, Staudinger HW, Schuijt C (1992). Asthma deaths in New Zealand. BMJ 304: 1634 (letter).

Hunt LW, Silverstein MD, Reed C, et al (1993). Accuracy of the death certificate in a population-based study of asthmatic patients. JAMA 269: 1947–52.

Inman WHW, Adelstein AM (1969). Rise and fall of asthma mortality in England and Wales in relation to use of pressurized aerosols. Lancet 2: 279–85.

Jackson RT, Beaglehole R, Rea HH, et al (1982). Mortality from asthma: a new epidemic in New Zealand. BMJ 285: 771–4.

Jackson R (1985). Undertreatment and asthma deaths. Lancet 2: 500 (letter).

Jackson R, Sears MR, Beaglehole R, et al (1988). International trends in asthma mortality: 1970 to 1985. Chest 94: 914–8.

Jackson R (1993). A century of asthma mortality. In: Beasley R, Pearce NE (eds). The Role of Beta Agonist Therapy in Asthma Mortality. New York: CRC Press, pp 29–47.

Keating G, Mitchell EA, Jackson R, et al (1984). Trends in sales of drugs for asthma in New Zealand, Australia and the United Kingdom, 1975–81. BMJ 289: 348–51.

Kleinbaum DG, Kupper LL, Muller K (1988). Applied Regression Analysis and Other Multivariable Methods. 2nd ed. Belmont, CA: Wadsworth.

Korsgaard J (1983). Mite asthma and residency: a case-control study on the impact of exposure to house-dust mites in dwellings. Am Rev Respir Dis 128: 231–5.

La Vecchia C, Fasoli M, Negri E, Tognoni G (1992). Fall and rise in asthma mortality in Italy, 1968–84. Int J Epidemiol 21: 998–9 (letter).

Lambert PM (1981). Oral theophylline and fatal asthma. Lancet 2: 200–1 (letter).

Lanes SF, Walker AM (1987). Do pressurized bronchodilator aerosols cause death among asthmatics? Am J Epidemiol 125: 755–60.

MacDonald JB, Seaton A, Williams DA (1976a). Asthma deaths in Cardiff 1963–74: 90 deaths outside hospital. BMJ 2: 1493–5.

MacDonald JB, MacDonald ET, Seaton A, Williams DA (1976b). Asthma deaths in Cardiff 1963–74: 53 deaths in hospital. BMJ 2: 721–3.

Ormerod LP, Stableforth DE (1980). Asthma mortality in Birmingham 1975–7: 53 deaths. BMJ 1:687–90.

Osler W (1901). The Principles and Practice of Medicine. 4th ed. Edinburgh: Pentland.

Paterson JW, Musk AW (1987). Death in patients with asthma. Med J Aust 147: 53–5.

Pearce NE, Crane J, Burgess C, et al (1991). Beta agonists and asthma mortality: déjà vu. Clin Exp Allergy 21: 401–10.

Pearce NE, Beasley R, Crane J, Burgess C (1994). Epidemiology of asthma mortality. In: Busse W, Holgate S (eds). Asthma and Rhinitis. Oxford: Blackwell Scientific, pp 58–69.

Pearce N, Beasley R, Crane J, et al (1995). End of the New Zealand asthma mortality epidemic. Lancet 345: 41–4.

Read J (1968). The reported increase in mortality from asthma: a clinico-functional analysis. Med J Aust 1: 879–91.

Robertson CF, Rubinfeld AR, Bowes G (1990). Deaths from asthma in Victoria: a 12 month survey. Med J Aust 152: 511–7.

Sears MR, Rea HH, de Boer G, et al (1986). Accuracy of certification of deaths due to asthma: a national study. Am J Epidemiol 124: 1004–11.

Sirken MG, Rosenberg HM, Chevarley FM, Curtin LR (1987). The quality of cause-of-death statistics. Am J Public Health 77: 137–9.

Sly RM. Mortality from asthma, 1979–1984 (1988). J Allergy Clin Immunol 82: 705–17.

Speizer FE, Doll R (1968). A century of asthma deaths in young people. Br Med J 3: 245–6.

Speizer FE, Doll R, Heaf P (1968a). Observations on recent increase in mortality from asthma. BMJ 1: 335–9.

Speizer FE, Doll R, Heaf P, et al (1968b). Investigation into use of drugs preceding death from asthma. BMJ 1: 339–43.

Stolley PD (1972). Why the United States was spared an epidemic of deaths due to asthma. Am Rev Respir Dis 105: 883–90.

Stolley PD, Schinnar R (1978). Association between asthma mortality and isoproterenol aerosols: a review. Prev Med 7: 319–38.

Stolley P, Lasky T (1993a). Asthma mortality epidemics: the problem approached epidemiologically. In: Beasley R, Pearce NE (eds). The Role of Beta Agonist Therapy in Asthma Mortality. New York: CRC Press, pp 49–63.

Stolley PD, Lasky T (1993b). The bellman always rings thrice. Ann Intern Med 118: 158 (letter).

Venning GR (1983). Identification of adverse reactions to new drugs. I. What have been the important adverse reactions since thalidomide? BMJ 286: 199–202.

Weiss KB, Wagener DK (1990). Changing patterns of asthma mortality: identifying populations at high risk. JAMA 264: 1683–7.

Weiss KB, Gergen PJ, Wagener DK (1993). Breathing better or wheezing worse? The changing epidemiology of asthma morbidity and mortality. Annu Rev Public Health 14: 491–513.

Wilson JD, Sutherland DC, Thomas AC (1981). Has the change to beta-agonists combined with oral theophylline increased cases of fatal asthma? Lancet 1: 1235–7.

8

Studying the Causes
of Asthma Deaths

In this chapter we discuss the study design options and principles involved in studying the causes of asthma deaths. Most epidemiological studies of asthma deaths have focused on pharmacological risk factors, and we therefore give emphasis to the methodological issues involved in such studies, but we also consider studies of nonpharmacological risk factors. We begin by considering the various study design options theoretically available, including case series, randomized trials, cohort studies, and case-control studies, and we conclude that case-control studies are generally the most feasible approach. We then discuss in more depth the study design issues involved in case-control studies of asthma deaths.

Background

Until recently, epidemiological studies of asthma deaths had mostly involved analyses of time trends, supplemented by case series reports. However, time trend analyses provide relatively weak evidence as to the causes of asthma deaths, and a major problem with case series reports is the lack of a control group. Thus, if a certain proportion of patients are reported to have been prescribed a particular asthma drug, the lack of a control group means that it is very difficult to determine whether the patients who died had been prescribed the drug more or less often than might have been "expected." Similarly, it is very difficult to determine whether other factors such as overuse of medication, delays in seeking medical help, psychosocial factors, or underuse of corticosteroids occurred more often than expected. These issues can only be addressed with more formal epidemiological studies.

Study Design Options

In this section we consider the various formal epidemiological study design options theoretically available for studying the causes of asthma deaths, and the links between them. Most cohort and case-control studies of asthma deaths have focused on pharmacological risk factors, and we therefore give emphasis to methodological issues in studies of such factors. In particular we discuss the various study design options in the context of investigating the hypothesis that prescription of a particular drug increases the risk of asthma mortality (in comparison with other drugs within the same class). The discussion is loosely based on the studies of fenoterol and asthma deaths, which are discussed as an extended example at the end of this chapter, but in this section, we consider the more general principles involved in such studies.

The ideal approach to testing such a hypothesis would be a randomized controlled trial, but this is usually impractical and unethical. However, the randomized controlled trial remains the "gold standard" for epidemiological studies of asthma deaths (Pearce and Crane, 1993). We therefore first discuss the design of a hypothetical randomized trial to compare the death rate in patients prescribed a drug that is suspected to increase the risk of asthma death (drug A) to that in patients prescribed the standard treatment (drug B); next, we design a hypothetical cohort study to achieve the same objective; finally, we design a hypothetical case-control study to achieve the same objective more efficiently than the full cohort study.

A randomized trial of asthma mortality

In a randomized trial of asthma medication and asthma mortality, it would be most appropriate to study the effects of the asthma drugs in the clinical setting in which they are most commonly used (Elwood, 1993). Thus, the most reasonable approach would be to randomize patients to receive either drug A or drug B as their regular prescribed therapy. This approach is most feasible and appropriate irrespective of whether the hypothesis under study involves chronic or acute effects. Because asthma deaths are a rare event, it would also be important to base the randomized trial on a group of "high risk" asthmatics, rather than asthmatics in general. Patients recently hospitalized for asthma would be one suitable population for study because it is known that such patients are at increased risk for asthma death during the subsequent year (Crane et al, 1992).

Methodological issues. Figure 8.1 shows the design of a hypothetical study of this type. Patients would be identified at the time of hospitalization for asthma

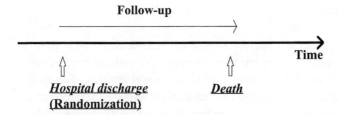

Figure 8.1. A hypothetical randomized trial or cohort study of asthma mortality.

and would be randomized to receive either drug A or drug B. They would then be followed over time, and any subsequent deaths from asthma would be identified from national death registrations (some deaths would be identified directly because they occurred in the hospital, but most would occur outside the hospital). There would be two major methodological issues.

First, for a variety of reasons, some patients would have changes to their therapy after they had been randomized. In particular, patients who were experiencing acute attacks with an increasing frequency or severity might have changes to their medication. However, in analyzing such a study, it would be incorrect to take such changes into account, because these might result in serious bias if the increasing severity was caused by the drug to which they had been randomized. The correct approach would be to analyze the data according to the "intention to treat" principle; that is, the study subjects would be classified according to the regular prescribed medication that they were originally randomized to, and subsequent changes to their medication would be ignored.

The second methodological issue is that although randomization should generally ensure that the two groups under study are similar with respect to their chronic asthma severity, this cannot be guaranteed in every instance. Thus, it would be important to gather information on recognized markers of chronic asthma severity at the time of randomization, such as frequency of previous hospital admissions for asthma and recent prescription of oral corticosteroids. The two groups would then be compared with respect to their average chronic asthma severity. If they were found to differ in this respect, then the analysis would be controlled for, or stratified on, chronic asthma severity. For example, the study might be split into two groups: those that had chronically severe asthma according to a particular severity marker, and those that did not; the comparison between drug A and drug B would then be conducted within each of these two subgroups, and an overall effect estimate adjusted for chronic severity would also be derived if this were appropriate. It is important to note that only the baseline severity at the time of randomization would be relevant in this regard. It would be incorrect to consider subsequent changes in acute or chronic severity, because

Table 8.1. Findings from a hypothetical
randomized trial or cohort study of asthma mortality

	Drug A	Drug B
Deaths	70	35
Survivors	39,930	39,965
Total	40,000	40,000
Risk	70/40,000	35/40,000
Relative risk (95% CI)	2.0 (1.3–3.0)	

these could be a result of treatment. Thus, only the baseline severity (at time of randomization) should be used when considering the potential for confounding by severity.

A hypothetical randomized trial. Table 8.1 shows data from such a hypothetical randomized trial. This involved enrolling 80,000 patients aged 5 to 34 years who had been admitted to the hospital with asthma over a 5-year period. The study subjects were randomized to receive either drug A or drug B in equal numbers, and each study subject was followed for a period of one year after randomization. There were 70 deaths in group B and 35 deaths in group B, yielding a relative risk of 2.0 (95% CI 1.3–3.0). However, there would be considerable problems with conducting a randomized trial of this type, particularly because of the large numbers of patients required. Thus, although some notable randomized trials have been conducted of beta agonists and nonfatal hazardous outcomes (e.g., Sears et al, 1990), it is usually impractical (see Example 8.1), and sometimes unethical, to conduct such a trial involving a fatal outcome (e.g., a trial of isoprenaline forte or fenoterol would now be unethical).

Example 8.1

Castle et al (1993) conducted a double-blind randomized clinical trial to assess the safety of salmeterol, a new long-acting beta agonist. The study involved 25,180 patients, recruited through general practitioners, who were considered to require regular treatment with bronchodilators. They were randomized (two patients to the salmeterol group for each patient to the salbutamol group) to receive either salmeterol (50 μg twice daily) or salbutamol (200 μg four times daily), and then followed for 16 weeks. The two groups were found to be similar in terms of their demographic and clinical characteristics at time of randomization, and there was therefore no need to control for these characteristics in the data analysis. There were only 14 asthma-related deaths in the study (table 8.2), but the risk of death was higher in the salmeterol group (RR = 3.0). The authors argued that the observed excess was not statistically significant, there was no excess risk of other serious events such as asthma hospital admissions, and the overall number of deaths was "in line

Table 8.2. Findings from a clinical trial of salmeterol or salbutamol and asthma deaths

Deaths	Treatment		Relative risk	95% CI
	Salmeterol	Salbutamol		
Asthma related	12	2	3.0	0.7–13.5
Other obstructive airways disease	4	1	2.0	0.2–18.0
Other respiratory	2	1	1.0	0.1–11.1
Cardiovascular	29	10	1.5	0.7–3.0
All other causes	6	6	0.5	0.2–1.6
Not known	1	0	—	—
Total deaths	54	20	1.4	0.8–2.3
Total persons	14,113	7,082		

Source: Derived from Castle et al, 1993.

with that which would have been expected of a sample of patients with asthma of this size in the United Kingdom." Nevertheless, the data show that there were three times as many asthma-related deaths (proportionally) in the salmeterol group than in the salbutamol group. These findings illustrate the difficulties of undertaking a randomized trial (or prospective cohort study) of asthma deaths. Even with 25,180 patients followed for 16 weeks it was not possible to draw firm conclusions because of the small number of deaths occurring in the study.

A cohort study of asthma mortality

Thus, a randomized trial of asthma deaths is impractical, because death from asthma is such a rare event, even among patients with severe asthma, and an epidemiological (observational) approach is required. One obvious option would be to conduct a cohort study. The design of such a hypothetical cohort study would be identical to that of the hypothetical randomized trial shown in Figure 8.1, except that the subjects would not be randomized into treatment groups. Instead, their regular prescribed medication (either drug A or drug B) would be ascertained (rather than randomly allocated) at time of discharge. Once again, they would be followed for one year (or until their next admission) to ascertain subsequent asthma deaths.

Methodological issues. The two major methodological concerns of the hypothetical randomized trial would also apply to this hypothetical cohort study. First, some patients would change their medication after leaving the hospital, particularly if their asthma subsequently became more troublesome or severe, but it would be inappropriate to take such changes into account in the analysis. Although the "intention to treat" principle does not apply as a general rule in nonrandomized studies, the specific biases discussed above in the context of clinical trials would also apply to a cohort study, and it would once again be necessary to analyze the data according to the regular prescribed medication at time of discharge.

Second, group A and group B might differ according to their chronic asthma severity at time of discharge. This problem would be of potentially greater concern in the cohort study than in the clinical trial because since patients had not been randomized to treatments. However, the solution would be the same: to gather information on various markers of chronic asthma severity at time of hospitalization and to conduct analyses of subgroups defined by these severity markers. Once again, only the baseline chronic asthma severity at the time of commencement of follow-up (at time of hospitalization) would be relevant, and it would be incorrect to consider subsequent changes in severity. In particular, subsequent changes in acute or chronic asthma severity could well be a result of treatment, and it would be incorrect to control for this. Assuming that there was little difference in the baseline chronic asthma severity of those prescribed drug A and those prescribed drug B, then the findings of the hypothetical cohort study would be similar to those of the hypothetical clinical trial shown in Table 8.1; if there were differences in baseline chronic severity between group A and group B, then this could be controlled for with the severity subgroup analyses described above.

A hypothetical cohort study. Thus, a hypothetical cohort study might involve enrolling 80,000 patients aged 5 to 34 years who had been admitted to the hospital with asthma over a given period and recording their regular prescribed medication from hospital notes at the time of discharge (Table 8.1). Assume for simplicity that when this was done, it was found that 50% of patients had been prescribed drug A and 50% prescribed drug B. Each study subject was followed for a period of one year after randomization. Once again, there were 70 deaths in group A and 35 deaths in group B, and the relative risk was 2.0 (95% CI 1.3–3.0).

Such a hypothetical cohort study would have two major advantages over a clinical trial: it would not have the same ethical problems and it could be conducted historically rather than prospectively. However, it would still have one major problem: the need to enroll a large number of patients and to collect information on prescribed medication for all of them. Although this is occasionally possible (see Example 8.2), it is rare to have historical records available in sufficient numbers for a historical cohort study to be conducted.

Example 8.2

Suissa et al (1994a) conducted a historical cohort study of patients who had been prescribed asthma medications in the Canadian province of Saskatchewan. They

Table 8.3. Rates of asthma death by use of fenoterol or salbutamol during the previous 12 months: findings from a cohort study of asthma deaths in Saskatchewan during 1980–1987

	Both	Fenoterol only	Salbutamol only	Neither
Asthma deaths	8	15	21	2
Person-years	1245	2493	28,348	15,755
Death rate per 10,000 per year	64.3	60.2	7.4	1.3
Rate ratio (95% CI)	8.7 (3.8–19.6)	8.1 (4.2–15.8)	1.0* —	0.2 (0.0–0.7)

*Reference category.

identified 12,301 patients aged 5 to 54 years who had received at least 10 prescriptions for asthma medication during 1978–1987. The patients were then followed (retrospectively) over the period 1980–1987 and all asthma deaths were identified, and death certificates, coroners' reports, autopsy reports, and hospital-discharge summaries were reviewed. Of the 180 deaths, no documents were found for seven. Three physicians reviewed the available information for the remaining 173 deaths, and classified 46 deaths as probably due to asthma. Table 8.3 shows that the death rate among those prescribed fenoterol (in the dose in which it was marketed) was about eight times that among those prescribed salbutamol, whereas there was a very low death rate among those who were not prescribed either medication.

A case-control study of asthma mortality

As noted in Chapter 2, when a disease outcome is rare, as is the case with asthma deaths, the case-control approach is usually more efficient than a cohort study. In a case-control study, a group of persons with a disease (or an event, such as asthma death) is compared to a control group of persons without the disease (or event) with respect to their past exposure to a particular factor. The first modern case-control study was published in 1926 (Cole, 1979; Lane-Claypon, 1926), and this method is now perhaps the predominant form of epidemiological research. It is thus surprising that the first case-control study of asthma deaths was not published until 1985 (Strunk et al, 1985), and the first case-control study of the role of specific asthma drugs in asthma deaths was not published until 1989 (Crane et al, 1989).

Methodological issues. Figure 8.2 shows the design of a case-control study intended to achieve the same results as the cohort study in a more efficient manner. This would involve studying all the cases of asthma mortality generated by the cohort, and a control group sampled at random from the same cohort. Once again, the same major methodological considerations would apply as in the clinical trial and cohort study.

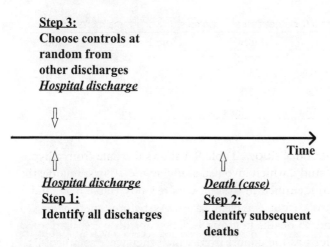

Step 3:
Choose controls at
random from
other discharges
Hospital discharge

Time

Hospital discharge   *Death (case)*
Step 1:   **Step 2:**
Identify all discharges **Identify subsequent**
                            deaths

Figure 8.2. A hypothetical case-control study of asthma mortality.

First, the data would be analyzed according to the regular prescribed medication at time of discharge, and changes in medication that occurred after discharge from hospital would not be considered (Elwood, 1993).

Second, the potential for bias due to differences in baseline chronic asthma severity would be exactly the same as in the full-cohort study. The solution would also be exactly the same: to collect information on chronic asthma severity at time of hospitalization (i.e., at baseline). Once again, it would be incorrect to control for subsequent changes in acute or chronic severity, because these might be a result of treatment. It should also be noted that the subsequent acute severity of the controls would, by design, be different from that of the cases because the cases died and the controls did not. In this context, it should be emphasized that the controls are, in general, intended to be representative of the cohort (source population) that generated the cases, and are not required to be identical with the cases in every respect. It is also important to note the appropriate approach to assessing whether a drug (e.g., drug A) was selectively prescribed to patients with more severe asthma. In a full cohort study, this would be assessed by examining the full cohort (not just those who died) and comparing the baseline chronic severity of group A and group B. Because the control group (in the case-control study) is a sample of the full cohort, the same conclusions can be drawn (as would have been drawn from examining the full cohort) by comparing the average chronic severity of the controls prescribed drug A to the average chronic severity of the controls prescribed drug B. The cases are not relevant in this context, and incorrect results may be obtained if they are considered (Burgess et al, 1990).

Table 8.4. Findings from a hypothetical case-control study of asthma mortality

	Drug A	Drug B	Odds
Deaths (cases)	70	35	70/35
Controls	210	210	210/210
Odds	70/210	35/210	
Odds ratio (95% CI)			2.0 (1.3–3.2)

A hypothetical case-control study. Table 8.4 shows the data from a hypothetical case-control study, which involved studying the 105 asthma deaths that would have been identified in the full-cohort study (table 8.1), and a sample of 420 controls (four for each case). As before, there were 70 deaths in group A and 35 deaths in group B. The controls were distributed in the same proportions as the cohort from which they were sampled: 210 (50%) were on drug A, and 210 (50%) were on drug B. In fact, the proportion will not be exactly 50:50 if the controls were sampled from the survivors (Table 8.1), but this minor bias is trivial because asthma deaths are so rare, and it is avoided if controls are selected by density sampling rather than cumulative incidence sampling (Checkoway et al, 1989). Also, the proportion of controls on drug A may be different from 50% merely by chance, but on the average the control distribution will be similar to that shown in Table 8.4.

The odds ratio is then the ratio of the odds of being a case in group A (70/210) to the odds of being a case in group B (35/210). This, once again, yields a relative risk of 2.0 (95% CI 1.3–3.2); exactly the same answer can be obtained by taking the ratio of the odds of being prescribed drug A in the case group (70/35) to that of being prescribed drug A in the control group (210/210). Thus, such a case-control study would achieve the same findings as the full-cohort study, but would be considerably more efficient because it would involve ascertaining the prescribed medication of 525 patients (105 cases and 420 controls) rather than 80,000. This remarkable gain in efficiency is achieved with only a very minimal reduction in the precision of the relative risk estimate (reflected in the slightly wider confidence interval for the odds ratio estimate).

Example 8.3

Spitzer et al (1992) nested a case-control study within the cohort study described in Example 8.2. Up to eight controls for each case were selected randomly within the cohort after they were matched for region of residence, receipt of social assistance, age at entry into cohort, date of entry, and hospitalization at least once in the 2 years before the event. The controls were also required to have been at risk for the

Table 8.5. Odds ratios for asthma death by use of fenoterol or salbutamol during the previous 12 months: findings from a case-control stury of asthma deaths in Saskatchewan during 1980–1987

	Both	Fenoterol only	Salbutamol* only	Neither
Deaths	7	14	21	2
Controls	11	26	145	51
Odds ratio	4.4	3.7	1.0*	0.3
95% CI	1.6–11.8	1.7–8.0	—	0.1–1.1
Estimated death rate per 10,000 per year[+]	31.0	26.2	7.1	1.9

*Reference category.
[+]Based on 233 controls sampled from 47,842 person-years at risk.

outcome at the time of the event in the corresponding case. Because this was a nested case-control study, it was possible to estimate the death rates for each group in the overall cohort (Table 8.5). This yields estimates that are similar to those obtained in the full-cohort analysis (Example 8.2), although the fenoterol relative risks were higher in the full-cohort analysis, possibly because this includes two additional deaths, both of patients who were prescribed fenoterol; and the matching process used in the case-control study has yielded a higher proportion of controls on fenoterol (37/233 = 15.9%) than in the person-years used in the cohort study (3738/47842 = 7.8%). However, the overall patterns of risk are very similar in the cohort and the case-control study; in both studies there were higher risks of death in patients who had been prescribed fenoterol than in those prescribed salbutamol, and the group that was not prescribed either drug had a relatively low death rate.

Another hypothetical case-control study. A case-control study of the type shown in Figure 8.2 could be nested within a formal cohort, created by

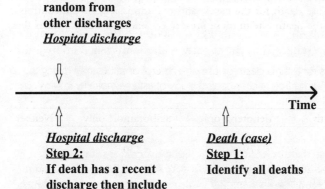

Figure 8.3. Alternative design for a hypothetical case-control study of asthma mortality.

listing all hospital admissions for asthma in a country or region over a period of time. However, the same result could be achieved more efficiently in the manner illustrated in Figure 8.3. This shows a study in which the first step is to identify asthma deaths from national death registration records. For each death, the records of hospitals to which the patient was likely to have been admitted in an acute attack were then searched to identify any admission for asthma in the previous 12 months. If such an admission was identified, the death was included in the study, and the admission closest to death was used. For each death, one or more controls were then selected at random from patients discharged from the same hospital with the diagnosis of asthma at the time that the case's discharge occurred. The prescribed medication at discharge was then ascertained for cases and controls from hospital records (for the admission prior to death for the cases and for the corresponding admission for the controls). This would yield the same findings as the case-control design shown in Figure 8.2 (and the cohort/clinical trial design shown in Fig. 8.1) but would have the advantage that it would not be necessary to enumerate the entire cohort before selecting controls.

Example 8.4

Grainger et al (1991) conducted a case-control study of asthma deaths in the 5 to 45 years age group in New Zealand during August 1981–December 1987. The study design was similar to that depicted in Figure 8.3. The study was based on 32 hospitals throughout New Zealand, and the potential cases comprised all patients aged 5 to 45 years who died of asthma during that period, and who had been admitted to one of these hospitals during the 12 months before death. Controls (referred to as control group B in the original publication) were selected at random from all asthma admissions to these major hospitals in this age group and time period, matched for hospital, year of admission, and age. Prescribed medication at discharge was recorded from hospital notes for the index admission (the admission in the 12 months before death for the cases, and the admission for the controls). Table 8.6 shows that the death rate in those prescribed fenoterol was 2.5 times that

Table 8.6. Odds ratios for asthma death by use of fenoterol or salbutamol during the previous 12 months: findings from a case-control study of asthma mortality in New Zealand during 1981–1987

	Both	Fenoterol only	Salbutamol* only	Neither
Deaths	9	64	33	6
Controls	6	179	230	33
Odds ratio	10.5	2.5	1.0	1.3
95% CI	4.2–26.3	1.6–3.9	—	0.5–3.3

*Reference category.
Source: Derived from Grainger et al, 1991.

in those prescribed salbutamol; this is similar to the estimate of 3.7 in the Saskatchewan study described in Example 8.3 (Table 8.5).

It should also be noted that in some situations, the control group might not be chosen as a completely random sample of the source population. For example, it is common to ensure that the control group has an age distribution similar to that of the cases (i.e., age-matching) in order to make it easier to control for potential confounding by age. Similarly, it might be considered desirable to ensure that the control group had an average chronic severity similar to the cases at the time of hospitalization (it would be impossible for the controls to have the same acute severity at the time of the final attack because the cases died and the controls did not). This would not be necessary if there was in fact no tendency for drug A to be selectively prescribed to more severe asthmatics. However, if this was not known with certainty, then it might be considered appropriate to match for chronic asthma severity, either directly or indirectly. A direct match for severity ("pair matching") would involve taking each case and ensuring that the matched controls were identical to the case with respect to certain markers of chronic asthma severity. An indirect approach (analogous to frequency matching) might involve requiring potential controls to have had a further hospital admission within a 1-year period, so that the cases had had an admission followed by death within 1 year and the controls had had an admission followed by another admission within a year (Fig. 8.4).

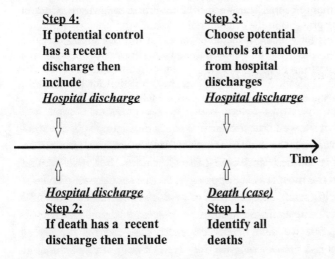

Figure 8.4. A further alternative design for a hypothetical case-control study of asthma mortality.

Table 8.7. Odds ratios for asthma death by use of fenoterol or salbutamol during the previous 12 months: findings from a case-control study of asthma mortality in New Zealand during 1981–1987

	Both	Fenoterol only	Salbutamol* only	Neither
Deaths	9	64	33	6
Controls	12	189	196	30
Odds ratio	4.5	2.0	1.0	1.2
95% CI	1.8–10.7	1.3–3.2	—	0.5–3.1

*Reference category.
Source: Derived from Grainger et al, 1991.

Example 8.5

The study of Grainger et al (1991), described in Example 8.4 above, included a further control group (control group A) that was selected from the same group of asthma hospital admissions on which the study was based but that involved an additional restriction. For each case, controls were selected from patients discharged from the same hospital, with the diagnosis of asthma, in the calendar year in which the death occurred, and who had also had a previous hospital admission during the 12 months prior to the admission under consideration. This control selection procedure, which is similar to that in Figure 8.4, was adopted to achieve an indirect match for asthma severity. Once again, for both groups, information on prescribed asthma medication was obtained from hospital records for the index admission (the admission prior to death for the cases and the corresponding admission for the controls). Once again the death rate in the fenoterol group was about twice that in the salbutamol group (Table 8.7), but the odds ratio (2.0) was slightly lower than that obtained with the "unmatched" control group (2.5) shown in Example 8.4 and Table 8.6, indicating that there had been weak confounding in the analysis based on the "unmatched" controls.

Case-Control Studies of Asthma Deaths

The presentation of the study design issues in the previous section was relatively "generic"; it showed that the various study design options theoretically available for studying the causes of asthma deaths include case series, clinical trials, cohort studies, and case-control studies, but case-control studies are generally the most feasible approach. In this section we discuss in more depth the specific study design issues of case-control studies of asthma deaths. The focus is once again on studies of pharmacological risk factors for asthma deaths, but we also briefly consider case-control studies of nonpharmacological risk factors because they are not only of importance in themselves (particularly to clinicians who wish to identify patients who are at increased risk for death) but are also of importance to epidemiologists who wish to control for potential confounders in studies of pharmacological risk factors for asthma deaths.

General principles

Case-control studies, like other types of epidemiological studies, are based on the experience of a particular population (the study population, source population, or base population) over a particular period of time (the study period or risk period). In a *nested case-control study*, the source population is explicitly defined and enumerated and controls are sampled directly from this base; usually, the source population is a defined geographical population, and therefore the study is *population-based*. In a *registry-based study*, cases may be drawn from one or more registries (e.g., death registries or hospital records); the task is then to ascertain the source population that generated the cases and to sample controls from this source population. In practice, case-control studies of asthma deaths usually involve all deaths in a particular region, or in a well-defined population within a region. Thus, the source population is usually well-defined, and the distinction between nested and registry-based studies is not of major importance.

Selection of cases. The first step in a case-control study is usually to attempt to ascertain all cases generated by the source population—that is, to identify all asthma deaths occurring within the base population over the study period. These can usually be identified in a straightforward manner from death registration records for the area. It may be necessary to gather further information to confirm the diagnosis and to eliminate false positive (and if possible false negative) cases. However, in studies involving the 5 to 34 years age group, the certification of asthma deaths appears to be very accurate in most countries for which information is available. Thus, it is usually reasonable to accept as cases all deaths in this age group that have been coded as being due to asthma.

Selection of controls. The purpose of selecting a control group is to estimate the "typical" exposure of the source population that generated the deaths. Thus, the most obvious and straightforward approach is to select controls as a random sample of the source population. For example, if the case group involves all asthma deaths in a particular region and time period, then the source population comprises all asthmatics in that region and time period, and the most obvious method of selecting controls is to sample from all asthmatics living in the region at that time. This may not be straightforward, because a list of all asthmatics in the region may not be available.

However, an appropriate sample might be obtained through a general population survey to identify asthmatics.

In some instances, it may be appropriate to restrict the source population in order to make it more clearly defined. For example, it might be reasonable to restrict the study to asthmatics who had been diagnosed and who had a general practitioner. This would make it appropriate to select controls through general practitioner records; a similar restriction would be applied to the deaths, but almost all asthma deaths would fall into this category and only a few would be excluded because of this restriction (see example 8.6).

Example 8.6

In the study of Rea et al (1986), the source population comprised all asthmatics aged 0 to 59 years who were normally resident in the Auckland region during 1981–1982, and all of the asthma deaths generated by this source population were identified. Controls were selected by asking a random sample of Auckland general practitioners to submit lists of all patients known to have asthma who consulted them over a 4-week period. Thus, the controls were sampled from asthmatics who had been diagnosed and treated by a general practitioner. An alternative approach would have been to carry out a general population survey to identify a random sample of all asthmatics. However, this would have been more expensive, and would have identified many mild asthmatics who had not been recently treated by a general practitioner. Thus, it is reasonable to restrict the source population to asthmatics who have been diagnosed and treated by a general practitioner. Ideally, a similar restriction should have been applied to the cases; apparently this was not done, but only two of the 44 cases did not have a general practitioner.

Exposure information. Once the cases and controls have been selected, the next step is to obtain exposure information for both groups. The most important principle is that this information should be of similar accuracy in cases and controls, and should ideally be collected from the same sources in the same manner in order to ensure that any misclassification is nondifferential (see Chapter 3).

Example 8.7

Crane et al (1989) conducted a case-control study of asthma deaths in New Zealand in the 5 to 45 years age group during 1981–1983. For each of the 117 cases, four controls were selected from hospital records of patients discharged from the hospital with the diagnosis of asthma in the period during which the case died. The study was restricted to an examination of the regular prescribed medication from general practitioners and hospital records. Information an actual drug use was generally not available. Some information was available from incidental anecdotes during interviews with the next-of-kin of those who had died, although this information was not collected systematically and was of doubtful accuracy. It was deemed inappropriate to use this information because it was only available for the cases and not for the controls. Therefore, using the information could have introduced substantial differential information bias. Restricting the study to examining the regular prescribed medication involved some loss of information, but it meant that comparable information was collected for cases and controls (i.e., any information bias was nondifferential).

Studies of nonpharmacological risk factors

Nonpharmacological risk factors for asthma deaths can be categorized as involving characteristics of the disease (asthma severity) and characteristics of the patient (such as phychosocial factors). The investigation of nonpharmacological factors for asthma deaths is relatively straightforward because the aim is usually to ascertain which factors are associated with asthma deaths without attributing causality. If a particular factor (e.g., previous hospital admissions) is associated with asthma deaths, then this is of interest in itself, both as a means of identifying high-risk patients and as a means for controlling for confounding by asthma severity, irrespective of whether the association is causal. Thus, there is no need to match for asthma severity when selecting controls, and it is in fact inappropriate to do so because this would distort the association between some of the factors of interest and asthma deaths. Thus, controls should usually be selected as a random sample of the source population in a study of nonpharmacological risk factors for asthma death.

Characteristics of the disease. Four studies have examined the association between markers of asthma severity and risk of asthma death in adults (Table 8.8). Rea et al (1986) studied deaths among asthmatics aged 0 to 59

Table 8.8. Case-control studies of asthma severity and asthma deaths

	Rea et al. (1986)	Ryan et al. (1991)	Crane et al.* (1992)	Spitzer et al. (1992)
Location	Auckland	Perth	New Zealand	Saskatchewan
Time period	1981–1982	1976–1980	1981–1987	1980–1987
Source population	Asthmatics	Asthmatics with recent hospital admission	Asthmatics with recent hospital admission	Asthmatics with 10+ prescriptions in 1978–1987
Period at risk	1+ years	2–6 years	1 year	1–8 years
Deaths	44	186	39	44
Controls	44	452	263	233

*Cases and controls who were prescribed fenoterol were excluded.

Table 8.9. Case-control studies of markers of chronic asthma severity and subsequent risk of death

	Rea et al (1986)		Ryan et al (1991)		Crane et al* (1992)		Spitzer et al (1992)	
	Odds ratio	95% CI	Odds ratio	95% CI	Odds ratio	95% CI	Odds ratio	95% CI
Three or more categories of asthma drugs	3.0	1.0–11	—	—	1.7	0.9–3.3	—	—
Oral corticosteroids	—	—	2.3	1.6–3.3	1.3	0.6–2.8	3.1	1.5–6.5
Admission in previous 12 months	16.0	2.5–666	—	—	3.5	1.8–6.9	—	—
5+ admission in previous 12 months	—	—	—	—	8.8	1.2–56	—	—
A&E visit in previous 12 months	8.5	2.0–76	—	—	—	—	—	—

*Cases and controls for whom fenoterol was prescribed were excluded.

years in the Auckland region during 1981–1982; Ryan et al (1991) studied deaths during 1976–1982 among asthmatics with a recent hospital admission in Perth during 1976–1980; Crane et al (1992) studied deaths among asthmatics aged 5 to 45 years in asthmatics with a recent admission to a major hospital in New Zealand during 1981 to 1987; and Spitzer et al (1992) studied deaths during 1980–1987 among asthmatics in Saskatchewan with 10 or more prescriptions for asthma medications during 1978–1987. The studies primarily involved four markers of chronic asthma severity: (1) a hospital admission during the previous 12 months, (2) prescription of three or more categories of asthma drugs, (3) prescription of oral corticosteroids, and (4) hospital emergency room visits. All of the markers of chronic asthma severity were associated with an increased risk of subsequent asthma death (Table 8.9).

For example, in the study of Rea et al (1986) 17 of the 44 cases, compared with two of the 44 community controls, had had a hospital admission for asthma in the previous 12 months. The crude odds ratio for this factor was 13.2, and the matched pairs odds ratio was 16.0. Thus, a recent hospital admission for asthma is a strong marker of chronic asthma severity and risk of asthma death. The marker "three or more categories of prescribed asthma drugs" was also strongly associated with deaths (Table 8.9). The evidence was more equivocal for the marker "prescribed oral corticosteroids," which had had only a weak association with subsequent risk of death in the New Zealand study but showed a stronger association with

Table 8.10. Case-control studies of markers of acute asthma severity and subsequent risk of death

	Rea et al (1986)		Ryan et al (1991)		Crane et al* (1992)		Spitzer et al† (1992)	
	Odds ratio	95%CI	Odds ratio	95% CI	Odds ratio	95% CI	Odds ratio	95% CI
Blood gases‡	—	—	1.9	1.1–3.1	4.0	0.9–21	3.1	1.3–7.6
PaO₂<60	—	—	1.2	0.7–1.9	—	—	—	—
FEV₁§	—	—	0.8	0.3–1.9	1.5	0.1–34	—	—
FVC<40% pred	—	—	1.6	0.8–3.0	—	—	—	—
PEFR<100	—	—	—	—	1.9	0.7–5.4	—	—
K⁺<3.5	—	—	—	—	0.4	0.1–1.5	—	—
Loss of consciousness	—	—	—	—	—	—	10.2	3.9–26.7

*Cases and controls for whom fenoterol was prescribed were excluded.
†As reported in Ernst et al (1993).
‡PCO₂>=45 (Ryan et al, 1991; Crane et al, 1992)) or poor blood gas score (Spitzer et al, 1992).
§FEV1<40% predicted (Ryan et al, 1991) or FEV1<1.0 (Crane et al, 1992).

death in the studies in Perth (Ryan et al, 1991) and Saskatchewan (Spitzer et al, 1992). The equivocal findings for oral corticosteroids may be because this class of drugs may be beneficial in the severe group of patients for whom it is prescribed; thus it may identify a high-risk group of patients, whose risk is then lowered by use of oral corticosteroids.

Three studies have examined the association between acute severity markers and risk of death in a subsequent asthma attack (Table 8.10). In all three studies, an elevated PaCO₂ was associated with a three- to fourfold risk of subsequent death, and in one study a PEFR of less than 100 L/min was associated with an approximately twofold risk of subsequent death. The use of markers of acute asthma severity is difficult because of the poor quality and paucity of available data. Nevertheless, it would appear that a PEFR of less than 100 L/min, a PaCO₂ of greater than 45 mmHg, or loss of consciousness are markers of an increased risk of death in a subsequent attack of asthma. These factors are essentially markers of a near-fatal attack.

Characteristics of the asthmatic. Several studies have examined characteristics of the asthmatic that may be associated with an increased risk of death (Table 8.11). In particular, Rea et al (1986) have noted that the risk of asthma death in adults is associated with psychosocial problems, and other psychological characteristics of the patient, as well as the underlying severity of the asthma (Joseph, 1997). Similarly, Ryan et al (1991) and Crane et al (1992) have noted an association between asthma deaths and prescription of psychotropic drugs, which is a marker of psychosocial or psychiatric problems. Strunk et al (1985) have reached similar conclusions in a small

Table 8.11. Case-control studies of markers of characteristics of the asthmatics and risk of death

Characteristics	Rea et al (1986)		Ryan et al (1991)		Crane et al (1992)		Spitzer et al (1992)	
	Odds ratio	95% CI	Odds ratio	95% CI	Odds ratio	95% CI	Odds ratio	95% CI
Prescribed medication for psycho-social problems	—	—	1.7	1.2–2.5	3.7	1.3–10.8	3.2	1.4–7.5‡
Noncompliance	—	5.2–UH	—	—	—	—	2.0	1.1–3.8†
Below average medical care	2.9	1.2–8.0	—	—	—	—	—	—
Conflict	—	—	—	—	—	—	1.6	0.8–3.3†
Depression	—	—	—	—	—	—	1.6	0.8–3.4†
Psychiatric illness	—	—	—	—	—	—	1.6	0.8–3.2†
Cardiovascular disease	—	—	2.0	1.4–2.9	—	—	—	—

*Cases and controls for whom fenoterol was prescribed were excluded.
†As reported in Ernst et al (1993).
‡As reported in Joseph et al (1997).
UH: unquantifiably high.

study of children that found that various psychosocial factors were associated with an increased risk of asthma death, including conflicts between the patient's parents and hospital staff regarding medical management, depressive symptoms, and disregard of asthma symptoms. However, the proportion of patients with serious psychosocial problems is relatively low, and there is little evidence of selective prescribing of asthma medications to these patients (Grainger et al, 1991); therefore, psychosocial problems appear unlikely to be a major source of confounding in studies of pharmacological risk factors for asthma death.

Severity markers. On the basis of these studies, it is possible to consider a crude index of asthma severity. Rea et al (1986) have proposed a severity index based on a combination of empirical and clinical observations: asthma was defined as *moderate* if the patient had been frequently prevented from working, often woke at night, or needed to visit the doctor urgently because of asthma once or twice in the past year (or any combination of these); patients were classified as having *severe asthma* if there had been one or more hospital admissions or three or more urgent general practitioner or accident and emergency department visits in the previous 12 months. The category of severe asthma can be further divided into a subgroup of patients with *very severe asthma,* comprising those severe asthmatics (according to the classification of Rea et al, 1986) who had had three or more admissions in the previous 12 months or a near-fatal attack in the previous 12 months (Crane et al, 1992; McFadden and Warren, 1997). The most reliable and valid routinely recorded markers of the severity of an acute attack (e.g., one requiring an intensive care unit (ICU) admission) would appear to be a raised $PaCO_2$, a low or unrecordable peak expiratory flow rate, or loss of consciousness. These may therefore be useful supplements to markers of chronic asthma severity in historical epidemiological studies when appropriate data are available, provided that these factors (which are essentially markers of a near-fatal attack) are not themselves part of the causal pathway. The characteristic of the asthmatic that is most strongly and consistently associated with an increased risk of asthma death is the existence of psychosocial problems.

Methodological issues in studies of pharmacological risk factors

In this subsection we consider the various methodological issues involved in case-control studies of pharmacological risk factors for asthma deaths. Such studies are more complex than those investigating nonpharmacological risk factors because the aim is usually to assess causality, rather than just to observe associations. Thus, there is a much greater need to assess the potential for confounding, and to attempt to control such confounding.

The hypothesis under study. The first issue to consider in designing case-control studies of asthma drugs and asthma deaths is whether the objective is to examine the association of asthma deaths with drugs prescribed or used in a severe attack, or the association with regular prescribed medication. As Elwood (1993) points out, the former hypothesis is almost impossible to study. A possible comparison group would be patients experiencing near-fatal attacks, but even in this case it would not be possible to obtain a control group whose attacks had been as severe as the cases, because the cases, by definition, had died. Furthermore, information on drug use would be difficult to obtain and would probably be very inaccurate. This general approach is analogous to conducting a clinical trial in which patients are randomized at the time of a very severe attack. This approach would be completely impractical in the situation of a clinical trial, and it is also inappropriate in epidemiological studies.

The alternative approach (Elwood, 1993) is to restrict the study to the examination of the regular prescribed medication that the patient is likely to use in a severe attack. This is analogous to the clinical trial approach described above in which patients are randomized to receive a particular drug as their regular prescribed medication. This situation is much more straightforward and practicable, in that it is much easier to obtain cases and controls of similar severity (i.e., to match on chronic asthma severity). Furthermore, it is much easier to obtain accurate and comparable information on the regular prescribed medication (from routine medical records) than it is to obtain information on actual drug use. Of course, other asthma drugs may be administered during the acute attack, both in those who die and those who are admitted to the hospital, and this will not be ascertained by considering prescribed drug therapy. However, such nondifferential differences in drug information will bias the relative risk toward the null value of 1.0; that is, they will cause us to underestimate the true relative risk (Copeland et al, 1977). Thus, restricting the study to examining the regular prescribed medication will introduce some misclassification of the exposure information if a drug is primarily hazardous when overused in an acute attack. However, the misclassification will (in a well-designed study) apply equally to cases and controls, and the resulting bias will be in a known direction (toward the null value).

Baseline data. A related issue is that because the focus is on the regular prescribed medication, it is therefore the chronic asthma severity (rather than the acute asthma severity) that is the focus of concern in terms of assessing confounding by severity, because this is more likely to be associated with changes in the regular prescribed medication. Furthermore, it is the chronic asthma severity at the time that the medication was prescribed that is relevant. This is analogous to the situation in a clinical trial, where it is the baseline severity at time of randomization that is important, rather than subsequent severity. In fact, taking into account subsequent changes in asthma severity (after randomization in the case of a clinical trial, or after entry into the study in the case of a cohort study) may introduce serious bias because an increase in severity may be an effect of taking (or not taking) a particular drug. In particular, the severity of the final attack is irrelevant because this will have usually occurred several months after the prescription was written.

Example 8.8

In the study of Grainger et al (1991) of asthma deaths in the 5 to 45 age group in New Zealand during 1981–1987, the source population comprised asthmatics who had had a hospital admission for asthma in the previous 12 months. This previous admission was termed the *index admission.* All information on prescribed medication and asthma severity was collected at the time of the index admission, and information on subsequent changes in prescribed medication or asthma severity were not considered. In particular, information was collected on three measures of chronic asthma severity at the time of the index admission (three or more categories of prescribed asthma drugs, a hospital admission for asthma in the 12 months prior to the index admission, and prescribed oral corticosteroids at time of index admission), and on four measures of acute asthma severity at time of index admission (arterial carbon dioxide tension ($PaCO_2$), plasma potassium concentration (K^+), forced expiratory volume in one second (FEV_1), and peak expiratory flow rate (PEFR)).

Matching for severity. There is therefore a need to collect information on the markers of chronic asthma severity (reviewed above) and to use these to assess the potential for confounding by severity (see below), and to attempt to control for such confounding. There are, however, particular problems in such analyses when controls are sampled at random from the source population because very few of the controls will have severe asthma whereas most of the cases will. This situation makes it almost impossible to adequately stratify on, or control for, chronic asthma severity. Furthermore, because the available markers of chronic asthma severity are imperfect, residual confounding is likely to remain even after control for these markers.

For example, in the case-control study of Rea et al (1986), 39% (17/44) of the patients who died of asthma had had an admission in the previous year, but only 5% (2/44) of the community asthmatic control group identified through general practitioners had an admission in the previous year. Thus, very few of the controls had severe asthma (using this marker of asthma severity), making it almost impossible to adequately stratify on, or control for, chronic asthma severity.

It is therefore usually preferable to match for chronic severity when selecting controls. However, it is often difficult to obtain adequate information on markers of chronic asthma severity at the time of control selection, thus making it difficult to directly match for chronic asthma severity. An alternative approach is suggested by the observation that several studies, have found that controls selected from hospital admissions for asthma had a chronic asthma severity similar to that of cases of asthma death. For example, Rea et al (1986) also included an additional control group of asthma hospital admission controls. This control group was very similar to the deaths with respect to the major markers of chronic asthma severity. In particular, a similar percentage of cases (39%) and hospital admission controls (44%) had had a hospital admission for asthma in the previous 12 months, whereas only 5% of the community asthma controls had had a previous admission. Thus, using hospital controls not only appeared to produce an indirect match for chronic asthma severity but would also enable the results to be stratified on chronic asthma severity. The authors concluded that "the similarity between cases and hospital controls is in accord with the common experience that patients admitted to hospital have more troublesome asthma than those with no previous admissions. . . . Asthmatic patients who are admitted to hospital and those who die appear to come from a similar portion of the asthmatic population—that is, they have troublesome disease (admissions to hospital), are non-compliant, and use accident and emergency departments for treatment of acute attacks" (Rea et al, 1986). Thus, Crane et al (1989) have argued that an indirect match for chronic asthma severity can be obtained by sampling controls from the subset of the source population with a hospital admission for asthma in the previous 12 months.

Assessing confounding by severity. Even when controls have been matched for chronic asthma severity (directly or indirectly), it is still necessary to assess the potential for conflunding by severity by stratifying on markers of asthma severity. In particular, if an elevated risk is due to confounding by severity, then the elevated risk should reduce (toward the null value of 1.0) when confounding is reduced, either by directly controlling for chronic asthma severity, or by focusing the analysis on the most severe subgroups of asthmatics (see Example 8.9). Both approaches involve stratifying on recognized markers of chronic asthma severity.

Example 8.9

Crane et al (1989) conducted a case-control study of asthma deaths in the 5 to 45 years age group in New Zealand during 1981–1983. The overall fenoterol odds ratio was 1.6. However, the fenoterol odds ratio increased from 1.6 to 2.2 when the analysis was restricted to more severe asthmatics (those with a hospital admission for asthma in the previous 12 months). The authors commented that if the elevated fenoterol relative risk had been due to confounding by severity, it would have decreased toward 1.0 when the analysis was restricted to the most severe asthmatics (and the potential for confounding was therefore reduced). The fact that this did not occur effectively excluded confounding by severity as an explanation for the observed association between prescribed fenoterol and asthma deaths.

Although stratification is the most direct method for assessing the potential for confounding by asthma severity, indirect methods can be used to supplement this approach; for example, by examining co-prescribing with other medications, or changes to prescribing occurring as a result of a severe attack resulting in hospitalization (see Example 8.10).

Example 8.10

Beasley et al (1994) examined prescribing of fenoterol and salbutamol in 1102 hospital admission controls from two New Zealand case-control studies of feno-

Table 8.12. Markers of asthma severity in patients prescribed fenoterol and those prescribed salbutamol

Severity marker	Time period	Salbutamol prescribed (n=534)	Fenoterol prescribed (n=446)
Three or more categories of	Total	46%	63%
asthma drugs on admission	1977–1981	47%	54%
	1981–1987	46%	65%
Admission in previous 12	Total	46%	44%
months	1977–1981	63%	51%
	1981–1987	41%	43%
Oral corticosteroids on	Total	25%	36%
admission	1977–1981	25%	31%
	1981–1987	25%	37%

Source: Beasley et al (1994).

terol and asthma deaths (Pearce et al, 1990; Grainger et al, 1991). For the major marker of asthma severity (a hospital admission in the previous year), there was little difference in the proportion with this marker among those prescribed salbutamol and those prescribed fenoterol (Table 8.12). Compared with salbutamol, there was greater co-prescribing of fenoterol with oral corticosteroids and other classes of asthma drugs, but these differences were minor in the early years of the epidemic (1977–1981). Beasley et al (1994) also reviewed the admission and discharge medication for the 1102 hospital admissions. They found that 5% of patients were switched to fenoterol as a result of the admission, whereas 8% were taken off the drug as a result of the admission (Table 8.13). Thus, there was no evidence that patients were switched to fenoterol as a result of a severe attack. In contrast, there were substantial changes for other classes of asthma drugs, with increased prescribing of oral theophyllines, inhaled corticosteroids, and oral corticosteroids (Table 8.13).

Table 8.13. Changes in prescribed medication in 1102 asthma admissions in New Zealand, 1977–1987

Drug	Prescribed drug at time of admission		Prescribed drug on discharge		Drug changed		Drug discontinued	
Oral beta agonists	23%	(251)	22%	(242)	8%	(91)	9%	(100)
Inhaled beta agonists	92%	(1013)	93%	(1025)	5%	(57)	4%	(45)
Fenoterol	46%	(502)	43%	(469)	5%	(57)	8%	(90)
Salbutamol	50%	(546)	51%	(557)	9%	(97)	8%	(86)
Oral theophyllines	60%	(660)	74%	(814)	20%	(218)	6%	(64)
Sodium cromoglycate	17%	(184)	20%	(215)	8%	(85)	5%	(54)
Inhaled corticosteroids	52%	(569)	62%	(685)	17%	(185)	6%	(69)
Oral corticosteroids	30%	(326)	72%	(790)	44%	(483)	2%	(19)
Three or more categories of asthma drugs	53%	(546)	79%	(870)	29%	(324)	4%	(39)

Source: Beasley et al (1994).

Studies of near-fatal attacks

Finally, it should be noted that fatal and near-fatal attacks of asthma may have common causes and that studying near-fatal asthma attacks (as well as being of value in itself) may provide useful information on the factors associated with fatal asthma attacks (Beasley et al, 1993). In particular, the study of near-fatal attacks has some practical advantages in that detailed information of the circumstances of the severe attack can sometimes be obtained, which is usually not available for fatal asthma attacks. Furthermore, if hospital admission controls are used it is possible to interview both cases and controls and to obtain information from hospital records using similar procedures.

However, there are also reasons for caution in studies of near fatal asthma attacks (Beasley et al, 1993). First, some factors may increase the risk of both fatal and near-fatal attacks, whereas other factors may solely affect whether a particular attack is fatal. For example, if there are changes in prehospital care that reduce delays in receiving urgent medical treatment, there may be an increase in hospital and intensive care unit admissions and a corresponding decrease in asthma deaths. Second, obtaining appropriate controls may be difficult in case-control studies of near-fatal attacks. Previous studies have shown that asthma deaths and asthma hospital admissions are very similar with respect to recognized markers of chronic asthma severity (e.g., Rea et al, 1986), but the same may not be true in case-control studies of near-fatal attacks. Patients experiencing near fatal attacks to some extent are a population of "survivors" who have frequent hospital admissions and high usage of asthma drugs; these factors may be responsible for the survival of this subgroup rather than for the occurrence of the severe attacks themselves. Thus, although there are some practical advantages in studying near-fatal asthma attacks, there may well be greater problems of interpretation of the findings than in studies of fatal asthma (Beasley et al, 1993).

Example 8.11

Burgess et al (1994) conducted a case-control study of near-fatal asthma attacks in the Wellington region during 1977–1988. The cases comprised 155 intensive care unit (ICU) admissions for asthma and 305 controls were selected from asthma admissions to the same hospitals (but not to ICU) during the same period. The relative risk of a near-fatal asthma attack in patients prescribed inhaled fenoterol was 2.0. This supported the hypothesis that fenoterol increases the risk of near-fatal as well as fatal asthma. However, the authors noted that the findings were not conclu-

Table 8.14. Studies of fenoterol and asthma deaths

	First New Zealand study	Second New Zealand study	Third New Zealand study	Saskatchewan study
Study period	1981–1983	1977–1981	1981–1987	1980–1987
Age group	5–45 years	5–45 years	5–45 years	5–54 years
Source population	Asthmatics	Patients with a hospital admission for asthma in previous year	Patients with a hospital admission for asthma in previous year	Patients with 10 different asthma prescriptions during 1978–1987
Study design	Case-control study	Case-control study	Case-control study	Nested case-control study
Matching for severity?	Yes	Yes	Yes	Partial
Source of drug information	General practitioner (cases); hospital records (controls)	Hospital records	Hospital records	Pharmacy records
Main exposure information	Prescribed* medication	Prescribed* medication	Prescribed* medication	Dispensed medication
Additional information	Nil	Nil	Nil	Number of units per month
Information on use?	No	No	No	No
Severity markers	Hospital admissions, oral steroids, 3+ categories of drugs	Hospital admissions, oral steroids, 3+ categories of drugs	Hospital admissions, oral steroids, 3+ categories of drugs	Hospital admissions, oral steroids

*Prescribed beta agonists were free during the study period.

Table 8.15. Findings from studies of fenoterol and asthma deaths

	First New Zealand study		Second New Zealand study		Third New Zealand study				Saskatchewan study	
					Group A		Group B			
	Odds ratio	95% CI	Odds ratio	95% CI	Odds ratio	95% CI	Odds ratio	95% CI	Odds ratio	95% CI
Fenoterol	1.6	1.0–2.3	2.0	1.1–3.6	2.1	1.4–3.2	2.7	1.7–4.1	4.8	2.5–9.3
Salbu-tamol	0.7	0.5–1.1	0.7	0.4–1.2	0.6	0.4–1.0	0.5	0.4–0.8	0.9	0.4–1.7
Fenoterol only	1.6	0.1–2.5	1.9	1.0–3.7	2.0	1.3–3.2	2.5	1.6–3.9	3.7	1.7–8.0
Salbuta-mol only*	1.0		1.0		1.0		1.0		1.0	

*Reference category.

sive because the ICU admissions (cases) had been prescribed more asthma drugs than the hospital admission controls and appeared to have more severe asthma. Thus, unlike the situation in the case-control studies of asthma deaths (see Example 8.10), the possibility of confounding by severity could not be excluded.

Summary of studies of fenoterol and asthma deaths

The study designs of the key case-control studies of fenoterol and asthma deaths are summarized in table 8.14 and the findings for fenoterol and salbutamol are summarized in Tables 8.15 and 8.16.

In the first New Zealand study (considered in examples 8.7 and 8.9) the source population comprised all asthmatics in New Zealand aged 5–45

Table 8.16. Subgroup findings (for fenoterol odds ratios and 95% CIs) from studies of fenoterol and asthma deaths

Subgroup	First New Zealand study		Second New Zealand study		Third New Zealand study			
					Group A		Group B	
	Odds ratio	95% CI	Odds ratio	95% CI	Odds ratio	95% CI	Odds ratio	95% CI
Total	1.6	1.0–2.3	2.0	1.1–3.6	2.1	1.4–3.2	2.7	1.7–4.1
Three or more categories of asthma drugs	2.2	1.3–3.9	3.0	1.2–7.7	2.2	1.3–3.9	2.8	1.6–4.9
Hospital admission in last year	2.2	1.1–4.1	3.9	1.8–8.5	2.5	1.4–4.2	2.7	1.5–4.8
Prescribed oral corticosteroids	6.5	2.7–15.3	5.8	1.6–21.0	3.2	1.5–6.8	3.8	1.7–8.5
Hospital admission in last year and prescribed oral corticosteroids	13.3	3.5–51.2	9.8	2.2–43.4	2.8	1.1–6.9	4.0	1.5–11.0

years during 1981–1983 (Crane et al, 1989). Controls were sampled from the subset of asthmatics who experienced a hospital admission for asthma during this period, in order to obtain an indirect match with respect to chronic asthma severity. In the second and third New Zealand studies (Pearce et al, 1990; Grainger et al, 1991) the source populations comprised asthmatics who had had an asthma admission to a major hospital during the previous year. Controls were sampled from the subset of asthmatics who had a further hospital admission within 12 months of the first admission, once again to obtain an indirect match for chronic asthma severity. In the third study an additional control group (group B) was sampled at random from the source population, i.e. without indirect matching for severity, in response to criticisms of the previous two studies (Poole et al, 1990). All three studies showed an increased risk of asthma death in patients pre-scribed fenoterol (Table 8.15) and this risk did not decrease, and in fact tended to increase, as the analysis was restricted to more severe asthmatics (Table 8.16). Although the data sources were different, the Saskatchewan case-control study (Spitzer et al, 1992) and the cohort study in which it was nested (Suissa et al, 1994) was similar in many respects to the New Zealand studies (Table 8.14), and yielded similar findings (Table 8.15), with little evidence of confounding by severity (Ernst et al, 1993).

Overall, this series of studies in New Zealand and Saskatchewan using a variety of study designs, together with the supporting evidence from Germany (Crieé et al, 1993) and Japan (Matsui, 1996), consistently suggests that the prescription of fenoterol (in the high-dose formulation in which it was marketed) increases the risk of asthma death in comparison with the prescription of other beta agonists (Table 8.17). The most persistent criticism of these studies relates to the potential for confounding by severity (Buist et al, 1989; O'Donnell et al, 1989; Blais et al, 1996; Garrett et al, 1996; Rea et al, 1996). It has been suggested that fenoterol was marketed for more severe asthmatics and selectively prescribed to this group, or that since fenoterol was the newer drug, then asthmatics might be switched to

Table 8.17. Proportions of asthma deaths (cases) and controls prescribed fenoterol in studies in New Zealand, Saskatchewan, and Japan

	Total deaths	Percent cases on fenoterol	Percent controls on fenoterol	Odds ratio	95% CI
First New Zealand study	117	51.3%	40.4	1.6	1.0–2.3
Second New Zealand study	58	51.7%	35.7%	1.9	1.1–3.4
Third New Zealand study	112	59.8%	45.9%	1.8	1.2–2.7
Saskatchewan study	44	47.7%	15.9%	4.8	2.5–9.3
Japan	30	53.4%	18.3*	5.1	2.6–9.9

*Market share (this study did not include a formal control group).

fenoterol as a result of deteriorating asthma (e.g. Buist et al, 1989). In fact, there is little or no evidence that fenoterol was selectively prescribed to more severe asthmatics in the population of recently hospitalized asthmatics on which the New Zealand studies were based (see Example 8.10 and Beasley et al (1994)). Furthermore, the findings from the three New Zealand studies show that the fenoterol relative risk did not decrease markedly, and in fact tended to increase, when the analysis was restricted to more severe asthmatics (Table 8.16). This is the most important piece of evidence that the case-control findings are not due to confounding by severity (Elwood, 1993; Sackett et al, 1990; Hensley, 1992). Further support for this interpretation comes from Cox and Elwood (1991), who reported that the results observed in the New Zealand case-control studies could not be produced by random misclassification in the severity markers used.

Thus, the fenoterol studies illustrate how carefully designed epidemiological studies can investigate the role of specific drug therapy in asthma mortality, addressing the major potential problem of confounding by severity, and obtaining similar findings in both cohort and case-control studies in several different countries.

Studies of a Class Effect of Beta Agonists

Although most attention has focused on the role of particular beta agonists (isoprenaline forte and fenoterol) in the mortality epidemics of the 1960s and 1970s, attention has more recently shifted to the possible role of a class effect of beta agonists in the gradual increase in asthma mortality that has been occurring in many countries around the world (Sears et al, 1990; Taylor and Sears, 1994). This research question involves very different methodologic issues than studies of specific beta agonists. In particular, in most western countries virtually all asthmatics are using beta agonists, and there is no appropriate comparison group (this is analogous to a clinical trial in which there is no valid placebo group). This situation is illustrated in Figure 8.5, which shows a typical situation in which virtually all asthmatics use either of two particular beta agonists (fenoterol or salbutamol) and there is only a very small group of asthmatics who do not use beta agonists at all. There are at least three questions that could be addressed in studies of this type:

1. Is the death rate of those prescribed fenoterol higher than those prescribed other beta agonists?
2. Is the death rate of those prescribed beta agonists higher than those not prescribed beta agonists?
3. Is there a dose-response according to the number of units of beta agonist prescribed on a regular basis?

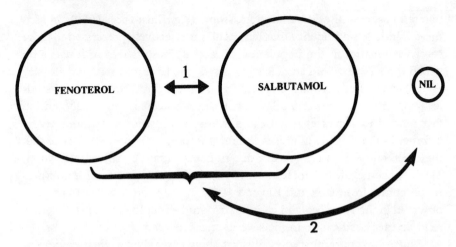

Figure 8.5. Comparisons involved in analyses of case-control studies of fenoterol, salbutamol, and asthma deaths

The fenoterol case-control studies considered above relate to question 1 and essentially involved a comparison of fenoterol with other drugs within the same class (see Fig. 8.5). Some analyses involved direct comparisons between patients prescribed fenoterol and those prescribed salbutamol, whereas others involved a comparison between those on fenoterol and those not on fenoterol; however, the fenoterol findings are similar whichever definition is used (Table 8.15) because almost all of these who were not prescribed fenoterol were prescribed another beta agonist. It is much more difficult to determine whether all beta agonists (including salbutamol) are hazardous (question 2), and the comparison problems are even more intractable when attempting to ascertain whether there is a dose-response according to the amount prescribed on a regular basis (question 3) because patients for whom several units per month are prescribed are very likely to have more severe asthma.

Is the death rate of those prescribed beta agonists higher than those not prescribed beta agonists?

Only one epidemiologic study has attempted to directly address the question of a role of a class effect of beta agonists in asthma deaths. This is the study of asthma deaths in Saskatchewan (Spitzer et al, 1992). Although the primary hypothesis of the study centered on fenoterol (Hensley, 1992; Horwitz et al, 1991), the authors also reported that prescription of beta agonists as a class may also be associated with an increased risk of death. By examining the design and analysis of the Saskatchewan study it is possible to illustrate the difficulties involved in examining such a class effect.

The Saskatchewan study was based on patients who had received 10 or more prescriptions for one or more asthma drugs over a 10-year period (Table 8.14) and their medication was then assessed for the previous 12 months (prior to death for the cases, and prior to the corresponding date for the controls). The diagnosis of asthma was confirmed for the patients who died (cases) but not for the controls. Some of the asthma drugs may have been used for patients with wheezing secondary only to an upper respiratory tract infection, or for patients with bronchitis or emphysema; in other instances, patients may have had asthma earlier in the 10-year period but may have no longer had the disease at the time that their drug therapy was assessed. This may partly explain why most asthma drugs were prescribed more frequently for cases than for controls, and why all of the patients who died had been prescribed beta agonists during the previous 12 months but 18% of the controls had not (Table 8.18).

These methodological problems are unlikely to be of major importance in analyses comparing two drugs within a class. However, they are of more concern when investigating a class effect (Crane et al, 1995). For example, in the Saskatchewan study analysis, salbutamol and fenoterol were entered simultaneously into a logistic regression model, and this essentially involved the comparison of the fenoterol and salbutamol groups with the very small group who were not prescribed either drug (Pearce et al, 1992). The latter group had a very low mortality rate in the Saskatchewan study and included some patients who were not prescribed any asthma drugs and who may have had very mild asthma or no longer had asthma (Pearce et al, 1992, 1994). This is shown in Table 8.19 where the data have been further subdivided into those prescribed other beta agonists and those not prescribed any beta agonists. There were no asthma deaths in the latter group, which is consistent with the hypothesis that many in this group may not have had asthma (or may not even have been prescribed any asthma drugs during the relevant period). If these controls are excluded, then the death rate on salbutamol is

Table 8.18. Case-control studies of beta agonists and asthma deaths

	Total deaths	Percent cases on β-agonists	Percent controls on β-agonists	Odds ratio	95% CI
First New Zealand study	117	91.5%	87.8%	1.5	0.7–3.0
Second New Zealand study	58	86.2%	83.3%	1.3	0.6–2.9
Third New Zealand study	112	90.2%	92.5%	0.7	0.4–1.5
Saskatchewan study	44	100%	82.4%	inf	7.8–inf
Miller and Strunk	30	58.3%	91.7%*	0.1	0.0–1.1

inf = infinity

Table 8.19. Odds ratios for asthma death by use of fenoterol or salbutamol during the previous 12 months: findings from a case-control study of asthma deaths in Saskatchewan during 1980–1987

	Both	Fenoterol only	Salbutamol only	Other beta agonists	No beta agonists
Deaths	7	14	21	2	0
Controls	11	26	145	10	41
Odds ratio	3.2	2.7	0.7	1.0*	0.0
(95% CI)	(0.5–18.7)	(0.5–13.7)	(0.1–3.5)		—

*Reference category.

similar to that on other beta agonists, whereas the death rate on fenoterol is substantially higher. These methodological problems may explain why a recent meta-analysis (Mullen et al, 1993) found that the results of Spitzer et al (1992) are significantly different from those reported by all other researchers (Table 8.18), whereas the findings of the New Zealand case-control studies are consistent with those of other researchers (Miller and Strunk, 1989; Strunk et al, 1985).

Is there a dose-response according to the number of units of beta agonist prescribed on a regular basis?

This issue poses even greater methodological problems because the number of units prescribed per month is likely to be a very strong marker of chronic asthma severity and it is likely to be impossible to control for confounding by severity. Suissa (1995) attempted to circumvent this apparently intractable confounding using a case-time-control design, but this approach only controls for bias due to time trends and can introduce new confounding in itself; thus case-time-control results may end up either more or less confounded than more standard analytic approaches (Greenland, 1996). There are also major problems of confounding with analyses (Suissa et al, 1994b) that take into consideration patterns of increasing beta agonist use, including increasing use over a 1-year period. Once again, such analyses are heavily confounded by (increasing) asthma severity (however, even in these analyses, the relative risk of death associated with heavy fenoterol use (5.2, 95% CI 1.2–23.7) was higher than the risk for heavy salbutamol use (2.6, 95% CI 1.4–5.1)).

A related problem is that of comparing the dose-response curves for specific beta agonists. For example, Spitzer et al (1992) also performed a "dose adjustment" in which an exponential dose-response curve was fitted to the fenoterol and salbutamol data, and it was estimated that the fenoterol and salbutamol dose-response curves would have been similar if fenoterol had been marketed in 100 μg doses (i.e., one half the dose actually marketed). However, this dose adjustment involves comparing two dose-response curves, both of which are likely to be strongly confounded by asthma severity. A further problem is that an exponential dose-response curve was assumed; this led to the conclusion that the fenoterol curve would have been similar to the salbutamol curve if fenoterol had been marketed in one half the actual dose (i.e., 100 μg per puff). Assuming a linear dose-response relationship (which is the more orthodox approach) would have resulted in comparability of the curves at a level of about one quarter of the actual dose (i.e., 50 μg per puff), a dose level that is more compatible with the findings of experimental studies (Beasley et al, 1991).

Summary

Until recently, epidemiological studies of asthma deaths had mostly involved analyses of time trends, supplemented by case series reports. However, time trend analyses provide relatively weak evidence as to the causes of asthma deaths, and a major problem with case series reports is the lack of a control group. More formal epidemiological studies are therefore needed to study the causes of asthma deaths. The ideal approach would be a randomized controlled trial, but this is usually impractical and unethical. Similarly, cohort studies are usually impractical because of the large numbers involved, and case-control studies are the method of choice. Nevertheless, in designing a cohort or case-control study of the causes of asthma deaths, it is important to keep in mind the clinical trial that ideally would have been done, and to design the cohort or case-control study with the aim of obtaining the same findings that would have been obtained in a randomized trial. In this context, it should be emphasized that different research questions involve very different methodological issues and require different methodological approaches. For example, studies of nonpharmacological risk factors usually involve sampling controls at random from the source population, whereas studies of pharmacological risk factors usually require some form of matching for nonpharmacological risk factors. Similarly, studying a class effect is generally more difficult and involves study design and analysis issues different from those involved in comparing drugs within the same class. Although epidemiology has a role to play in investigating class effects, the findings should be regarded with considerable caution and interpreted carefully together with other available information. The emphasis should be on using "appropriate technology" to address the question under consideration, and on using all the available evidence when interpreting the study findings.

References

Beasley R, Pearce NE, Crane J, et al (1991). Asthma mortality and inhaled beta agonist therapy. Aust N Z J Med 21: 753–63.

Beasley R, Pearce N, Crane J (1993). The use of near-fatal asthma for investigating asthma deaths. Thorax 48: 1093–4.

Beasley R, Pearch NE, Burgess C, et al (1994). Confounding by severity does not explain the association between fenoterol and asthma death. Clin Exp Allergy 24: 660–8.

Blais L, Ernst P, Suissa S (1996). Confounding by indication and channeling over time: the risks of β_2-agonists. Am J Epidemiol 144: 1161–9.

Buist AS, Burney PGJ, Feinstein AR, et al (1989). Fenoterol and fatal asthma. Lancet 1: 1071 (letter).

Burgess C, Beasley R, Pearce NE, Crane J (1990). Prescribing of fenoterol and severity of asthma. N Z Med J 103: 22 (letter).

Burgess C, Pearce NE, Thiruchelvam R, et al (1994). Prescribed drug therapy and near-fatal asthma attacks. Eur Respir J 7: 498–503.

Castle W, Fuller R, Hall J, Palmer J (1993). Serevent nationwide surveillance study: comparison of salmeterol with salbutamol in asthmatic patients who require regular bronchodilator treatment. BMJ 306: 1034–7.

Checkoway HA, Pearce NE, Crawford-Brown DJ (1989). Research Methods in Occupational Epidemiology. New York: Oxford University Press.

Cole P (1979). The evolving case-control study. J Chron Dis 32: 15–27.

Copeland KT, Checkoway HA, McMichael AJ, Holbrook RH (1977). Bias due to misclassification in the estimation of relative risk. Am J Epidemiol 105: 488–95.

Cox B, Elwood JM (1991). The effect on the stratum-specific odds ratios of nondifferential misclassification of a confounder measured at two levels. Am J Epidemiol 133: 202–7.

Crane J, Pearce NE, Flatt A, et al (1989). Prescribed fenoterol and death from asthma in New Zealand, 1981–1983: a case-control study. Lancet 1: 917–22.

Crane J, Pearce NE, Burgess C, et al (1992). Markers of risk of asthma death or readmission in the 12 months following a hospital admission for asthma. Int J Epidemiol 21: 737–44.

Crane J, Pearce N, Burgess C, Beasley R (1995). Asthma and the β-agonist debate. Thorax 50: S5–S10.

Crieé CP, Quast CH, Ludtke R, et al (1993). Use of beta agonists and mortality in patients with stable COPD. Eur Respir J 6: 426S (abstract).

Elwood JM (1993). Review of studies relating prescribed fenoterol to deaths from asthma in New Zealand. In: Beasley R, Pearce NE (eds). The Role of Beta Agonist Therapy in Asthma Mortality. New York: CRC Press, pp 85–123.

Ernst P, Habbick B, Suissa S, et al (1993). Is the association between inhaled beta-agonist use and life-threatening asthma because of confounding by severity? Am Rev Respir Dis 148: 75–9.

Garrett JE, Lanes SF, Kolbe J, Rea HH (1996). Risk of severe life threatening asthma and β agonist type: an example of confounding by severity. Thorax 51: 1093–1099.

Grainger J, Woodman K, Pearce NE, et al (1991). Prescribed fenoterol and death from asthma in New Zealand, 1981–1987: a further case-control study. Thorax 46: 105–11.

Greenland S (1996). Confounding and exposure trends in case-crossover and case-time-control designs. Epidemiology 7: 231–9.

Hensley MJ (1992). Fenoterol and death from asthma. Med J Aust 156: 882 (letter).

Horwitz RI, Spitzer WO, Buist S, et al (1991). Clinical complexity and epidemiologic uncertainty in case-control research: fenoterol and asthma management. Chest 100: 1586–91.

Joseph KS (1997). Asthma mortality and antipsychotic or sedative use. What is the link? Drug Safety 16: 351–4.

Joseph KS, Blais L, Ernst P, Suissa S (1997). Increased morbidity and mortality related to asthma among asthmatic patients who use major tranquillisers. Br Med J 312: 79–83.

Lane-Claypon JE (1926). A further report on cancer of the breast. Reports on Public Health and Medical Subjects 32. London: HMSO.

Matsui T (1996). Asthma death and β_2-agonists. Current Advances in Pediatric Allergy and Clinical Immunology: 161–4.

McFadden ER, Warren EL (1997). Observations on asthma mortality. Ann Internal Med 127: 142–7.

Miller DB, Strunk RC (1989). Circumstances surrounding the deaths of children due to asthma: a case-control study. Am J Dis Chest 143: 1294–9.

Mullen M, Mullen B, Carey M (1993). The association between β-agonist use and death from asthma. JAMA 270: 1842–5.

O'Donnell TV, Holst P, Rea HH, Sears MR (1989). Fenoterol and fatal asthma. Lancet 1: 1070–1 (letter).

Pearce NE, Grainger J, Atkinson M, et al (1990). Case-control study of prescribed fenoterol and death from asthma in New Zealand, 1977–1981. Thorax 45: 170–5.

Pearce NE, Crane J, Burgess C, et al (1991). Beta agonists and asthma mortality: déjà vu. Clin Exp Allergy 21: 401–10.

Pearce NE, Crane J, Burgess C, et al (1992). Fenoterol, beta agonists and asthma deaths. N Engl J Med 327: 355–6 (letter).

Pearce NE, Crane J (1993). Epidemiological methods for studying the role of beta agonist therapy in asthma mortality. In: Beasley R, Pearce NE (eds). The Role of Beta Agonist Therapy in Asthma Mortality. New York: CRC Press, pp 67–83.

Pearce N, Crane J, Burgess C, Beasley R (1994). Re: The association between beta agonist use and death from asthma. JAMA 271: 822–3 (letter).

Poole C, Lanes SF, Walker AM (1990). Fenoterol and fatal asthma. Lancet 1: 920 (letter).

Rea HH, Scragg R, Jackson R, et al (1986). A case-control study of deaths from asthma. Thorax 41: 833–9.

Rea HH, Garrett JE, Lanes SF, et al (1996). The association between asthma drugs and severe life-threatening attacks. Chest 100: 1446–51.

Ryan G, Musk AW, Perera DM, et al (1991). Risk factors for death in patients admitted to hospital with asthma: a follow-up study. Aust N Z J Med 21: 681–5.

Sackett DL, Shannon HS, Browman GW (1990). Fenoterol and fatal asthma. Lancet 1: 46 (letter).

Sears MR, Taylor DR, Print CG, et al (1990). Regular inhaled beta-agonist treatment in bronchial asthma. Lancet 336: 1391–6.

Spitzer WO, Suissa S, Ernst P, et al (1992). Beta agonists and the risk of asthma death and near fatal asthma. N Engl J Med 326: 501–6.

Strunk RC, Mrazek DA, Wolfson Fuhrmann GS, LaBrecque JF (1985). Physiologic and psychological characteristics associated with deaths due to asthma in childhood. JAMA 254: 1193–8.

Suissa S, Ernst P, Boivin J-F, et al (1994). A cohort analysis of excess mortality in asthma and the use of inhaled β-agonists. Am J Respir Crit Care Med 149: 604–10.

Suissa (1995). The case-time-control design. Epidemiology 6: 248–53.

Taylor DR, Sears MR (1994). Regular beta-adrenergic agonists: evidence, not reassurance, is what is needed. Chest 106: 552–9.

Index